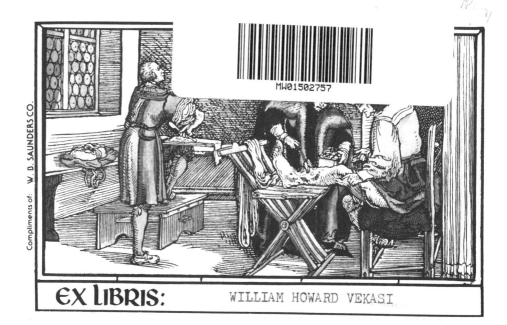

MW01502757

EX LIBRIS: WILLIAM HOWARD VEKASI

Quick Reference to
CLINICAL NUTRITION

Quick Reference to
CLINICAL NUTRITION
A Guide for Physicians

edited by
Seymour L. Halpern, M.D.
Clinical Assistant Professor of Medicine
New York Medical College;
Attending Physician
Department of Internal Medicine
Flower and Fifth Avenue Hospitals;
Associate Attending Physician
Beth Israel Hospital Medical Center;
Associate Attending Physician
Metropolitan Hospital Center; and
Attending Physician in Medicine
(Nutrition and Metabolism)
Cabrini Medical Center
New York, New York

with 36 Contributors

J. B. Lippincott Company
PHILADELPHIA · TORONTO

ISBN 0-397-50404-7

Library of Congress Catalog Card Number 78-12175

Printed in the United States of America

3 5 6 4 2

Library of Congress Cataloging in Publication Data
Main entry under title:

Quick reference to clinical nutrition.
Bibliography: p.
Includes index.
1. Nutrition. 2. Diet therapy. 3. Diet in disease.
I. Halpern, Seymour Lionel. [DNLM: 1. Nutrition.
2. Diet therapy. WB400.3 Q6]
QP141.Q54   613.2   78-12175
ISBN 0-397-50404-7

Dedicated to

Casimer Funk,
Osborne, Mendel, McCollum,
Goldberger, and the other
pioneers in clinical nutrition
whose work revolutionized
the practice of medicine

Contributors

Louis V. Avioli, M.D.
Shoenberg Professor of Medicine and Director,
Division of Bone and Mineral Metabolism
Washington University School of Medicine and
  the Jewish Hospital of St. Louis
St. Louis, Missouri

Jorge A. Bassi, M.D.
Postdoctural Fellow
Institute of Human Nutrition
Columbia University College of Physicians and
  Surgeons
New York, New York

Bruce R. Bistrian, M.D., M.P.H., Ph.D.
Clinical Assistant Professor of Medicine
Harvard Medical School
Boston, Massachusetts;
Research Associate
Department of Nutrition and Food Science
Massachusetts Institute of Technology
Cambridge, Massachusetts;
Associate Staff and Co-Director
Nutrition Support Service
New England Deaconess Hospital
Boston, Massachusetts

George L. Blackburn, M.D., Ph.D.
Associate Professor of Surgery
Harvard Medical School;
Director, Hyperalimentation Unit
New England Deaconess Hospital
Boston, Massachusetts

Henry Buchwald, M.D., Ph.D.
Professor of Surgery
University of Minnesota
  Medical School—Minneapolis
Minneapolis, Minnesota

Rafael A. Camerini-Davalos, M.D., D.Sc.
Professor of Medicine
Director, Metabolism and Diabetes Division
New York Medical College
New York, New York

Jerry G. Chutkow, M.D.
Professor and Chairman
Department of Neurology
State University of New York at Buffalo
  School of Medicine
Buffalo, New York

Harold S. Cole, M.D.
Professor of Pediatrics and
Chief, Sections of Metabolism and Diabetes
Department of Pediatrics
New York Medical College;
Visiting Pediatrician and
Chief, Pediatric Emergency Room
Metropolitan Hospital Center
New York, New York

George D. Ferry, M.D.
Assistant Professor of Pediatrics
Section of Nutrition-Gastroenterology
Baylor College of Medicine;
Chief, Section of Pediatric Gastroenterology
Kelsey Seybold Clinic;
Deputy Director of Clinical Nutrition and
  Gastroenterology
Texas Children's Hospital
Houston, Texas

Richard M. Freeman, M.D.
Professor of Medicine and
Associate Chairman for Educational Programs
University of Iowa College of Medicine
Iowa City, Iowa

Seymour L. Halpern, M.D.
Clinical Assistant Professor of Medicine
New York Medical College;
Attending Physician
Department of Internal Medicine
Flower and Fifth Avenue Hospitals;
Associate Attending Physician
Beth Israel Hospital Medical Center;
Associate Attending Physician
Metropolitan Hospital Center; and
Attending Physician in Medicine
  (Nutrition and Metabolism)
Cabrini Medical Center
New York, New York

Denham Harman, M.D., Ph.D.
Millard Professor of Medicine and
Attending Physician in Medicine
  (Nutrition and Metabolism)
Cabrini Medical Center
Professor of Biochemistry
University of Nebraska College of Medicine
Omaha, Nebraska

Herbert Jaffin, M.D.
Clinical Associate Professor of Obstetrics and
    Gynecology
Mount Sinai School of Medicine of the City University
    of New York;
Associate Attending Obstetrician and Gynecologist
The Mount Sinai Hospital
New York, New York

William J. Klish, M.D.
Associate Professor of Pediatrics
The University of Rochester School of Medicine and
    Dentistry;
Chief, Division of Gastroenterology and Nutrition
Department of Pediatrics
The Strong Memorial Hospital
Rochester, New York

Joel D. Kopple, M.D.
Associate Professor of Medicine and Public Health
University of California, Los Angeles (UCLA), School
    of Medicine;
Medical Investigator for the Veterans Administration
Veterans Administration Wadsworth Hospital Center
Los Angeles, California

Peter T. Kuo, M.D.
Professor of Medicine and
Chief of Cardiology
Department of Medicine
College of Medicine and Dentistry of New Jersey,
    Rutgers Medical School
Piscataway, New Jersey

Albert M. Lefkovits, M.D.
Clinical Associate
Mount Sinai School of Medicine of the City University
    of New York;
Senior Clinical Assistant and
Chief, Phototherapy Clinic
The Mount Sinai Hospital
New York, New York

Carroll M. Leevy, M.D.
Professor of Medicine and
Director, Division of Digestive Diseases
College of Medicine and Dentistry of New Jersey,
    New Jersey Medical School
Newark, New Jersey

Robert D. Lindeman, M.D.
Professor of Medicine and
Associate Dean for Veterans Administration Affairs
University of Louisville School of Medicine;
Chief of Staff
Louisville Veterans Administration Hospital
Louisville, Kentucky

Leo Lutwak, M.D., Ph.D.
Professor of Medicine and
Professor and Program Chief of Nutrition
Northeastern Ohio Universities College of Medicine
Rootstown, Ohio;
Chairman, Department of Medicine
Akron City Hospital
Akron, Ohio

Baltej S. Maini, M.D.
Junior Associate in Surgery
Peter Bent Brigham Hospital
Boston, Massachusetts

Shaul G. Massry, M.D.
Professor of Medicine
University of Southern
    California School of Medicine;
Chief, Division of Nephrology
Los Angeles County-University of Southern
    California Medical Center
Los Angeles, California

Roger G. Mazlen, M.D.
Senior Clinical Instructor of Medicine
Mount Sinai School of Medicine of the City University
    of New York;
Adjunct Assistant Professor of Medicine
New York Medical College
New York, New York;
Adjunct Associate Professor of Biology
Rensselaer Polytechnic Institute
Troy, New York

Corinne Mamo Montandon, M.P.H., R.D.
Assistant Professor of Nutrition and
Administrative Nutritionist
Section of Nutrition and Gastroenterology
Departments of Pediatrics and Community Medicine
Baylor College of Medicine;
Consulting Nutritionist
Junior League Outpatient Department
Texas Children's Hospital
Houston, Texas

Leonard J. Newman, M.D.
Assistant Professor of Pediatrics and Community and
   Preventive Medicine
Chief, Section of Pediatric Gastroenterology and
   Nutrition
New York Medical College
New York, New York

Paula Peirce, M.S., R.D.
Clinical Nutritionist
Department of Pediatrics
University of Chicago
The Pritzker School of Medicine
Chicago, Illinois

Dennis Philip Quinlan, M.D.
Assistant Professor of Medicine
College of Medicine and Dentistry of New Jersey
New Jersey Medical School
Newark, New Jersey

Edward H. Reisner, Jr., M.D.
Assistant Clinical Professor of Medicine
Columbia University College of Physicians and
   Surgeons;
Associate Attending Physician
St. Luke's Hospital Center
New York, New York

Pedro Rosso, M.D.
Associate Professor of Pediatrics
Institute of Human Nutrition
Columbia University College of Physicians and
   Surgeons
New York, New York

Catherine Schneider, M.S., R.D.
Instructor, Cupid Program
Department of Human Nutrition and Foods
College of Home Economics
Virginia Polytechnic and State University
Blacksburg, Virginia

Philip D. Schneider, M.D.
Medical Fellow
Department of Surgery
University of Minnesota Hospitals of the University of
   Minnesota Health Sciences Center
Minneapolis, Minnesota

James H. Shaw, Ph.D.
Professor, Department of Nutrition
Harvard School of Dental Medicine
Boston, Massachusetts

Carlo H. Tamburro, M.D.
Professor of Medicine and
Chief, Division of Digestive Diseases and Nutrition
Department of Medicine
University of Louisville School of Medicine
Louisville, Kentucky

Athanasios Theologides, M.D., Ph.D.
Professor of Medicine
University of Minnesota
   Medical School—Minneapolis
Minneapolis, Minnesota

Frank K. Thorp, M.D., Ph.D.
Associate Professor and
Joseph P. Kennedy, Jr., Scholar
Department of Pediatrics and
Member, Interdisciplinary Committee on Human
   Nutrition and Nutritional Biology
University of Chicago
The Pritzker School of Medicine;
Director of Clinical Services
Sylvain and Arma Wyler Children's Hospital
Chicago, Illinois

Joanne E. Wade, R.D.
Clinical Dietitian Specialist
Nutrition Support Service
New England Deaconess Hospital
Boston, Massachusetts

Edward Wasserman, M.D.
Professor and Chairman
Department of Pediatrics
New York Medical College
New York, New York

Preface

There can be no reasonable doubt concerning the universal role that nutrition plays in the maintenance of a positive state of high grade health and the prevention and treatment of disease. The nutrients supplied to the tissues exert powerful influences as structural essentials for synthetic processes and as regulators of all biochemical processes involved in the body metabolism. Furthermore, diet therapy has become the cornerstone of treatment of many disease states and is of utmost importance in the therapy of other medical and surgical disorders. An awareness by the physician of the continuous and important role of nutrition has become a prerequisite for first-rate medical practice.

The intent of this book is to make available to the physician the clinically significant parts of the new knowledge of nutrition and metabolism in a way that enables him to utilize it in his daily practice. It is not designed to be an encyclopedia of the nutritional sciences and does not contain certain details which can be found in any standard biochemistry textbook. An effort has been made to include that which is clinically significant or which may become so in the near future and to omit that which is solely of academic interest.

Clinical nutrition is no longer an empirical science. During the past few decades many new facts have been learned relative to the clinical consequences of the deprivation of the basic constituents of food and the importance of altered pathways of utilization. Nutrition still is important in the prevention and treatment of nutritional disorders, but in addition, it has become a major factor in safeguarding against many illnesses. The new knowledge acquired by systematic studies has made clear that the nutrient intake and the nutritional state of the body exercise a vital role in the etiology, course, and prognosis of the acute and chronic illnesses that now have become the primary causes of morbidity and mortality in our population.

The ability of a person to recover from an illness or from surgery and even the successful use of many newly introduced pharmaceutical agents frequently are dependent on both the person's previous and current nutrient supply. Proper application of the new knowledge of nutrition can make food a valuable adjuvant to the specific therapy of many illnesses.

Information on diet advice to the healthy patient, a design for the clinical evaluation of nutritional status based on the problem-oriented method, and recommended approaches to the use of nutrition in the treatment of medical problems of everyday importance are based on the latest available data. Many chapters are devoted to diet therapy of specific systemic diseases. Appropriate diet plans are given for special clinical problems.

Authors have been selected with great care in order that the subject matter covered will carry the weight of their authority and special expertise. Their expenditure of time and effort has made this manual possible.

Nutrition continues to be one of the most important environmental factors continually affecting health and disease. Rare indeed is the person who cannot be aided by the proper application of nutrition knowledge. Yet many physicians have not had formal training in nutrition. This quick reference to applied clinical nutrition will enable them to utilize diet therapy so as to enhance the quality of the medical care they deliver to their patients.

It is not possible for a quick reference to contain every recent advance in the science of nutrition, although an attempt has been made to include the new knowledge that is of greatest importance in medical practice. It is hoped that this new work will be of value not only to the practicing physician but also to medical students, house officers, nurses, dieticians, public health workers, and all those who are concerned with caring for people.

SEYMOUR L. HALPERN, M.D.

Acknowledgments

Many people deserve thanks for their assistance during the period that it took to give birth to this book, especially my secretary, Joanne Marinos, and other members of my staff who have helped with typing and the handling of manuscripts and proofs. Too, I wish to acknowledge the efforts and assistance of the able staff of the J. B. Lippincott Company. Finally, I wish to thank my wife, Anafred N. Halpern, M.D., and children, Adrienne, Vivienne, and Ronald, for their tolerance, understanding, and cooperation.

Contents

Quick Reference to
CLINICAL NUTRITION

1. EVALUATION OF NUTRITIONAL STATUS

Leo Lutwak, M.D., Ph.D.

I. Population at Risk

A. Virtually every patient with acute or chronic illness should be evaluated nutritionally by his physician.

B. There are certain populations, in which the risk of malnutrition is much higher. These groups, therefore, should be considered prime candidates for a nutritional evaluation.

1. The obese patient is one who suffers primarily from overnutrition, which is a form of malnutrition, but who also may be suffering from particular aspects of undernutrition.

a. The chronically obese patient frequently has subjected himself to a series of diets over the years that may have produced aspects of protein malnutrition superimposed on the caloric surplus.

b. Many of these patients may have undergone fad reducing regimens for varying periods of time, with chronic sequelae.

2. Cachexia may occur as a result of social psychiatric conditions such as anorexia nervosa, malignancy, and gastrointestinal malabsorption syndromes.

a. Although the malnutrition in these patients is apparent on observation, further documentation is necessary to follow the course of therapy and to predict the severity of accompanying complications.

3. Protein-calorie malnutrition

a. This is far from rare in the U.S.

b. Although no estimates are available of the incidence of protein-calorie malnutrition in the general population, surveys in various large hospitals in the U.S. indicate that:

(1) Approximately 50% of general medical-surgical admissions have some evidence of protein-calorie malnutrition.

(2) Approximately 25% may have functional disease related to protein-calorie deficiency.

(3) About 10% may have far advanced evidence of malnutrition.

c. Protein-calorie malnutrition should be suspected in patients with some degree of intellectual or physical impairment who are living in nursing homes.

4. Elderly persons who live alone, who may have economic and physical problems in obtaining adequate food or preparing it, or who may be psychologically depressed may show evidence of malnutrition.

5. Patients with chronic diseases such as arthritis, orthopaedic problems, gastrointestinal disease, endocrine disorders such as thyroid or adrenocortical disease, diabetes, and alcoholism will frequently show evidence of protein-calorie malnutrition.

6. The adolescent who eats and diets in an erratic fashion may, as a consequence, be suffering from some degree of malnutrition.

C. Patients who may develop potential problems of malnutrition as a result of their presenting complaints should be carefully evaluated.

1. The pregnant adolescent

a. Although she has not yet satisfied her own nutritional needs for growth and development, the pregnant adolescent may be superimposing the stress of pregnancy on the normal stresses of this age group and, consequently, may develop complicating malnutrition.

2. The otherwise healthy young adult with multiple trauma, acute burns, or who has undergone gastrointestinal surgery presents a potential for subsequent nutritional problems.

3. Newly diagnosed patients with malignancy

a. Patients who are placed on a regimen of chemotherapy and radiation therapy should be evaluated prior to the onset of nutritional difficulties and followed through the course of therapy.

II. Reasons for Concern about Nutritional Status

A. In many chronic diseases, such as hypertension, diabetes, obesity, atherosclerotic heart and cerebral vascular disease, metabolic bone disease, and alcoholism, deteriorated nutritional status may contribute to the etiology of the disease process and may prevent effective recovery unless it is corrected in the course of a therapeutic regimen.

B. In still other conditions such as malignancies, arthritis, and chronic gastrointestinal disease, malnutrition may result as a consequence of the underlying pathology and must be diagnosed and treated as part of the total care of the patient.

C. Protein-calorie malnutrition produces progressive weight loss, weakness, and apathy.

1. This combination leads to a further decrease in food intake and further exacerbation of the malnutrition.

D. The metabolic effects of protein-calorie malnutrition can become superimposed on any underlying disease process, preventing recovery from infection, surgery, and injury, even in a previously healthy person.

E. The result of protein-calorie malnutrition may be impairment of wound healing, exacerbation of decubitus ulcers at pressure points, increased wound disruption, and increased fistula formation following bowel surgery.

F. Fluid and electrolyte imbalances become more difficult to correct as a result of imbalances in protein distribution.

G. Endocrine imbalances may result as a consequence of the impairment of synthesis of polypeptide hormones when protein deficiency is present.

H. Depressed ventilatory response to hypoxia has been reported with protein-calorie malnutrition and thus may make it difficult to wean the patient from a respirator post-operatively.

I. A long-standing protein deficiency can lead to impairment of immune mechanisms.

1. This impairment of immune mechanisms results in increased wound infections, increased incidence of pneumonitis and of urinary tract infections, and impaired responses to chemotherapy used against infection and cancer.

J. Particularly in patients with malignancies, protein-calorie malnutrition leads to markedly decreased tolerance to therapeutic regimens such as chemotherapy and radiation therapy (see Chap. 18).

K. The social consequences of malnutrition are equally important in these days of increasing concern with the cost of medical care delivery systems.

1. Because of the delayed responses to various therapies, malnutrition increases the need for critical care facilities and for special nursing care.

2. It increases the duration of hospital stay and convalescent care in most instances.

3. These special needs and the long duration of the treatment of malnutrition produce stresses on the family environment of the patient and delay the patient's return to work.

CLINICAL EVALUATION

I. Basic Principles

A. Relatively simple procedures for quantitative measurement of nutritional states are available to every physician.

B. It is not sufficient to merely evaluate nutritional status as thin, fat, obese, normal, cachectic, or well-nourished.

C. More complex tests are easily obtained in hospital situations, in which evaluation of nutritional status is an essential part of the care of the patient.

II. History

A. Medical History

1. Contributory factors to malnutrition may be uncovered from the history of chronic illness, weight loss, and weight gain.

2. This information can be obtained by direct questioning as well as by indirectly asking for the weight at different key points in the patient's history, such as entry into high school, graduation from high school, marriage, and after the birth of children.

3. Overnutrition can be diagnosed from historical information concerning weight reduction regimens: nature of weight reduction regimens, frequency of use, degree of weight loss, and rate at which weight was regained.

B. Diet History

1. A diet history is of extreme importance but must be obtained accurately. When available, completely trained persons should do this.

2. Simply asking a patient what he ate is usually insufficient.

3. A diet history can be obtained more accurately by questioning food intake for specific meals within the past 24 hours.

4. Diet history by recall can be corroborated by asking specific questions about the patient's consumption and the family's purchases of individual food items, such as bread and other grain products, meat, milk, vegetables, fruit, eggs, alcoholic beverages, and desserts.

5. More accurate estimates of nutritional history can be obtained, when time permits, by having the patient maintain a one-week diet diary.

    a. All foods and liquid ingested, with approximate quantities, should be recorded at the time of actual consumption.

6. The data obtained from all of these mechanisms should then be evaluated.

    a. The U.S. Department of Agriculture's Handbook No. 8, can aid in estimating the intake of a given nutrient.*

III. Physical Examination

A. Routine Examination

1. The presence of edema may be suggestive of protein deficiency.

2. Certain skin changes offer additional evidence of possible malnutrition.

    a. Cheilosis and tongue changes, while associated with many other disorders, may be suggestive of vitamin B-complex deficiencies.

    b. Petechiae may be related to ascorbic acid deficiency.

    c. Folliculitis has been reported in association with vitamin A deficiency.

3. Eyes may provide evidence of

    a. Vitamin A deficiency—conjunctival transluscence, dryness, and opacity; night blindness; and with serious vitamin A deficiency, keratomalacia.

    b. Vitamin B-complex deficiency—circumoral and bulbar conjunctival vascularity, angular conjunctivitis, and blepharitis.

4. The tongue should be examined for signs of

    a. Iron deficiency—glossitis with papillary atrophy →smooth tongue

    b. B-complex deficiency—glossitis and angular stomatitis

5. Examination of the gingivae offers additional information.

    a. Hemorrhages are seen in vitamin C deficiency.

    b. Gingival recession may be associated with chronic calcium deficiencies.

6. Hepatomegaly is common in chronic protein-calorie malnutrition.

7. Abnormalities of the ribs and

---

*Composition of Foods—Raw, Processed, Prepared. Available from U.S.D.A., Washington, D.C. 20250. This book is the largest, most detailed source of food information ever prepared.

bowing of the legs may be seen with osteomalacia or vitamin D deficiency.

8. Pallor of the mucosa may suggest iron deficiency.

9. Muscle wasting, associated with neurologic diseases and endocrine abnormalities, may also suggest protein deficiency.

10. The presence of an ostomy or fistula indicates a source of chronic protein loss and, hence, deficiencies.

B. Anthropometry

1. Height

a. This should be measured by the observer.

b. The patient should be without shoes, heels together, against a straight surface, and with the head level and erect.

2. Weight

a. This should be measured by the observer, with the patient in a gown or in underwear.

3. Height-Weight Indices

a. Height and weight alone are grossly inaccurate in the estimation of chronic malnutrition.

b. Various ratios have been proposed as indices that relate body proportions to body fat.

c. The simplest is a weight for height index, which is the basis for most insurance company standard tables (see Table 17-1).

d. Somewhat more accurate is the weight to height squared index.

e. Any index of weight and height, however, may be erroneous in the presence of edema, and this should be carefully considered.

4. Skin-Fold Thickness

a. A skin fold consists of two layers of subcutaneous fat without any muscle or tendon included.

b. This may be measured with standard calipers, such as the Lange skin fold caliper, used at standardized sites, with at least three measurements made at each site.

c. About 50% of body fat is subcutaneous. The measurement of skin-fold thickness, therefore, offers a rough estimate of total body fat.

d. Measurements of skin-fold thickness at certain points of the body have been found to be reproducibly correlated with body fat content as measured in the research laboratory with underwater weighing.

e. The measurements of skin-fold thickness are of value in longitudinal studies of a single patient and as an approximation for evaluation of overnutrition and undernutrition.

(1) In men, values less than 12.5 mm. suggest undernutrition, and values greater than 20 mm. suggest excess fat and overnutrition.

(2) In women, values less than 16.5 mm. suggest undernutrition, while values greater than 25 mm. indicate excessive body fat and overnutrition.

f. Generally, the more points that are measured, the more valid an estimation of total body fat is achieved.

(1) The simplest to use and the best correlated point is the triceps skin fold, obtained over the posterior upper arm at the midpoint. This value is particularly good for adult men.

(2) Almost as valuable in both men and women is the subscapular fold.

(3) In women under age 35, the upper abdominal skin fold is most reliable.

(4) In women over age 35, the lower abdominal skin fold, obtained midway between the umbilicus and the pubis, is valuable.

(5) Other points that have been used include the skin folds over the pectoralis major, the mid-abdominal region in the anterior axillary line, below the chin, the gluteal fold, and the back of the knee. These values taken alone are of relatively little value. However, if they are measured along with the others listed above, these points offer additional information.

(6) The skin-fold thickness mea-

surements may be used most effectively as follows:

(a) Several skin-fold thicknesses may be measured in a patient, and the average of these should be calculated.

(b) If the average is below or exceeds the normal values suggested above, the diagnosis may be undernutrition or overnutrition.

5. *Circumferences*

a. Head circumference in the infant is an index of growth and development, which may be related to both nutrition and genetics.

b. The mid-upper arm circumference is an index of muscle mass.

c. The mid-calf circumference is also an index of muscle mass.

d. "True" muscle mass circumference can be calculated from skin fold thickness and mid-upper arm circumference because the total circumference includes two layers of skin fold (see Table 27-1). It is assumed that the upper arm is a perfect cylinder.

(1) Within limits of error, this assumption is relatively valid.

(2) Absolute values for normal muscle mass circumference cannot be given because this is a function of total body dimensions.

(3) Average standard values for arm and muscle circumference are given in Table 27-1.

(4) The values can be used to diagnose the development of malnutrition and the reversal of muscle mass problems.

(5) Muscle mass is an indicator of protein nutrition.

IV. Laboratory Studies

A. *Complete Blood Count*

1. Hematocrit, hemoglobin, and red cell indices will offer diagnostic evidence of iron deficiency or megaloblastic anemia (vitamin B_{12} and folate; see Chapter 14).

2. Examination of white blood cells

may suggest other aspects of malnutrition.

a. The presence of multilobular granulocytes suggests vitamin B_{12} and folate deficiencies.

b. A total lymphocyte count of less than 1500 may be suggestive of protein-calorie malnutrition.

B. *Routine Biochemistry*

1. Serum albumin concentration less than 3.5 g./dl. suggests protein malnutrition.

2. Serum calcium and phosphorus levels below the normal range for the laboratory suggest vitamin D deficiency. Elevation of alkaline phosphatase in association with this substantiates the suspicion.

3. Blood urea nitrogen concentration below the normal range suggests inadequate intake of protein.

4. In the absence of renal disease, serum creatinine concentration is an index of lean body mass. Within the normal range of 0.7 to 1.5 mg./dl, the lower values are seen in small persons, and the higher values are seen in those with larger muscle mass. The proportionality, however, is very poorly correlated, and, therefore, no indices can be calculated based on this.

5. Serum cholesterol and serum triglyceride concentrations are indices of fat nutrition.

a. Serum triglycerides should be measured in a blood sample that is obtained after a 12-hour fast.

b. Values in excess of 150 mg./dl. are indicative of abnormality in lipid handling but do not differentiate between persons whose hypertriglyceridemia is dietary lipid sensitive and persons whose hypertriglyceridemia is dietary carbohydrate sensitive (see Chap. 10).

c. The range of normal values for serum cholesterol is quite wide and depends on the age and sex of the patient.

d. Generally, values in excess of 230 to 250 mg./dl. are considered abnormally high and indicate metabolic problems in lipid metabolism.

e. Serum cholesterol values below

160 mg./dl. are suggestive of either chronic liver disease or malnutrition.

6. Table 27-2 summarizes the normal range for biochemical tests used in assessing nutritional status.

C. Special Blood Tests

1. In semi-starvation, 2-hour postprandial blood glucose values may be in the diabetic range.

2. Serum iron values below 60 μg./dl. are indicative of chronic iron deficiency.

3. Serum folic acid levels below 6 ng./ml. indicate deficient intake or abnormal metabolism of folate.

4. Serum vitamin B_{12} values below 200 pg./ml. are seen in patients who have been consuming diets totally deficient of animal protein as well as in those with pernicious anemia.

5. Serum magnesium values below 1.5 mEq./L. may be found in chronic generalized malnutrition as well as in some patients with parathyroid disease.

6. Red blood cell transketolase is a highly specialized test that is only performed in selected laboratories. It serves as a sensitive indicator of thiamine concentration.

7. Red cell riboflavin nucleotide concentrations are indicative of riboflavin nutritional status but are also available only in specialized laboratories.

8. Serum ascorbic acid and leukocyte ascorbic acid concentrations are indicative of the ascorbic acid saturation of the organisms.

a. Serum levels less than 0.5 mg./dl. are highly suggestive of vitamin C deficiency.

b. If such values are obtained, these should be substantiated by performing an ascorbic acid loading test and by measuring excretion in the urine under defined conditions.

9. Serum vitamin A and serum carotene concentrations can serve as indices of malabsorption of fat and fat-soluble vitamins.

a. They also are accurate indicators of the vitamin A status of the patient.

b. A normal range for serum vitamin A is between 0.15 and 0.6 μg./ml.

10. Serum transferrin can be readily estimated in routine laboratories by measurement of serum iron-binding capacity.

a. Values for iron-binding capacity below 250 μg./dl. are highly suggestive of deficiencies of transferrin.

b. Transferrin is a liver-synthesized protein whose concentration is extremely sensitive to systemic protein deficiency.

c. Decreases in transferrin occur early in protein deficiency and are measurable before significant changes occur in serum albumin.

11. Serum zinc is becoming of increasing interest. Normal ranges have not been established for the general population as yet. Deficiencies in zinc appear to be related to protein deficiencies of the organism.

12. Table 27-4 contains what are considered to be normal blood levels for essential vitamins.

13. Table 27-5 lists the normal range in blood and urine for essential minerals.

D. Urine Tests

1. Twenty-four-hour creatinine excretion

a. In patients with normal renal function, 24-hour urinary creatinine excretion is related to lean body mass.

b. In the normal adult, 23 mg. of creatinine are excreted per kilogram of body weight per 24 hours.

c. This value may be used in conjunction with the anthropometric measurements for estimations of malnutrition.

2. Urea nitrogen per gram of creatinine

a. Approximate nitrogen balance can be estimated in patients without complete metabolic collections by measurement of urea nitrogen excretion.

b. Usually, if the total urea nitrogen excretion per 24 hours is known, addition of 3.5 g. of nitrogen for non-urea nitrogen and stool and cutaneous nitrogen losses permits an estimation of nitrogen balance.

c. From the height and weight of the patient and the predicted urinary creatinine excretion, an approximate nitrogen balance measurement can be attained from the ratio of urinary urea to creatinine excretion.

3. Twenty-four-hour excretion of calcium and phosphorus can give information concerning the possible presence of adult osteomalacia or rickets.

a. The excretion of calcium and phosphorus are significantly below normal in these conditions.

b. Usually urinary 24-hour calcium excretion is 100 to 200 mg./day, and phosphorus excretion is proportional to dietary phosphorus.

c. Normal urinary phosphorus is equal to approximately 50% of the dietary phosphorus and thus can be used as an index of dietary intake as well.

E. Special Urine Tests

1. Hydroxyproline

a. Urinary hydroxyproline is derived from the synthesis of collagen.

b. During a person's period of active growth, urinary hydroxyproline excretion is elevated.

c. The range of normal values is dependent on the technique used in the individual laboratory.

d. In chronic protein-calorie malnutrition, these values are usually depressed, particularly in adolescence.

2. Urinary thiamine can be measured by specialized techniques in laboratories that are equipped to perform this determination and can yield an index of thiamine nutrition.

3. Urinary N-methylnicotinamide is the primary metabolite of niacin and has been utilized as an index of the nutrition status of this vitamin.

4. Urinary riboflavin excretion is related to the intake of this vitamin.

V. Immune Reactivity Studies

A. Cell-mediated immunity is an important host defense system against infection.

1. In chronic malnutrition, the thymus-derived lymphocytes are impaired in function and in number.

2. Depressed cellular immunity occurs very rapidly in malnutrition and returns to normal with even short-term nutritional repletion.

B. When the development of nutritional impairment is expected, tests for cell-mediated immunity should be performed at weekly intervals using a portion of the battery of tests available.

C. Initially, all tests that are available to the observer should be recorded.

D. In the course of nutrition repletion, selected tests should be performed at frequent intervals.

E. Tests for Immune Reactivity

1. Serum complement level. Components of complement have been shown to be influenced by nutritional status.

2. Skin tests with recall antigens

a. The most commonly used antigens are those for Candida, Varidase (streptokinase/streptodornase), and for mumps.

b. Most persons have been sensitized to these antigens in the course of normal living and should give positive responses.

c. The responses disappear very rapidly in protein malnutrition and return very rapidly with realimentation.

d. These skin tests and the serum complement test are easily performed at all levels of medical care.

3. Dinitrochlorobenzene (DNCB) sensitization by the Catalona technique. This tests the general inflammatory response by the appearance of a prominent blister 24 hours after sensitization. It is a highly sensitive test for cell-mediated immunity.

4. Identification of relative proportions of thymus-derived lymphocytes and B-lymphocytes indicate the effect of under-

nutrition on T cells as compared with the effect of immune deficiency diseases on B cells. This technique is a highly specialized procedure, which is usually available only in teaching hospitals.

5. Lymphocyte transformation to antigens and mitogens. This is a highly specialized test, which is available only as a research technique.

VI. Severe Protein-Calorie Deficiency Presentations

A. Protein Deficiency or Kwashiorkor

1. This is characterized by normal skin fold, normal height, and normal weight. (Obesity may even be present.)

2. Decreased visceral protein is indicated by decreased serum albumin, decreased transferrin, and decreased immune competence.

3. Decreased muscle mass is indicated by decrease of urinary creatinine, urinary BUN, serum creatinine, and of arm circumference.

B. Calorie Deficiency or Marasmus

1. This is characterized by decreased anthropometric measurements, such as weight and skin folds, accompanied by normal visceral protein, normal immunity, and normal muscle mass.

C. Protein-Calorie Malnutrition or PCM

1. This condition is characterized by decreased anthropometric measurements as well as decreased visceral proteins, immune competence, and muscle mass.

METHODOLOGY OF NUTRITIONAL EVALUATION

I. Initial Evaluation

A. Certain patients must be considered as suspect of malnutrition on admission or suspect to develop malnutrition in the course of hospitalization. These include

1. Elderly patients from nursing homes

2. Patients with stroke

3. Patients with chronic diseases such as arthritis, with associated anorexia

4. Patients with acute massive trauma

5. Patients with acute burns

6. Patients with malignancies

7. Patients undergoing chronic chemotherapy and radiation therapy

8. Patients admitted for gastrointestinal surgery who may remain on parenteral fluids postoperatively

9. Patients with massive infections

10. Patients with psychiatric disorders

11. Patients with gastrointestinal disorders who require special diets or patients with malabsorption

II. Follow-up Evaluations

A. Clinical judgment must determine the frequency of follow-up evaluations.

B. Malnutrition can occur within 7 to 10 days in a previously healthy person and more rapidly in a partially malnourished person.

C. If the predisposing condition progresses or does not improve, follow-up measurements should be performed at weekly intervals.

D. If preexisting malnutrition is being corrected, a similar schedule for follow-up should be devised.

III. Prevention and Correction of Malnutrition

A. The simplest causes of decreased food intake should be sought and corrected.

1. Dental Evaluation

a. Patients who lack dentures or who have ill-fitting dentures may have difficulty eating a routine hospital diet.

b. Correction of the dental problem or the administration of a diet of appropriate texture may be sufficient.

2. Food Preferences

a. For sociological and religious reasons, patients will frequently refuse to eat a routine hospital diet.

3. Careful evaluation by the dietitian, with substitution of appropriate foods, can often correct this.

B. Supplemental Feedings

1. Many patients will have difficulty in completely consuming the diet trays at prescribed meal hours.

2. The provision of appropriate between-meal feedings can increase the intake of both calories and protein.

a. Normal foods provided between meals

b. Hospital-designed and -prepared milkshakes and eggnogs.

c. Commercially available high-calorie, high-protein liquid formula supplements (see Tables 12-1, 12-3, and 12-5).

3. Complete oral nutrition using liquid formulas

a. The commercial and hospital-prepared preparations mentioned above can be utilized for complete oral nutrition, particularly if they are provided in refrigerated vacuum jugs at the bedside for self-administration.

b. The preparations come in many flavors and can be further modified by the addition of flavoring agents.

c. Because of the monotonous texture of these preparations, it is sometimes desirable to permit the patient to select different flavors and to offer the preparations in small quantities.

4. Tube feedings. The same preparations can be administered by tube feeding to patients with anorexia and swallowing difficulties and to patients who are uncooperative in eating.

a. Because of the dangers of aspiration, these preparations should not be administered by tube feeding without continuous supervision.

b. For further discussion of the use and problems associated with tube feeding, see Chapter 20.

5. Defined elemental formulas

a. In patients with gastrointestinal disorders, in which malabsorption plays a large role or in which a residue-free diet may be desired (as in patients with rectal fistulae, Crohn's disease, or ulcerative colitis), a defined elemental formula, containing amino acids, medium-chain triglycerides, simple sugars, minerals, and vitamins, may be administered either orally with a flavor pack or by tube feeding (see Tables 12-1 to 12-4 and Chap. 11 to 13).

6. Parenteral nutrition. As a last resort, when oral feeding and tube feeding are impossible, nutrition supplementation or total nutritional requirements may be administered parenterally (see Chap. 20).

VII. Delivery of Nutritional Support Service

A. A well-trained team is required for effective delivery of nutritional support.

B. The team should be prepared to conduct nutritional evaluation, to prescribe preventive and therapeutic nutrition modalities, to follow-up the effect of this therapy, and to monitor the delivery.

C. Ideally, in hospital situations, the team should consist of a physician-clinical nutritionist, a therapeutic dietitian, a nurse, and a pharmacist.

D. House staff should be assigned to work with the nutritional support service to improve their own training in clinical nutrition.

2. NUTRITIONAL ADVICE TO THE HEALTHY PATIENT

Richard M. Freeman, M.D.

Giving nutritional advice to the healthy patient sounds like a simple task. Let us assume, however, the following:

1. A healthy patient's 54-year-old father died of coronary artery disease.

2. A 24-year-old patient has an identical twin sister in whom the diagnosis of diabetes mellitus has recently been made.

3. A 35-year-old woman has a history of hypertensive cardiovascular disease in both parents as well as one sibling.

4. A 43-year-old male spontaneously passed a calcium-containing kidney stone five years ago.

The patients in all of the circumstances above may well be healthy and asymptomatic on the basis of all the usual tests and a physical examination. The nutritional advice to these patients, however, will not necessarily be the same.

1. If cholesterol-restricted diets are of benefit to patients prone to coronary artery disease, they should probably be instituted long before the vascular disease is symptomatic.

2. A patient with a high likelihood of developing diabetes mellitus may deserve a discussion of the carbohydrate content of the diet.

3. Early stages of hypertension are often controlled by moderate reduction of salt intake.

4. A calcium-restricted diet in a stone-forming patient may be an appropriate undertaking despite the present asymptomatic status of the patient.

I. Discussing Diet With the Asymptomatic Patient

A. Asymptomatic patients who request nutrition advice are generally concerned about one or more aspects of their diet.

1. This may be due to disease in one or more family members, an illness or death of a neighbor or acquaintance, or perhaps a television show which the patient viewed the previous week.

B. Critical to an appropriate discussion of nutrition with the healthy patient are a thorough history and physical examination.

C. It is up to the physician to determine why the patient is concerned about diet in the first place. Having done so, the doctor may be able to give some psychological support, as well as nutritional advice, to the worried patient.

D. In the absence of definitive problems, the nutritional aspects of the following factors might theoretically be discussed with the asymptomatic patient:

1. Undernutrition
2. Overnutrition
3. Alcoholism
4. Dental caries
5. Allergies
6. Bone disorders
7. Cardiovascular disease
8. Endocrine disorders, especially diabetes
9. Gastrointestinal disorders
10. Hereditary disorders
11. Kidney disorders including uremia and renal calculi
12. Liver disease

E. From a practical point of view, the list above is impossible to review with a patient.

1. It is probably more valuable to discuss the major food groups with the healthy patient and answer specific questions about the list of topics should they arise.

II. General Considerations

A. Before discussing the nutritionally adequate diet, a few comments regarding ideal weight and calorie requirements may be appropriate.

1. Tables listing desirable weights for men and women will be found in Chapter 17.

B. Healthy patients will frequently ask the physician, "How much should I weigh?" Doctors have a tendency to respond on the basis of a superficial glance at the patient, with perhaps palpation of a mid-abdominal skin fold. The charts in Chapter 27 give somewhat more definitive data.

1. One must keep in mind, however, that the heights listed in height-weight tables were measured with the patients' shoes on, in contrast to the usual practice today.

C. Doctors may not automatically discuss caloric intake with healthy patients. Some patients are curious about this information, however.

1. As a general guideline, the adult female will require 35 cal./kg. of desirable body weight.

2. The adult male generally will need 40 cal./kg. of desirable body weight per day.

3. The range of caloric intake, however, varies widely.

4. Thirty calories per kg. is probably adequate for the sedentary individual.

5. Up to 55 cal./kg. of desirable body weight per day may be required for persons who regularly engage in strenuous physical activity.

III. Nutritional Requirements

A. Basic Food Groups*

1. Milk and milk products
2. Meat and meat substitutes

---

*A table of Recommended Daily Dietary Allowances designed for the maintenance of good nutrition of practically all healthy persons in the U.S. has been published by the National Research Council, Food and Nutrition Board (see Table 2-1). These recommendations can be fulfilled by eating a variety of food-stuffs from the four basic food groups.

3. Vegetables and fruits
4. Breads and cereals

The actual amounts to be eaten will, of course, depend upon the size of the patient as well as his daily energy expenditure. The number of servings from each food group which should be included in the daily diet is listed below.

Include Each Day

Milk
Two or more glasses daily or an equivalent amount of other milk products

1 slice American cheese	= $\frac{3}{4}$ glass milk
$\frac{1}{2}$ cup cottage cheese	= $\frac{1}{3}$ glass milk
$\frac{1}{4}$ pint ice cream	= $\frac{1}{4}$ glass milk

Meat
Two or more servings daily of meat, fish, poultry, eggs, or cheese. Dry beans, peas, nuts, or peanut butter are acceptable alternatives.

Vegetables and Fruits
Four or more servings daily. A serving of citrus fruit or tomato daily for vitamin C. Dark green leafy or deep yellow vegetables or yellow fruit three to four times weekly for vitamin A.

Bread and Cereals
Four or more servings daily

B. Milk

1. Milk is needed primarily as a source of calcium, although $\frac{1}{2}$ pint of milk also contains approximately 8 to 9 g. of protein.

2. Milk is also a good source of riboflavin, vitamin D, B_{12}, and phosphorus.

3. Two glasses of milk daily will satisfy the nutritional needs of healthy adult patients.

4. A surprising number of patients dislike milk.

   a. For these individuals, cheese, ice cream, and many foods containing milk are available.

5. Pasteurized whole milk is also an excellent source for fat. If one consumes 1 pint of milk daily, 5840 g. of fat will be ingested from this source over 1 year.

   a. Most Americans do not need this extra source of calories.

   b. Therefore, skim or low-fat milk
   (Text continues on p. 14)

Table 2-1. **Food and Nutrition Board, National Academy of Sciences-National**

	Age (years)	Weight (kg.)	Weight (lbs.)	Height (cm.)	Height (in.)	Energy (Cal.)[2]	Protein (g.)	Vitamin A Activity (RE)[3]	Vitamin A Activity (I.U.)	Vitamin D (I.U.)	Vitamin E Activity (I.U.)	Ascorbic Acid (mg.)	Folacin[6] (µg.)
								Fat-Soluble Vitamins					
Infants	0.0–0.5	6	14	60	24	kg. × 117	kg. × 2.2	420[4]	1,400	400	4	35	50
	0.5–1.0	9	20	71	28	kg. × 108	kg. × 2.0	400	2,000	400	5	35	50
Children	1–3	13	28	86	34	1300	23	400	2,000	400	7	40	100
	4–6	20	44	110	44	1800	30	500	2,500	400	9	40	200
	7–10	30	66	135	54	2400	36	700	3,300	400	10	40	300
Males	11–14	44	97	158	63	2800	44	1,000	5,000	400	12	45	400
	15–18	61	134	172	69	3000	54	1,000	5,000	400	15	45	400
	19–22	67	147	172	69	3000	54	1,000	5,000	400	15	45	400
	23–50	70	154	172	69	2700	56	1,000	5,000		15	45	400
	51 +	70	154	172	69	2400	56	1,000	5,000		15	45	400
Females	11–14	44	97	155	62	2400	44	800	4,000	400	10	45	400
	15–18	54	119	162	65	2100	48	800	4,000	400	11	45	400
	19–22	58	128	162	65	2100	46	800	4,000	400	12	45	400
	23–50	58	128	162	65	2000	46	800	4,000		12	45	400
	51+	58	128	162	65	1800	46	800	4,000		12	45	400
Pregnant						+300	+30	1,000	5,000	400	15	60	800
Lactating						+500	+20	1,200	6,000	400	15	60	600

[1]The allowances are intended to provide for individual variations among most normal persons as they live in the U.S. under usual environmental stresses. Diets should be based on a variety of common foods in order to provide other nutrients for which human requirements have been less well defined.
[2]Kilojoules (KJ) = 4.2 × Cal.
[3]Retinol equivalents
[4]Assumed to be all as retinol in milk during the first 6 months of life. All subsequent intakes are assumed to be 50% as retinol and 50% as β-carotene when calculated from international units. As retinol equivalents, 75% are as retinol and 25% as β-carotene.

Research Council Recommended Daily Dietary Allowances,[1] Revised 1974

Water-Soluble Vitamins					Minerals					
Niacin[7] (B_1) (mg.)	Riboflavin (B_2) (mg.)	Thiamine (mg.)	Vitamin B_6 (mg.)	Vitamin B_12 (µg.)	Calcium (mg.)	Phosphorus (mg.)	Iodine (µg.)	Iron (mg.)	Magnesium (mg.)	Zinc (mg.)
5	0.4	0.3	0.3	0.3	360	240	35	10	60	3
8	0.6	0.5	0.4	0.3	540	400	45	15	70	5
9	0.8	0.7	0.6	1.0	800	800	60	15	150	10
12	1.1	0.9	0.9	1.5	800	800	80	10	200	10
16	1.2	1.2	1.2	2.0	800	800	110	10	250	10
18	1.5	1.4	1.6	3.0	1200	1200	130	18	350	15
20	1.8	1.5	1.8	3.0	1200	1200	150	18	400	15
20	1.8	1.5	2.0	3.0	800	800	140	10	350	15
18	1.6	1.4	2.0	3.0	800	800	130	10	350	15
16	1.5	1.2	2.0	3.0	800	800	110	10	350	15
16	1.3	1.2	1.6	3.0	1200	1200	115	18	300	15
14	1.4	1.1	2.0	3.0	1200	1200	115	18	300	15
14	1.4	1.1	2.0	3.0	800	800	100	18	300	15
13	1.2	1.0	2.0	3.0	800	800	100	18	300	15
12	1.1	1.0	2.0	3.0	800	800	80	10	300	15
+2	+0.3	+0.3	2.5	4.0	1200	1200	125	18[8]	450	20
+4	+0.5	+0.3	2.5	4.0	1200	1200	150	18	450	25

[5]Total vitamin E activity, estimated to be 80% as α-tocopherol and 20% other tocopherols.

[6]The folacin allowances refer to dietary sources as determined by *Lactobacillus casei* assay. Pure forms of folacin may be effective in doses less than one-fourth of the RDA.

[7]Although allowances are expressed as niacin, it is recognized that on the average 1 mg. of niacin is derived from each 60 mg. of dietary trytophan.

[8]This increased requirement cannot be met by ordinary diets; therefore, the use of supplemental iron is recommended.

(Reproduced from Recommended Dietary Allowances. ed. 8. With the permission of the National Academy of Sciences, Washington, D.C.)

should be recommended to the healthy patient in the belief that the decreased fat may reduce the likelihood of the patient developing atherosclerosis.

6. A normal serving of skim milk ($\frac{1}{2}$ pint) contains 1 g. of fat in comparison to 8 g. in $\frac{1}{2}$ pint of pasteurized whole milk.

C. Meat

1. The meat group is the primary source of protein in the diet of most Americans.

2. The amount ingested usually far exceeds the amount needed to maintain positive nitrogen balance.

3. Approximately 1 g. of protein/kg. of body weight per day is adequate for maintaining positive nitrogen balance.

4. Two daily servings of meat, fish, poultry, or eggs are adequate for the normal healthy person.

5. A patient should be reminded that meat is a relatively expensive source of calories.

6. Meat is also an excellent source of fat.

a. With the high incidence of coronary artery disease in the U.S., moderation in fat intake should be suggested to healthy patients, especially if there is a family history of coronary artery disease.

b. Limiting egg consumption to two to four weekly can be suggested for the same reasons.

7. The physician should remind patients that the average American breakfast of fried eggs, bacon, and buttered toast may have been appropriate for the farmer who needed 5000 cal./day, but it is likely to lead to increased weight in patients with more sedentary occupations.

8. For those persons who lean towards vegetarianism, dry beans, peas, and nuts are reasonable alternatives to the meat group.

D. Vegetables and Fruits

1. Vegetables and fruits are particularly valuable as sources of vitamin A and vitamin C.

2. Four or more servings should be taken from this group daily.

3. This is the area in which a teen-ager's diet may become nutritionally inadequate.

4. A source of vitamin C should be ingested daily (oranges, grapefruits, tomatoes, strawberries).

5. While potatoes have nutritional merit, the physician should emphasize the need for green leafy or yellow vegetables because of their higher vitamin content.

6. The vitamin content of cooked vegetables depends upon the method of preparation.

a. Vegetables which are cooked quickly in a small volume of water will have retained most of their vitamins.

b. In vegetables cooked slowly in a large volume of water which is discarded, a substantial amount of vitamins will be lost down the drain.

E. Breads and Cereals

1. The popularity of breads and cereals as dietary components has, in the past, largely been due to their low cost.

2. In contrast to the three other food groups, breads and cereals are a cheap source of calories.

3. Many of the commercial bread products have been further enriched with vitamins and minerals.

4. The ultimate value of cereals may depend less on low cost and more upon its high fiber content.

a. Increasing epidemiologic evidence suggests that diets with high fiber content are protective against constipation, diverticular diseases, hemorrhoids, and cancer of the colon.

b. The relationship between these factors is presently associative rather than cause and effect.

c. Nonetheless, the recommendation of four or more servings daily from this food group seems most reasonable.

d. An excellent symposium about the interrelationship between the diet and the colon has recently been published.*

---

*Flock, M.D. (ed.): Diet, bacteria and the colon. Am. J. Clin. Nutr., *29:*1409, 1976.

F. General Advice

1. In addition to these general guidelines, certain clinical problems occur with such statistical frequency that general advice even to the healthy patient may be appropriate. These are in the areas of control of body weight, ingestion of sodium chloride, food faddism, and vitamin intake.

IV. Control of Body Weight

A. Details regarding the treatment of obesity appear in Chapter 17.

B. The difficulties in "curing" obesity are known to all.

1. Physicians seldom emphasize the prevention of the problem.

C. In practice, physicians are commonly faced with the 40-year-old man or woman who is 40 lbs. overweight. It is likely that this patient has added 2 lbs. each year since age 20. Had this patient been given proper nutrition advice at 25 years (when he was "only" 10 lbs. overweight) perhaps better nutritional habits would have been developed over the subsequent 15 years.

1. Unfortunately, it is difficult for the physician to get properly motivated when the weight excess is mild.

2. It is at this time, however, that the dietary intake of a patient should be reviewed, and advice should be given.

D. In addition to any specific advice given after reviewing a patient's dietary intake, the following nutritional guidelines should be stated:

1. Do not skip meals.

2. Avoid overemphasis on any one component of the diet (i.e., protein, carbohydrate, or fat).

3. Avoid bizarre diets. Such diets cannot be maintained for prolonged periods of time, and weight gain will often occur when they are discontinued.

4. Calorie restriction without obvious dieting is the only way to permanently control weight.

V. Ingestion of Sodium Chloride

A. The necessity for regulating salt intake is so common for patients over the age of 50 because of heart failure and hypertension that a few comments regarding salt intake to the healthy patient may be appropriate.

B. From a practical standpoint, the patient should be asked whether he salts food before he tastes it.

C. Many patients get so accustomed to massive salt intake during the first few decades of their lives that adjusting such intake later becomes extremely difficult.

D. While the merits of discussing sodium intake with the 25-year-old asymptomatic patient can be argued, it is the author's feeling that the patient who eats 20 to 25 g. of sodium chloride daily will have more difficulty in adjusting to restricted salt intake in the future than the patient who ingests 10 g.

E. One can point out that the interesting tastes of many foods may be minimized or suppressed by the use of large amounts of salt.

F. Figure 2-1 gives data on 78 untreated male hypertension patients between the ages of 24 and 49 studied in 1976.

1. The average urinary sodium excretion was 200 mEq./24 hours with a range from 35 to 465. Twenty-eight of 78 (36%) excreted more than 256 mEq. of sodium daily.

2. Ignoring the minimal extrarenal losses of sodium in most situations, this excretion would require the intake of 15 or more g. of sodium chloride to maintain a reasonable sodium balance.

3. Four of these subjects actually excreted more than 426 mEq./24 hours. These latter patients were presumably ingesting in excess of 25 g. of sodium chloride daily, or approximately 0.88 oz.

4. In practical terms, a 1-lb. carton of Morton's salt should last about 3 weeks.

5. This point is obviously oversimplified because it ignores the natural sodium

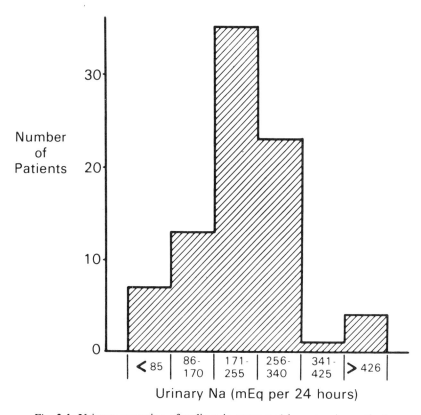

Fig. 2-1. Urinary excretion of sodium in untreated hypertensive patients.

content of certain foods which contributes to the total sodium content of the diet.

6. Comparatively large urinary sodium excretion has been observed in non-hypertensive patients.

VI. Food Faddism

A. A discussion with the healthy patient about food faddism frequently is in order.

B. This is particularly true in today's society in which eccentric diets appear to be particularly popular.

C. There are several reasons why food faddism should be avoided.

1. Unusual diets are generally more expensive than the regular nutritionally sound diets.

2. Many of these diets are unbalanced or inadequate by today's standards.

3. There is a tendency to be falsely secure about one's nutrition when one is on any special diet.

VII. Vitamins

A. The potential pharmacologic uses of vitamins are listed in Chapter 8.

B. If the general dietary instructions already given are followed, supplemental vitamins will not be needed by the healthy patient.

C. Although the author does not seriously object to a daily multivitamin preparation, some of these preparations are surprisingly expensive, and patients should be alerted that they may be spending their money foolishly.

D. At the present state of knowledge, the use of megadose vitamins should be discouraged.

1. There is no good evidence that super doses of vitamins are of value in the healthy patient.

2. Although toxicity from high doses of water-soluble vitamins has not been proven, there are no long-term data to definitely exclude this possibility and there is evidence currently pointing to this potentiality (see Chap. 8).

3. Toxicity syndromes from overdosage of vitamin A or vitamin D are proven clinical entities.

3. NUTRITION IN PREGNANCY

Herbert Jaffin, M.D.

BASIC PRINCIPLES

I. Two generations of American physicians have been taught to impose caloric restriction in pregnancy with a view of limiting weight gain to between 16 and 18 lbs. This practice stemmed from faulty reasoning concerning the origin of weight gain exhibited by pregnant patients who develop preeclampsia/eclampsia, namely, a failure to distinguish between weight gain owing to extracellular fluid retention, one of the hallmarks of preeclampsia, and that resulting from tissue accretion, and a failure to realize that it is the pattern of weight gain rather than the total amount of gain that provides the significant clue for the recognition of preeclampsia.

II. Caloric restriction has no effect on the incidence of preeclampsia/eclampsia, and there is no evidence that these are caused by excessive weight gain either in the form of fat or water. On the other hand, there are clear indications that inadequate weight gain in pregnancy increases the incidence of low-birth-weight infants.

III. The National Institutes of Health (NIH) Collaborative Study revealed that of some 30 variables predictive of a high-risk pregnancy, next to a history of low-birth-weight (for height) infant, small weight gain during pregnancy and low prepregnancy weight are the most important etiological factors in the birth of growth-retarded babies. Further, evidence has been accumulating that maternal nutritional status both before and during pregnancy influences not only the birth weight but perhaps also brain development significantly.

IV. For all these reasons, the importance of an adequate weight gain for the pregnant woman and ample dietary resources to promote optimal nutrition of the mother and fetus cannot be overemphasized. The notion that the pregnant woman must eat for two has long been recognized as fallacious, but pregnancy does indeed make increased demands for both calories and specific nutrients that must be met. Although calorie restriction is ill-advised in pregnancy, a degree of weight control is desirable to prevent excessive fat deposition that may cause obesity.

V. Weight gain in normal pregnancies is highly variable. Young women tend to gain slightly more than older women, primigravidas more than multi-gravidas, and thin women more than fat women.

VI. A target of 24- to 26-lb. weight gain for healthy women is considered a reasonable average and consistent with the most favorable outcome of pregnancy. It is recommended that individual weight gain be kept reasonably close to this average. Asthenic or undernourished women should be encouraged to gain more than this.

VII. The RDA for the pregnant woman is 2500 cal./day, 300 cal./day more than the basic caloric requirement of the reference nonpregnant mature woman. This means that the expectant mother should receive 15% more calories per day than she needs to sustain her ideal body weight. The ideal or desirable body weight should be determined by reference to standard height and weight tables (see Table 2-1).

VIII. The pregnant woman synthesizes complex new tissues at a greater rate than at any other time in life. Because the efficiency of protein utilization is lower in pregnancy than has previously been assumed, the recommendations call for an additional 30 g./day over the basic allowance in the non-pregnant state, amounting to 1.3 to 1.7 g. of protein per kg. of body weight per day or 76 g. per day (see Table 2-1).

A. To ensure adequate utilization of protein during pregnancy, the energy intake must be kept above 36 Cal./kg./day. The usual recommendation is to give 40 Cal./kg./day in a balanced distribution: protein 9 to 16%, fats 33 to 45% (assuming satisfactory tolerance), and carbohydrate 35 to 55%.

B. The carbohydrate component of the diet should consist predominantly of complex polysaccharides (e.g., starch), but simple sugars are better tolerated by patients with hyperemesis.

IX. Notwithstanding its limitation, body weight is the best guide for estimating the nutrient needs, and weight gain during pregnancy is the best clinical parameter by which to judge the progress of pregnancy.

X. The rate of weight gain should parallel the physiologic pattern of fetal growth, which has an S shape, there being little gain in the first trimester, rapid increase in the second trimester, and some slowing in the third trimester. Thus weight gain should amount to 2 to 4 lbs. (about 1 lb./month) during the first trimester, and approximately 1 lb./week thereafter. A weight gain slightly above this rate, if proceeding at a regular rate, should not be criticized. Inadequate weight gain—2.2 lbs. (1 kg.) or less per month—or excessive weight gain—6.5 lbs. (3 kg.) or more per month—necessitates reevaluation of the patient's nutritional state.

XI. Mild generalized edema associated with gradual accumulation of fluid and edema in the lower limbs are not unphysiologic. Some women accumulate as much as 9 L. of fluid in normal pregnancies. The fluid is lost usually as a result of physiologic diuresis in the immediate postpartum days. A sudden increase in weight, however, especially after about the 20th week of gestation, is cause for suspecting that water is being retained at an inordinate rate and should be regarded as a warning sign of impending preeclampsia.

XII. The products of conception account for only 50% of the total weight gain during normal pregnancy, the expanded maternal blood volume plus the tissues added to the reproductive organs account for another 18%, and the remainder of the gain usually is fat with perhaps 1 or 2 kg. of "excess" body water at term. Thus, women tend to add to their body fat stores during pregnancy, which may not be entirely lost after delivery and can contribute to subsequent obesity. The permanent weight gain is lessened in mothers who nurse their babies as it is used up to provide energy for the production of milk.

XIII. Weight reduction programs for obese patients should not be initiated during pregnancy. Caloric restriction may not only result in deficient intake of essential nutrients, but it also exposes the patient to the hazard of starvation ketosis with serious consequences to the offspring. This is also true of diets emphasizing severe carbohydrate restriction. Weight gain in obese patients should generally be managed in accordance with the same general principles as in the nonobese; caloric intake should be adequate to support the customary weight gain.

XIV. The best diet for the pregnant woman consists of simple, balanced meals including properly prepared fresh foods to minimize the loss of essential vitamins and minerals.

A. It is wise to explain to the expectant mother the principles underlying the selection of a suitable diet. She should understand the need not only for sufficient total calories but also for specific nutrients, and she should know the foods that are the best sources for these nutrients.

B. The diet should include liberal amounts of citrus fruits and fruit juices and leafy green vegetables. Frequent servings of meat and fish are important because the presence of essential elements increases their value beyond simply serving as protein sources. Pastries and candies should not be eaten in quantity.

C. Fluid intake should at least replace daily losses. Water may be drunk freely. Coffee and tea may be taken in moderation. Intake of alcoholic beverages should be minimal. (Ingestion of 3 oz. of 80-proof liquor a day has been shown to have an adverse effect on the offspring.) Normal women do not have to restrict their salt intake.

XV. Although the worth of vitamin supplements may be debatable, it is fair to say that practically all obstetricians routinely prescribe prenatal multivitamin supplements. In addition all patients should receive iron supplements in the form of ferrous sulfate, 300 mg. three times a day, and a folic acid supplement, 1 mg. per day. One must be aware that polyvitamin capsules and tablets vary considerably in the number and concentration of the different constituents, and it is incumbent on the physician to know the contents of the preparation prescribed. For example, some prenatal supplements contain 50% of the iron supplement needed, whereas others may contain iron in amounts greater than the RDA. The same consideration applies to folic acid.

XVI. All pregnant women should have their nutritional status evaluated at the first prenatal visit. In addition to routine laboratory tests this should include a dietary history taken in the context of her life style, family situation, and dietary intake.

A. It is important that inappropriate dietary habits be recognized at the outset and that the patient receive assistance in correcting them. It is well to ask about alcohol consumption as patients do not usually volunteer this information.

B. The physician should also inquire about drugs that can be obtained without prescription, such as vitamin and mineral supplements, large doses of vitamin C, A,

or E, laxatives, or simple analgesics, because patients do not usually think of these products as drugs.

XVII. Pregnant women who need particular attention to their nutrient needs include:

A. Adolescents who may be biologically immature (less than 17 years old). The stresses of pregnancy are added to the nutrient needs for body growth and maturation.

B. Women in poor nutritional status on entering pregnancy. This compromises pregnancy outcome.

C. Women who have experienced a rapid succession of pregnancies, which often depletes maternal nutrient stores.

D. Overweight women, whose food selection is likely to emphasize foods high in fat and carbohydrate and low in essential vitamins and minerals.

E. Women who show limited weight gain during gestation. This may be caused by a limited food budget, a history of poor diet and suboptimal health, or concurrent disease conducive to impaired absorption of nutrients.

F. Women whose religious or other preferences limit food intake to certain varieties (e.g., vegetarian diets and food fads).

G. Healthy pregnant women besieged with confusing, conflicting, and misleading information that regularly appears in women's magazines or the popular press or media.

WEIGHT AND WEIGHT GAIN IN PREGNANCY—RELATION TO MATERNAL NUTRITION AND LOW-BIRTH-WEIGHT INFANTS

I. How Much Weight Should Be Gained?

A. The question of how much weight gain is desirable has been the subject of numerous studies and seemingly endless discussions. An attempt has been made to estimate the desirable weight gain from data concerning the average gain in normal pregnancies gathered from studies of large groups of women, presumably eating to appetite, and by calculating the physiologic gain from the average weights of identifiable components of the products of conception (see Table 3-1).

B. Based on such considerations, the Committee on Maternal Nutrition, National Research Council, concluded that the normal physiologic gain averages 11 kg. (24 lbs.). Other authorities suggest that an average weight gain of 12.5 kg. (27.5 lbs.) during the course of pregnancy is associated with lowered incidence of low birth weights, prematurity, preeclampsia, and perinatal mortality.

C. The pattern of weight gain is more significant than the total amount. Normally, weight gain is small in the first 10 to 12 weeks after conception. It then begins to accelerate and is relatively rectilinear during the second and third trimesters.

D. The components of weight gained in relation to the stage of pregnancy are presented in Figure 3-1.

1. Initially the growth of the uterus and breast and the increase in maternal blood volume account for the small gain.

2. During the second trimester, maternal compartments expand and nutrient stores (mainly fat, but also protein) are laid down in anticipation of the greatly increased energy requirement of the fetus in the last weeks of pregnancy.

3. The accumulated interstitial fluid in the pelvis and extremities (owing to the increased venous pressure created by the large pregnant uterus) amounts to at least 2 to 3 lbs. in the ambulatory woman.

4. Indirect indices (e.g., isotope dilution) show the increment in total body water as 7 L., of which 5 to 6 L. represent extracellular water (more in women with edema). Most of the growth in the third trimester involves the fetus placenta and amniotic fluid.

II. Management of Weight Gain

A. From the components and pattern of weight gain in normal pregnancy it can be surmised that the influence of maternal nutrition on fetal growth and, hence, birth weight could be expected to be particularly pronounced in the third trimester. This contention is supported by findings that

1. The effects of maternal malnutrition on birth weight, length, and head circumference are strongest when deprivation occurs late in pregnancy and that

2. Birth weights increased significantly when pregnant women on suboptimal calorie intake were given protein-calorie supplements during the last month of pregnancy.

Table 3-1. **Identifiable Components of Weight Gained at 40 Weeks' Gestation**

Tissue or Fluid	Weight	
	g.	*lb.*
Fetus	3,500	7.7
Placenta	650	1.4
Amniotic fluid	800	1.8
Uterus	900	2.0
Breasts	405	0.9
Interstitial fluid	1,200	2.7
Maternal blood	1,800	4.0
TOTAL	9,255	20.5
Total weight gained during average pregnancy	10,896	24.0
Weight gained but not accounted for	1,641	3.5

(Jacobson, H. N.: Weight and weight gain in pregnancy. Clinics in Perinatology, *2*:236, 1975)

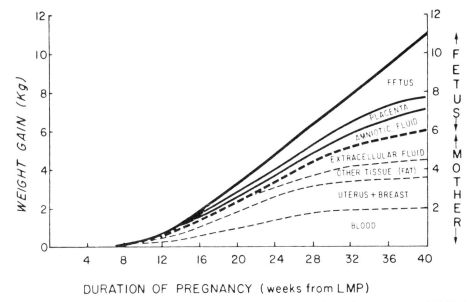

Fig. 3-1. Pattern and components of average maternal weight gain during pregnancy (*LMP*, last menstrual period). (Pitkin, R: Nutritional support in obstetrics and gynecology. Clin. Obstet. Gynecol, *19*:489, 1976)

B. Proper management of weight gain is tailored to individual needs and includes

    1. Calculation of the normal or desirable weight extrapolated from standard height and weight tables

    2. Estimation of the nutritional status, dietary habits, and activity patterns

    3. Determination of weight gain that would be best for the particular woman.

C. Most healthy women show weight gains of from 24 to 30 lbs. in normal pregnancies. Obviously a wide range is compatible with favorable pregnancy outcome and maternal health. It is possible, however, to define the upper and lower limits of desirable weight gain.

D. A woman who gains no more than 18 to 20 lbs. must catabolize her own tissues to produce an 8-lb. child. Healthy well-nourished women who enter pregnancy with ample nutrient stores will tolerate temporary deprivations without obvious harmful effects, but women in suboptimal health and nutritional state may be seriously compromised by further depletion of inadequate nutrient reserves.

E. Clearly the desirable weight gain cannot be achieved if deliberate efforts are made to restrict food intake. On the other hand, the recommendation "to eat to appetite" should not be taken as a license to overindulge in empty calories, which result merely in deposition of extra fat and an invitation to obesity. Guidance in the selection of foods that are both nutritious and appealing is conducive to adequate but not excessive weight gain. Calories should be distributed as about 10 to 15% protein, 33 to 45% fats, and 35 to 55% carbohydrates.

III. Clinical Problems in Weight Management

A. Weight management presents considerable clinical problems with patients who are seriously underweight or overweight on entering pregnancy and those who show inadequate or excessive weight gain during the course of pregnancy. The following arbitrary definitions have been suggested:

1. *Underweight* —prepregnant weight that is 10% or more below standard weight for height and age.

2. *Inadequate Weight Gain* —gain of less than 1 kg./month during the second and third trimesters.

3. *Overweight* —prepregnant weight that is 20% above standard weight for age and height.

4. *Excessive Weight Gain* —gain of 3 kg./month or more in the second and third trimesters.

B. The obstetrical hazards and difficult management problems presented by underweight obstetrical patients generally are underestimated.

1. Those who are seriously underweight on entering pregnancy or show inadequate weight gain during the course of gestation are more likely to deliver a low-birth-weight infant and, in addition, are at a greater risk of developing preeclampsia/eclampsia, antepartum hemorrhage, and other pregnancy complications.

2. The nutritional status of such patients deserves careful evaluation or reevaluation. A carefully supervised larger-than-normal increase in weight (as much as 40 lbs.) may be necessary to produce a normal offspring and still preserve the health of the mother. Studies have shown that protein-calorie supplements can correct for past nutritional deficits and depleted stores as well as provide for pregnancy needs and can be highly successful if accompanied by nutritional education and counsel.

3. Similarly, women who show inadequate gain after about the 20th week should be reevaluated. Their energy intake or specific nutrient intake may be deficient by reason of a limited food budget, unusual dietary habits, unwise choices in selecting foods, or an underlying condition impairing absorption.

4. It is customary to think that such problems are likely to arise in third-world countries, but the National Research Council's report estimated that one-third of prenatal patients in clinic practice are underweight, and increased perinatal mortality related to inadequate weight gain during gestation has been well documented in private practice in the U.S.

C. Excessive Weight Gain

1. The products of conception account for only 20 lbs. of the average weight gain. Much of the additional weight gain is likely to be deposited around the trunks and hips as fat and, unless used up at least in part in the production of milk, is likely to become a permanent contribution to obesity in susceptible subjects. It has been suggested that maternal overnutrition during pregnancy plays a role in the development of obesity in the offspring.

2. Weight gain owing to the accumulation of fat must be differentiated from weight gain owing to the retention of extracellular fluid. Extracellular fluid retention is one of the signs of preeclampsia and, in many cases, of a gain in weight. There is no firm evidence, however, that excessive weight gain, whether in the form of fat or water, causes preeclampsia.

3. Edema of the lower extremities owing to the accumulation of interstitial fluid as a result of the obstruction of pelvic veins is seen commonly. This responds to bed rest in the lateral recumbent position. Many women show mild generalized edema associated with gradual accumulation of fluid during the last weeks of pregnancy.

4. A large shift in water balance is likely to be reflected in a sudden increase in weight and should be regarded as a warning sign of impending toxemia. It should be noted that a considerable amount of fluid may accumulate and the total weight gain may be small if the edema fluid is exchanged for loss of fat and lean tissues.

5. Once nutrient and energy intake is adequate to fully meet the needs of the fetus and supporting tissues and to maintain the body weight of the mother, any additional

food intake will result in both increased excretion of some nutrients as well as storage of excessive fat. Moreover, if the diet consists of predominantly carbohydrates— usually in women who make unwise food choices or those on a limited food budget— the energy intake is more than sufficient, but protein intake is low so that the mother's lean body mass will be used to meet the protein needs of the fetus.

6. The aim of dietary counselling in the presence of excessive weight gain is not to restrict weight gain markedly but to restore the pattern toward normal.

7. Obesity in and of itself carries an increased risk of pregnancy complications including diabetes, chronic hypertension, and thromboembolic disease. These complications compromise maternal health and are responsible for increased perinatal morbidity and mortality.

8. Proper management of obese pregnant patients during pregnancy apparently is a matter of some controversy.

a. Some obstetricians advocate moderate caloric restriction with limited weight gain so that the patient will conclude pregnancy with a net weight loss.

b. Severe calorie restriction during pregnancy is generally opposed by most obstetricians and nutritional experts for several reasons:

(1) No convincing evidence has been presented that weight loss or limited weight gain has any effect on pregnancy complications of the obese patient.

(2) On the other hand, severe caloric restriction could be expected to be highly detrimental in pregnancy. Aside from the probability that restriction of calories will result in deficiency of some essential nutrients, the susceptibility to starvation ketosis during pregnancy would endanger both fetal and maternal health.

(3) Fetal glucose uptake in pregnancy results in an acceleration of the normal metabolic response to starvation, and blood ketone levels are two to three times greater than those observed after an overnight fast in the nonpregnant state. Caloric restriction in cases of obesity may further exaggerate this tendency to starvation ketosis.

(4) Furthermore, ketone bodies accumulate in the amniotic fluid, and uptake has been noted in the fetus who may utilize them when glucose supply is restricted for fuel, a utilization which may have an adverse effect on neuropsychologic development.

(5) A significant reduction in IQ has been reported in the offspring of mothers who have shown ketonuria whether owing to starvation or diabetes during pregnancy. Whether ketones per se or associated metabolic alterations (in amino acid levels) are responsible for the deleterious effects on brain development is not known.

9. Thus dietary management of the obese pregnant patient should emphasize the avoidance of severe caloric restriction as well as prevention of excessive weight gain. In particular, a minimal intake of 150 g. of carbohydrate should be maintained at all times. Energy intake should be sufficient to adequately support the desirable weight gain. The same general principles in management should be observed as in patients with normal weight (see Chap. 17).

MATERNAL NUTRIENT NEEDS

I. Energy Requirements (Calculations)

A. Adequate energy intake during pregnancy is important for the support of the growth and development of the fetus, as well as the growth of maternal tissues and the additional metabolism the new tissues incur.

B. The total energy cost of pregnancy calculated from the amounts of fat and protein accumulated by the mother and fetus and the additional metabolism incurred in this accumulation has been estimated at 75,000 or 80,000 Cal. Prorated over the period of gestation this amounts to a daily increment of 300 Cal./day throughout pregnancy. The allowance for the mature nonpregnant reference woman is 2,000 or

2,100 Cal. (depending on the age) thus the 300 Cal./day represents an increment of 15%. This figure does not take into consideration variables that influence caloric needs such as physical activity, ambient temperature, altitude, or growth requirements unrelated to pregnancy (e.g., adolescence).

C. Because body mass increases about 20% during pregnancy, work that requires a lot of movement will require as much as 20% more energy. Energy expenditures being variable (from 38 to 50 Cal./kg.), the best assurance of adequate intake is a satisfactory weight gain. Recommendations for energy intake per day, therefore, should be expressed in terms of enough calories (and other nutrients) to produce an optimal weight gain of between 24 to 30 lb. during pregnancy. Weight gain measures a relative adequacy of the energy level of the diet, which is independent of the actual amount of calories consumed. That is, a 24-lb. increase in weight may require only 1,800 Cal./day for a sedentary woman, whereas an active, growing teenager might require 3,000 Cal./day to produce the same 24-lb. weight increase.

D. Energy intake of healthy women should not be reduced below 36 Cal./kg. of pregnant body weight, the energy required for adequate utilization of protein during pregnancy.

MACRONUTRIENTS

I. Proteins and Amino Acids/Energy Interactions

A. Specific amino acid requirements for pregnancy and lactation are unknown.

B. The protein allowance for mixed proteins in the U.S. diet is 0.8 g./kg./day, which amounts to 46 g. per day for the healthy 58 kg. reference woman. The allowance is based on average protein requirement of 0.47 g./kg./day (as estimated from balance studies) increased by 30% to allow for individual variability and corrected for 75% efficiency of utilization.

C. The amount of protein deposited during gestation is uncertain. By measuring tissue composition, it has been estimated that on the average about 925 g. of protein is deposited in the fetus and accessory tissue of the mother at a rate of 0.6, 1.8, 4.8, and 6.1 g. per day during successive quarters of gestation. Protein may be stored in maternal tissues during the early stages of gestation to be mobilized later when demands for growth of the fetus are greatest. The observed nitrogen retention of the healthy, adequately fed pregnant woman is double the amount predicted from analysis of tissues.

D. Reports of benefit to the mother and infant from generous protein intakes are suggestive but controversial. Because low protein intakes (which impair reproductive performance) are commonly associated with low caloric intakes, epidemiologic data are not conclusive. Increased energy supplements alone or with protein were found to be beneficial when given to mothers who were consuming diets marginal in protein.

E. For the pregnant reference woman 30 g. of protein/day is added to the basic 46-g./day allowance from the second month to the end of gestation. This gives an allowance of 1.3 g./kg./day for the mature woman, 1.5 g./kg./day for pregnant adolescents age 15 to 18, and 1.7 g./kg./day for pregnant girls under age 15.

F. For lactation an additional 20 g. of protein/day above the maintenance allowance is recommended. The average daily milk yield is estimated at 850 to 1200 ml., with a protein content of 1.2%, yielding 10 to 15 g./day. The allowance is then adjusted for 70% efficiency of conversion of dietary protein to milk protein.

II. Carbohydrates

A. Sufficient carbohydrate in the diet is required to prevent ketosis, excessive breakdown of body protein, loss of cations especially sodium, and dehydration.

B. Usually 50 to 100 g. of digestible carbohydrate/day will offset the undesirable metabolic responses associated with high-fat diets and fasting. In pregnancy, a minimum amount of 150 to 200 g. of carbohydrate should be provided.

III. Fats and Essential Fatty Acids

A. Two polyunsaturated fatty acids, linoleic acid and arachidonic acid are the only fatty acids known to be essential for the human fetus and infant.

B. The diet must contain 1 to 2% essential fatty acids to prevent deficiency. Various edible vegetable oils contain linoleic acid in high concentration, for example, corn, cottonseed, peanut, safflower, soybean oil (but not olive oil or coconut oil). Arachidonic acid occurs in animal fats, albeit in rather small amounts.

MICRONUTRIENTS

I. Vitamins

A. Basic Principles
1. Vitamins are transported across the placenta by different mechanisms:
   a. Simple diffusion (fat-soluble vitamins)
   b. Facilitated diffusion (fat-soluble vitamins)
   c. Active transport (water-soluble vitamins)
2. Factors of storage, transport, and excretion are instrumental in determining the potential of vitamins to induce maternal deficiency or fetal toxicity.
3. Fat-soluble vitamins are stored in the liver where they are available for release when maternal intake is insufficient. Therefore, maternal deficiency is rare, but because urinary excretion is low, overdosage presents the potential risk of fetal toxicity.
   a. Maternal plasma levels tend to be increased in the pregnant as compared with the nonpregnant state, while fetal plasma levels generally are lower than maternal levels.

4. Water-soluble vitamins are not stored in the maternal organism and are excreted at a relatively high rate, thus they present a risk of maternal deficiency in times of deprivation, while the potential for fetal toxicity with overdosage is low.
   a. Maternal blood levels tend to be lower in the pregnant than in the nonpregnant state, while fetal plasma levels generally are higher than maternal levels.
5. Some causes of vitamin deficits during pregnancy are:
   a. INADEQUATE INTAKE OR DEFECTS IN ABSORPTION
      (1) Faulty nutrition
      (2) Improper food preparation
      (3) Malabsorption
   b. DEFECTS IN UTILIZATION AND METABOLISM
      (1) Inherent in pregnancy, owing to steroid effects on liver function and physiologic changes in pregnancy
      (2) Administration of drugs (e.g., vitamin antagonists) during pregnancy
   c. INCREASED DEMANDS BY
      (1) Placenta and fetus
      (2) Increased maternal metabolism of multiple pregnancies
      (3) Closely spaced pregnancies
      (4) Presence of associated conditions (e.g., hemoglobinopathies)

B. Thiamine (Vitamin B_1)
1. Thiamine requirement is influenced by carbohydrate intake and total energy expenditure. The recommended dietary allowances for pregnant women are increased by 0.3 mg./day over that recommended for nonpregnant women (1 mg./day), an amount that is readily provided in the usual diet.
2. Thiamine apparently is actively transported by the placenta as indicated by the 1.8 times greater concentration found in newborns as compared with that in maternal plasma.
3. No evidence has been presented that thiamine deficiency in pregnant females has an adverse effect on the course of gestation or the status of the neonate.

Using erythrocyte transketolase activation to assess thiamine status, some 30% of 600 women at various stages of gestation were judged to be thiamine deficient (by standards in nonpregnant women), but the incidence of neonatal complications was no greater than in vitamin-sufficient women.

C. Riboflavin

1. Studies of urinary excretion in humans indicate that tissue reserves cannot be maintained with riboflavin intakes of 0.5 mg./1000 Cal. or less, and the riboflavin allowances have been computed as 0.6 mg./1000 Cal. for persons of all ages.

2. In order to transfer riboflavin from the maternal to the fetal circulation, the placenta takes flavin adenine dinucleotide (FAD) from the maternal blood and splits it to free riboflavin which then is secreted into the fetal circulation.

3. Maternal riboflavin deficiency has been confirmed by a number of studies. As pregnancy progresses women tend to excrete less riboflavin and to require more of the vitamin than nonpregnant women eating similar diets. In one study, the proportion of women deficient in riboflavin increased from 25% during the first trimester to 40% at term.

4. Because pregnancy increases energy requirements, the RDA calls for 0.3 mg./day of riboflavin in addition to the normal allowances for females (1.4 mg. for 15 to 22-year-old women and 1.2 mg. daily for older women).

D. Niacin

1. Niacin requirements in pregnancy are slightly increased. The normal requirement of 13 to 14 mg./day is increased to 15 to 16 mg./day.

2. These amounts are easily supplied by the diet.

E. Vitamin B_6 (Pyridoxine)

1. Naturally occurring dietary vitamin B_6 deficiency has rarely been described in humans, although seizures in infants have been ascribed to absence of pyridoxine in feeding formulas, and a pyridoxine-responsive anemia is recognized.

2. Reduction of vitamin B_6 in maternal tissues and correction of the biochemical abnormality by pyridoxine intake have been demonstrated by a variety of biochemical procedures.

3. The occurrence of vitamin B_6 deficiency during normal pregnancy is suggested by clinical studies showing increased xanthurenic acid excretion or depressed pyridoxal phosphate levels in pregnant women consuming an apparently adequate diet. These unfavorable biochemical changes could be normalized by administration of pyridoxine. In one study, blood levels were decreased to approximately one-fourth that found in nonpregnant women.

4. In another study, approximately 60% of gravidas presented biochemical evidence of B_6 depletion at the 19th or 20th week of gestation, although infants of such women exhibited no evidence of deleterious effects.

5. Vitamin B_6 coenzymes have been found to be three to four times higher in fetal than in maternal blood, suggesting that active transport of the vitamin and sequestration may be responsible for the maternal deficiency and that transport may be more efficient toward the end of pregnancy.

6. In one study, progressive decline in plasma pyridoxal phosphate levels was observed during the course of pregnancy in women receiving no supplement. The fall was less marked in those receiving 2-mg. supplements, and sustained raised levels were obtained in the group given 10-mg. doses.

7. The clinical significance of laboratory evidences of B_6 deficiency during pregnancy (when judged by standards for nonpregnant women) is not clear. Such data have been widely interpreted as evidence that pregnancy is associated with B_6 deficiency and possibly suggesting the need for supplementation of the maternal diets to be at levels at least five times greater than those recommended by the National Research Council (i.e., Recommended Dietary Allowances—1974).

8. More recently it was postulated that a poorly understood metabolic adjustment to pregnancy may be responsible for the biochemical abnormalities observed. However, late in pregnancy, a true deficiency state owing to fetal uptake is superimposed on these metabolically induced changes.

9. Because xanthurenic acid, an intermediary product of tryptophan metabolism, appears to bind insulin in vitro, findings that xanthurenic acid levels in pregnant women are lowered by pyridoxine gave rise to the suggestion that pyridoxine deficiency may be involved in the development of gestational diabetes.

   a. This view appears to be supported by the improved glucose tolerance observed, without change in insulin levels, in women with gestational diabetes given a large dose (25 mg. q.i.d.) of pyridoxine for two weeks.

   b. It has been suggested that some of the carbohydrate changes accompanying pregnancy, especially in obese women, may involve vitamin B_6 alterations, and that measurement of pyridoxine blood levels might be useful in identifying some women at risk of developing gestational diabetes.

   c. It has been suggested that the B_6 requirement might be reappraised at a higher daily intake, which might prevent some of the mild carbohydrate changes associated with perinatal mortality and death.

10. Supplementation: The recommended dietary allowance for vitamin B_6 is 2.5 mg./day, an increase of 0.5 mg. over that recommended for nonpregnant females. This is easily provided by the usual American diet. However, it is far below that necessary to normalize biochemical abnormalities. Estimates of requirements based on supplements necessary to correct abnormal laboratory findings suggestive of B_6 deficiency range from 10 to 20 mg., or at least five times the recommended allowance. These amounts are not attainable with diet and would necessitate supplementation.

F. Pantothenic Acid

1. Dietary intakes in adults range from 5 to 20 mg./day. In a study of pregnant teenagers, the average daily dietary intake was 4.7 mg., and blood levels were less in pregnant than in nonpregnant women. The RDA for adults is 5 to 10 mg., the upper level being suggested for pregnant and lactating women.

2. Pantothenic acid is widely distributed in food, particularly in meats, whole-grain cereals, and legumes. Isolated dietary deficiencies are unlikely, but marginal deficiencies may exist in generally malnourished persons, along with deficiency of other B-complex vitamins.

G. Folic Acid

1. Depletion of folic acid is the most frequent vitamin deficiency in pregnancy, and megaloblastic anemia owing to folic acid deficiency occurs most frequently in pregnant women.

2. Sources

   a. Folates are found in a number of foods. Particularly rich sources of folic acid are liver (300 μg./100 g.), spinach (50 to 100 μg./100 g.), lettuce (20 to 200 μg./100 g.), and asparagus (70 to 160 μg./100 g.); beef (5 to 18 μg./100 g.), fish, and fruits are relatively poor sources.

   b. Folate in foods is unstable on exposure to air and light, accounting for loss of the vitamin in storage. Folate is also heat-labile and from 50 to 90% of the vitamin may be destroyed by boiling foods in large volumes of water. The relative stability of folate in citrus fruits may be due to the presence of ascorbic acid which protects it from degradation.

3. The total amount of folate in the usual daily diet averages 700 μg. of which 270 μg. is absorbable.

   a. Folic acid is ubiquitously present in cells, and requirements are related to metabolic rate and cell turnover. Hence, an increased amount of folic acid is needed in pregnancy.

   b. Total body stores of folates, which are small (10 to 15 mg.), are located mainly in the liver and are sufficient to maintain normal body metabolism for 3 to 6 months. Thus, in normal women on a folate-deficient diet, megaloblastic anemia develops after 15 to 18 weeks and more rapidly in pregnant women.

    c. Folate depletion develops gradually. If deficiency persists megaloblastic (macrocytic) anemia with a fall in erythrocyte count and increased mean corpuscular volume of erythrocytes develops.

    d. During pregnancy urinary excretion of folate is decreased, and folate accumulates in the placenta. Serum and red cell folate levels gradually decline starting the 16th week of gestation. In the third trimester, folate levels as well as hemoglobin and hematocrit are higher in cord blood than in maternal plasma of well-nourished women.

    e. The need for folate increases during pregnancy mainly because of demands of maternal erythropoiesis and fetal-placental growth. Normal values in pregnancy are greater than 4 ng./ml. for serum folate and greater than 150 ng./ml. for red cell folate.

5. Daily folate requirements to maintain positive folate balance in pregnancy range from 150 to 300 μg./day as opposed to 50 to 100 μg./day in the nonpregnant state.

    a. To allow for variability of absorption, the RDA is set at 400 μg. in the nonpregnant state and 800 μg. in pregnancy.

    b. Folate deficiency results from increased requirement in hypermetabolic states (e.g., pregnancy, hyperthyroidism), inadequate dietary intake, or failure to absorb, utilize, or retain folic acid.

    c. The reported incidence of folate deficiency in pregnancy varies from 0.2 to 75%, depending on the population studied and method and criteria used for diagnosis.

    d. Several European studies reported an incidence of 25 to 30% of normal pregnancies with biochemical evidence of folate deficiency (reduced serum and red cell folate) and megaloblastic changes in the

blood, which could be corrected with small folate supplements of 300 to 350 μg. daily.

    e. Estimates of folate content in normal diet in the U.S. have been variable depending on the population studied. A high-cost diet contains 65 μg. free folate and 193 μg. total folate, as compared with 15 and 47 μg., respectively, in a poor diet, suggesting that many persons subsist on diets with suboptimal folate content.

    f. Recent surveys in the U.S. have shown that 30% of low-income pregnant mothers have red cell folate levels suggestive of deficiency. The growing fetus acquires folic acid from the mother; if she suffers from borderline depletion because of inadequate diet or impaired absoprtion, increased fetal demand can precipitate anemia in both mother and child.

    g. Prevention of folate deficiency is said to be important for normal fetal growth; gross deficiency in animals may lead to malformations and death.

    h. The need for routine folic acid supplementation during pregnancy has been a subject of controversy.

    i. Routine folate supplementation can be justified on the basis of an increased need in pregnancy and the frequent presence of additional factors conducive to folate deficiency (e.g., marginal folate intake as indicated by dietary surveys in large segments of the population, malabsorptive syndromes, and alcoholism). Routine supplementation with 1 mg./day will prevent megaloblastic anemia with its attendant risks in the majority of subjects.

6. Folic acid supplementation and preparations.

    a. Doses of 0.5 or 1 mg./day of folic acid are suggested for supplementation. Doses larger than 1 mg. are excreted in the urine and provide no advantage.

    b. Folic acid given without vitamin B_{12} to patients with pernicious anemia may correct hematologic abnormalities while accelerating the neurologic damage. For this reason OTC (over the counter) vitamin preparations are not permitted to contain

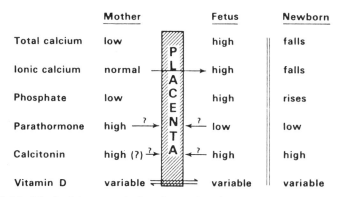

	Mother		Fetus	Newborn
Total calcium	low		high	falls
Ionic calcium	normal		high	falls
Phosphate	low		high	rises
Parathormone	high		low	low
Calcitonin	high (?)		high	high
Vitamin D	variable		variable	variable

Fig. 3-2. Model of calcium metabolism in mother, fetus, and the newborn. (Pitkin, R. M.: Vitamins and minerals in pregnancy. Clinics in Perinatology, 2:221, 1975)

more than 0.4 mg. of folic acid, except for those intended for pregnant and lactating women which may contain as much as 0.8 mg. folic acid.

c. Because folic acid and iron deficiency frequently coexist, routine administration of a prenatal multivitamin capsule containing 65 mg. of iron and 1 mg. of folic acid is suggested. If a patient is discovered with serum iron less than 42 μg./dl., she is treated with ferrous sulfate 320 mg., three times daily, in addition to the routine capsule.

H. Vitamin A

1. The recommended allowance for women is 4000 I.U. of vitamin A activity. The allowance during pregnancy is increased to 5000 I.U. to compensate for storage of the vitamin in the fetus, and an even greater allowance, 6000 I.U., is recommended during lactation to provide for vitamin A secreted in milk.

2. Vitamin A levels tend to fall during early pregnancy, then start to rise at the 13th to 16th week exceeding the normal range by the 21st week and reaching a concentration one-and-one-half times normal at the 37th week of gestation.

3. Preformed vitamin A in large doses is toxic. Hypervitaminosis A may result because of the availability of high-potency vitamin preparations without a prescription, the use of vitamin A in high doses for the treatment of adolescent acne, or the use

of bizarre highly fortified health foods.

4. The American Academy of Pediatrics advises against vitamin A supplements greater than 6000 I.U. for pregnant women. Central nervous system anomalies with hydrocephalus and other teratologic effects have been observed in the offspring of rats given large doses during gestation. There are many pediatricians who believe that excessive intake of Vitamin A by pregnant women is responsible for teratogenesis seen in human infants.

I. Vitamin D

1. Vitamin D regulates calcium and phosphorus metabolism. It promotes the intestinal absorption of calcium, and probably has a direct influence on bone mineralization. Vitamin D, together with parathyroid hormone, phosphate, and calcitonin, is involved in maintaining serum calcium homeostasis by controlling and regulating the movement of calcium across cell membranes. The relationship among various factors involved in calcium metabolism in the pregnant woman near term, fetus, and the newborn (first 48 hours) is illustrated in Figure 3-2.

2. In the presence of vitamin D deficiency, mineralization of the bone matrix is impaired, and collagen synthesis is defective, resulting in the disorder called rickets in children and osteomalacia in adults.

3. The recommended dose of vitamin D for pregnant women is 400 I.U., the same

as for nonpregnant women. It is necessary to promote the positive calcium balance needed during pregnancy and for neonatal calcium homeostasis.

J. Vitamin E

1. Except in low-birth-weight infants evidence of deficiency of vitamin E is not recognized in humans.

2. Vitamin E deficiency was observed to lead to abortion and stillbirth in rats, and the possible role of vitamin E in human reproduction has been investigated. Such studies, however, have failed to demonstrate a relation between vitamin E deficiency and spontaneous abortions or other reproductive pathology.

3. The gradual rise in plasma tocopherol levels throughout pregnancy to nearly double that in the nonpregnant state at term is said to probably reflect the normal hyperlipedemia of pregnancy as vitamin E travels in the blood bound to lipoproteins.

4. The transport mechanism for vitamin E from maternal to fetal circulation is unknown. Although fetal and maternal plasma levels are correlated, vitamin E levels amount to only one-third to one-fourth of the maternal levels in both preterm and term infants indicating limited placental transfer. This is also shown by the difficulty in raising fetal levels by oral administration of vitamin E to the mother and by the failure of injected vitamin E prior to delivery to prevent the hemolytic anemia of vitamin

E deficiency in premature infants. Because manifestations of vitamin E deficiency appear only 6 weeks after birth, oral supplementation to the infant is preferable.

5. The RDA of Vitamin E is 12 I.U./ day in nonpregnant women and 15 I.U./ day in pregnant women. The difference is intended to provide for fetal deposition.

II. Inorganic Nutrients

A. Iron

1. The National Research Council recommends a daily allowance in excess of 18 mg. of iron per day for pregnant (or nonpregnant) women. Because this requirement cannot be met by even the best diet, adequate prenatal care requires supplemental iron. If iron supplementation is not given, pregnant women even in a state of excellent nutrition will finish gestation with an iron store deficit, and if prepregnancy nutrition has been suboptimal, anemia will develop. Iron deficiency during pregnancy reduces iron stores in the infant.

2. Poor women are most prone to enter pregnancy in a state of iron undernutrition, but optimal iron nutrition is not invariably present even among economically well-off women. This is due most often to willfully reduced total intake of food, increased consumption of highly refined foods, or food fads (particularly among teenagers). Repeated infections or, more rarely, malabsorption syndromes may also

Table 3-2. **Iron Balance in Pregnancy**

Iron	Amount (mg.)	
	Mean	Range
Lost to fetus	270	(200–370)
Lost in placenta and cord	90	(30–170)
In blood lost at delivery	150	(90–310)
Normal body iron loss	170	(150–200)
Added to expanded red cell mass	450	(200–600)
TOTAL	1,130	(670–1650)
Returned to stores when red cell mass contracts after delivery	450	(200–600)
Net Loss mg./9 months	680	(470–1050)
mg./day	2.5	(1.7–4.0)

(Adapted from AMA Council on Food and Nutrition, Committee on Iron Deficiency: Iron deficiency in the U.S. J.A.M.A., *203*:407, Copyright 1968, American Medical Association)

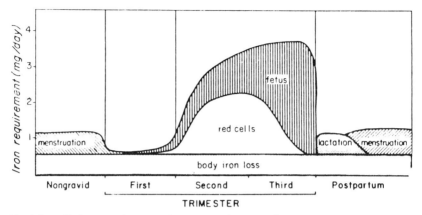

Fig. 3-3. Daily iron requirements in the adult female during pregnancy and postpartum. The requirement includes iron lost from the body and iron for the fetus, for the enlarging red cell mass during pregnancy, and for lactation after birth of the child. (Bothwell, T. H., and Finch, C. A.: Iron Metabolism. Boston, Little, Brown & Co., 1962)

contribute to the development of clinically recognized iron deficiency syndromes.

3. Total body iron store in women ranges from 200 to 400 mg. (35 mg./kg.) as opposed to approximately 1000 mg. in men. In addition to other body functions, women lose iron from menstruation, pregnancy, and lactation. Iron loss in normal menses may amount to 10 to 30 mg./month. Added to loss of iron from sweat, urine, and feces, the total iron loss in nonpregnant women averages 43 mg./month. With excessive menstrual loss (the most common single cause of iron deficiency in women), this can amount to 57 mg.

4. The only natural source of iron in pregnancy is diet. Because only 10% of food iron is absorbed (20% in iron deficiency states), the average gain in dietary iron in nonpregnant women is 39 mg. each month, in pregnant women 18 to 54 mg. per month, increasing as pregnancy approaches term.

5. Pregnancy constitutes a major drain on the iron reserves of women (see Table 3-2). Each pregnancy results in an average loss of 680 mg. of iron, the equivalent of 1300 ml. of blood. During pregnancy, iron must be available to meet the needs of an expanded red blood cell volume, averaging 450 to 550 ml., which requires 500 to 600 mg. of iron. This does not represent loss because after delivery the iron is returned to stores (see Fig. 3-3).

6. Parasitization by the fetus of the mother's iron stores (even when she is grossly deficient), maximal after the twentieth week of pregnancy, increases the iron need. The iron content of an average term infant is about 200 to 250 mg. Fetal blood, in the placenta and cord also contains about 50 mg. of iron.

7. Prorated over the second and third trimesters of pregnancy typical total maternal iron requirements have been put at 750 to 900 mg. or 5 mg. per day.

8. Iron deficiency designates a condition in which the total body iron content has been depleted. In latent iron deficiency, iron stores are exhausted, but blood hemoglobin levels remain above the lower limit of normal. This state can usually be detected by reduced serum iron level. A serum iron value below 42 μg./dl. may also reflect absence of marrow stores in the majority of pregnant women. This is suggested

by the numbers of pregnant women who show a hematocrit above 30% (as high as 34%) despite obviously low serum iron values.

    a. Anemia in pregnant women is defined as a hematocrit of less than 30% and hemoglobin of less than 11 g./dl. Using these values for screening cannot by definition detect latent iron deficiency.

    b. The amount of iron in the diet bears a rough relation to caloric content; in the U.S., the diet contains about 6 mg. iron per 1000 calories.

    c. Pica, the practice of eating starch (amylophagia), clay (geophagia), blocks of magnesia, numerous candy bars, ice (pagophagia), and perhaps even pickles and ice cream during pregnancy bears a special relationship to iron deficiency. The practice of pica is said to be rooted in custom, folklore and, superstition and appears to be common among pregnant black women in the South and West. Pica used to be interpreted as a cause of iron deficiency, but recent studies suggest strongly that the presence of iron deficiency is a factor for practicing pica. Clay eating may lead to iron deficiency by chelation or precipitation of iron in the gut.

    9. Supplements: For prophylaxis of iron deficiency, supplements should be given in the form of simple ferrous salts orally in an amount of 30 to 60 mg. daily throughout pregnancy and for 2 to 3 months postpartum. Larger amounts are needed for treatment of iron deficiency states.

    a. Only about 10% of an iron supplement is absorbed, the absorption increases to 20% in iron deficiency states.

    b. Iron is absorbed best when the stomach is empty. However, because a number of pregnant women may experience gastrointestinal irritation (heartburn, nausea, abdominal cramps, diarrhea), it is usually better to advise that the tablets be taken immediately after a meal. This can reduce the amount of iron absorbed by about 50%,

but the better patient acceptance promotes compliance.

    c. Parenteral iron therapy should only be used when the patient cannot tolerate oral preparations or absorption is impaired.

    d. Doses of 2 to 4 ml. of parenteral iron are administered intramuscularly, deep in the gluteal area, twice a week until the total calculated minimal iron deficit has been replaced. The formula used to replace iron stores is: hemoglobin deficit in g./dl. × body weight in lbs. = mg. iron necessary to correct the anemia, plus 1000 mg. iron.

    e. Constipation may be a side effect of iron therapy, which may be helped by a stool softener or bulk-forming laxative.

    f. The stools become black and tarry usually owing to the unabsorbed iron.

    g. Iron should not be given with antacids because the iron chelates formed are insoluble in alkaline duodenal contents.

    h. Prenatal vitamin capsules providing 65 mg. of iron and 1 mg. of folic acid are available commercially for supplementation.

    i. The effect of iron supplementation in pregnancy on hemoglobin and VPRC values is shown in Table 3-3.

B. Calcium and Phosphorus

    1. It is estimated on the basis of known sites of storage that at term the fetus has accumulated about 30 g. of calcium. Because this represents only 2.5% of maternal body calcium, it is suggested that it could be readily met from maternal stores without undue disturbance of maternal homeostasis. This view appears to be supported by results of radiographic studies of women with habitually low calcium intake showing no differences in bone density with increasing parity. However, the reported occurrence of osteomalacia with pregnancy is evidence that maternal calcium depletion is possible under certain circumstances.

    a. As the contents of both calcium and phosphorus in the fetus are linearly related to fetal weight, most calcium is deposited in the fetus late in pregnancy, averaging 200 to 300 mg. per day over the last trimester.

b. Calcium balance studies have indicated somewhat greater retention of calcium during pregnancy than would be anticipated on the basis of a total accumulation of 30 g. This has been interpreted as suggesting some degree of maternal storage starting early in pregnancy in anticipation of calcium needs for milk production.

c. The amount of calcium provided by the RDA—1200 mg. daily, 400 mg. more than the allowance for nonpregnant adults—is said to be adequate especially if the apparent capacity of the maternal organism to increase the absorption or decrease the excretion of calcium in response to immediate needs is taken into consideration.

d. It is possible that an intake of calcium of this magnitude is necessary only in late pregnancy, but, because storage in the maternal skeleton may normally occur earlier, it would seem advisable to have an adequate calcium intake throughout pregnancy.

e. The allowance for calcium during lactation is similarly 1200 mg./day, the increase being related to the amount of milk produced. Because milk contains 25 to 35 mg./dl. of calcium, depending on the amount of milk produced, the requirement during lactation ranges from 150 to 300 mg. calcium/day.

2. Dietary intake

a. The allowance for calcium can be met readily by consuming dairy products, especially milk. The calcium content of cow's milk is 120 mg./dl. Thus, 1 quart of milk or an equivalent amount of cheese (800 mg. calcium/100 g.) will supply a substantial proportion of the daily requirement. If milk is not tolerated or the dietary intake of calcium falls short of the recommended allowance, a calcium supplement (calcium gluconate, lactate, or carbonate,

Table 3-3. **Effect of Pregnancy, With and Without Iron Supplementation, on Values for VPRC and Hb**

Weeks of Gestation	VPRC‡ (Mean, I/I)			Hb§ (Mean, g./dl.)		
	No Supplement	*I.M.* Supplement*	*Oral† Supplement*	*No Supplement*	*I.M.* Supplement*	*Oral† Supplement*
0	0.420	—	—	13.4	—	—
12	0.383	0.406	0.357	12.5	13.1	11.4
16	0.395	0.379	0.363	12.4	12.1	11.4
20	0.364	0.370	0.371	11.7	11.8	11.8
24	0.356	0.363	0.371	11.4	11.8	11.8
28	0.346	0.369	0.368	11.0	11.8	11.8
32	0.341	0.372	0.370	10.6	12.1	11.8
36	0.343	0.375	0.375	10.7	12.1	12.0
40	0.349	0.385	0.387	10.9	12.7	12.4
Days Postpartum						
2	0.336	0.371	0.373	10.4	12.2	11.9
6	0.349	0.389	0.401	10.7	12.4	12.8
21	0.381	0.420	0.411	11.6	13.6	13.0
42	0.391	0.415	0.398	11.9	13.1	12.6
180	0.392	0.401	0.408	12.1	12.4	12.9

There were approximately 20 individuals in each group.
*1000 mg. Fe as iron dextran
†39 mg. elemental iron twice daily
‡Volume packed red cells
§Hemoglobin
(Wintrobe, M. M., *et al.*: Clinical Hematology. ed. 7. Philadelphia, Lea & Febiger, 1974, based on data from deLeevw, N. K. M., Lowenstein, L., and Hsieh, Y. S.: Medicine, *45*:291, 1966)

0.5 to 1 g., four times a day) should be considered.

b. The RDA of phosphorus can easily be obtained from food. The best sources of phosphorus are foods containing calcium and protein.

C. Fluoride

1. Fluoride prevents dental caries by forming a calcium-fluoride complex in dental enamel. Administration of fluoride to pregnant women has been suggested with a view of preventing caries in her offspring. However, the minimal amount of calcium in the pre-eruptive tooth would appear to limit the usefulness of fluoridated water for this purpose.

III. Trace Elements

The 1970s have witnessed a veritable explosion of published information on trace metals as a result of the expansion of basic knowledge concerning these elements, but the practical importance to human nutrition, in general, and pregnancy, in particular, has not yet been established.

Six trace elements are clearly essential for metabolism in mammals: zinc, copper, manganese, chromium, selenium, and magnesium. The roles of zinc in fetal development, copper in collagen formation, chromium in carbohydrate metabolism, and manganese in CNS function have been described.

A. Zinc

1. Although no teratologic effects of zinc deficiency have been demonstrated in man, strongly suggestive evidence for an association with congenital anomalies in humans has been cited:

a. Egypt and Iran, where zinc deficiency syndromes (e.g., hypogonadal dwarfism) have been clearly demonstrated, are among the four countries with the highest rate of CNS malformations.

b. Low serum zinc levels and hyperzincuria were found in cirrhotic and noncirrhotic alcoholics, and multiple congenital anomalies have been described in each of eight children of alcoholic mothers.

2. Zinc levels in serum and hair decline during gestation and in the first months of life. Whether these changes are physiologic or whether they reflect insufficient dietary intake is not known.

3. The average zinc content of a mixed diet consumed by American adults is between 10 and 15 mg.

4. The RDA for zinc is 20 mg. for pregnant women (an increase of 5 mg. over that for nonpregnant women) and 25 mg. for lactating women.

B. Copper, Iodine, and Manganese

1. In contrast to other trace elements, *copper* levels show a progressive rise in maternal serum during gestation, reaching levels at term that are considerably higher than those in nonpregnant women. At birth, maternal serum levels are five times greater than in the neonate, the difference being due to the high concentration of the copper-binding protein, ceruloplasmin, in maternal blood.

2. Simultaneous assessment of plasma levels during gestation showed a negative correlation between copper, and both magnesium and iron, which was interpreted as suggesting serial displacement in the metabolism of magnesium and iron by copper.

a. The average diet furnishes 2 to 5 mg. copper per day, and copper balance can be maintained on less than 2 mg./day.

3. *Iodine* is a component of the thyroid hormones thyroxine (T_4) and triiodothyronine (T_3). Prolonged iodine deficiency causes compensatory thyroid hypertrophy (endemic goiter). Large doses of potassium iodide given for prolonged periods to the mother have been reported to cause neonatal goiter with or without hypothyroidism. It is believed that a basic defect in iodine metabolism (in the organification of iodine) is present in such cases. The goiter usually regresses spontaneously after several months, but deaths have occurred rarely owing to compression of the trachea.

4. Vegetables that absorb iodine from the soil should provide the necessary iodine

intake of 140 µg./day for pregnant women. Surveys in the "goiter belt" (Texas, New Hampshire, Plain states) in the 1960s detected visible goiters in as many as 15% of women of child-bearing age. There are indications from clinical studies that iodine nutriture has improved in the last decade in the U.S.

5. *Manganese* is essential for normal bone structure, reproduction, and normal functioning of the CNS. Blood levels do not change in pregnancy, and manganese does not accumulate in fetal liver. Manganese deficiency is teratogenic in secondary animals. Overt manganese deficiency however is not known in humans, suggesting that the average dietary intake of 2.5 to 7.0 mg./day meets the requirements. Nuts and whole grains are excellent sources. Vegetables and fruits are other important sources.

C. Chromium

The interest in chromium in pregnancy derives from studies suggesting that relative chromium deficiency may be involved in gestational diabetes. Repeated pregnancies result in a reduction of hair chromium levels to approximately one-third that found in nulliparae suggesting depleted chromium stores.

PHYSIOLOGY OF PREGNANCY

I. Body Weight and Composition

A. The average total weight gain during a normal pregnancy, calculated on the basis of obvious pregnancy-induced physiologic changes, has been estimated at 22 to 26 lbs. (10 to 12 kg.) This would include an increase of about 11 lbs. for intrauterine contents including the fetus (7.5 lbs.), placenta and membranes (1.5 lbs.), and amniotic fluid (2 lbs.). A maternal contribution of 7 lbs. results from increases in the weight of the uterus (2.0 lbs.), blood (4.0 lbs.), and breast (1 lb.). Moderate expansion of interstitial fluid in the pelvis and extremities (attributable to the increased venous pressure created by the large pregnant uterus)

amounts to at least 2 to 3 lbs. in the ambulatory woman. Using indirect indices (e.g., isotope dilution), the increment in total body water has been found to be 7 L., of which 5 to 6 L. reflected the extracellular water. Pregnant women with edema may show substantially greater increases. The fat increase (skin-fold thickness) averages about 4 lbs. (2 kg.) but is highly variable. The total amount of protein added during pregnancy (calculated from nitrogen in the fetus, placenta, and expanded maternal components) is said to amount to about 2 lbs., (1 kg.). Whether protein is stored in additional sites, such as the liver or muscles, is unresolved (see Fig. 3-1).

B. Although there has been a tendency to over emphasize total weight gain, the pattern of weight gain is said to be of greater significance. Weight gain is minimal initially. It begins to accelerate toward the end of the first trimester and is relatively linear during the second and third trimesters, averaging about 400 g./week. During the second trimester maternal compartments expand, while most of the growth involves the fetus, placenta, and amniotic fluid during the third trimester.

II. Fuel-Hormone Metabolism in Normal Pregnancy

A. The substantial physiologic changes that characterize pregnancy are usually considered with respect to various organ systems (e.g., gastrointestinal and cardiovascular systems), but the function of virtually all systems is conditioned by changes in circulating body fuels (glucose, fatty acids, amino acids, and ketones).

B. The pattern of metabolic fuel availability in the maternal circulation is, in turn, dependent on:

1. The maternal hormonal milieu, notably the secretion of insulin, glucagon, and various placentally derived hormones and

2. The siphoning of metabolic fuels by the conceptus.

C. Under normal circumstances, these

various factors interact so as to provide adequate fuel storage by the mother and delivery of sufficient metabolic substrate to the conceptus, thus assuring normal fetal growth and development (see Table 3-4).

D. The metabolic events which culminate in starvation ketosis are explained below, with respect to the fasted and fed pregnant states.

1. The effects of pregnancy on metabolism in the fasted condition are primarily a consequence of the continuous withdrawal of glucose and amino acids from the maternal to the fetal circulation.

a. The fuel requirements of the developing fetus are believed to be met entirely by the consumption of glucose, which is utilized to provide energy necessary for protein synthesis and also as a precursor for the synthesis of fats and formation of glycogen.

b. Glycogen stores in the liver and muscle (per gram of tissue) are substantially greater in the fetus than in the adult.

c. The overall glucose uptake at 20 mg./minute at term represents a considera-

Table 3-4. **Hormonal Effects on Nutrient Metabolism in Pregnancy**

Hormone	*Primary Source of Secretion*	*Principal Effects*
Progesterone	Placenta	Reduces gastric motility; favors maternal fat deposition; increases sodium excretion; reduces alveolar and arterial P_{CO_2}; interferes with folic acid metabolism
Estrogen	Placenta	Reduces serum proteins; increases hydroscopic properties of connective tissue; affects thyroid function; interferes with folic acid metabolism
Human placental lactogen (HPL)	Placenta	Elevates blood glucose from breakdown of glycogen
Human chorionic thyrotrophin (HCT)	Placenta	Stimulates production of thyroid hormones
Human growth hormone (HGH)	Anterior pituitary	Elevates blood glucose; stimulates growth of long bones; promotes nitrogen retention
Thyroid stimulating hormone (TSH)	Anterior pituitary	Stimulates secretion of thyroxine; increases uptake of iodine by thyroid gland
Thyroxine	Thyroid	Regulates rate of cellular oxidation (basal metabolism)
Parathyroid hormone (PTH)	Parathyroid	Promotes calcium resorption from bone; increases calcium absorption; promotes urinary excretion of phosphate
Calcitonin (CT)	Thyroid	Inhibits calcium resorption from bone
Insulin	Beta cells of pancreas	Reduces blood glucose levels to promote energy production and synthesis of fat
Glucagon	Alpha cells of pancreas	Elevates blood glucose levels from glycogen breakdown
Aldosterone	Adrenal cortex	Promotes sodium retention and potassium excretion
Cortisone	Adrenal cortex	Elevates blood glucose from protein breakdown
Renin-angiotensin	Kidneys	Stimulates aldosterone secretion; promotes sodium and water retention; increases thirst

(Vermeersch, J.: Physiological basis of nutritional needs. *In* Worthington, B.S., Vermeersch, J., and Williams, S.R.: Nutrition in Pregnancy and Lactation. p. 35. St. Louis, C. V. Mosby, 1977)

ble excess of that observed in normal adults (6 mg./kg./minute as compared to 2 to 3 mg./kg./minute). The glucose level of fetal blood is generally 10 to 20 mg./dl. below the maternal level, so that diffusion would favor the net movement of glucose from mother to fetus, but a more rapid process, "facilitated diffusion," is also operative.

d. In contrast, maternal insulin does not traverse the placenta. Thus, fetal glucose utilization is independent of maternal insulin availability. On the other hand, fetal insulin is believed to play a central role in the development of the conceptus.

e. Insulin is present at 12 weeks of gestation and is stimulated (albeit sluggishly) by glucose availability, and much more effectively in response to aminogenic stimuli. While the fetus is dependent on insulin, it is capable of reaching full size in the total absence of maternal or fetal growth hormone.

2. In addition to the transfer of glucose to the fetus, amino acids are actively transported by the placenta from the maternal to the fetal circulation, resulting in maternal hypoaminoacidemia. The amino acids are utilized by the fetus for protein synthesis and are also catabolized serving as an energy-yielding fuel.

3. Because amino acids (notably alanine) are key precursors for gluconeogenesis by the maternal liver in the fasting state, the presence of the fetus drains the mother of both glucose and glucose precursors,

4. It has been noted that the conceptus may be viewed as an auxiliary brain (from the standpoint of maternal metabolism) both utilizing glucose independent of the maternal insulin, and continuously drawing amino acids from the maternal circulation. The result is that in the fasted state the mother is characterized by hypoglycemia, hyperketonuria, and hypoalaninemia (see Fig. 3-4 and Fig. 3-5).

5. The sequence of events is initiated by fetal glucose utilization leading to a reduction in maternal plasma glucose. As a consequence maternal plasma insulin falls, resulting in exaggerated starvation ketosis. At the same time maternal amino-acid levels are also reduced. Thus, the maternal hypoglycemia initiated by fetal glucose uptake is perpetuated and exaggerated by fetal siphoning of gluconeogenic precursors. The net effect on the mother is an increased response to starvation.

6. It should be noted that in association with maternal ketonemia, ketone bodies accumulate in the amniotic fluid and probably are available to the fetus since the enzymes necessary for oxidation of ketones are present. In contrast to ketones, free fatty acids are not transferred to the fetus. Ketone utilization is primarily determined by the rate of delivery of the substrate to the fetus. It is believed, therefore, that in circumstances of limited glucose availability, ketones synthesized by the maternal liver are transferred to the fetus and serve as an alternative to glucose in meeting fetal fuel requirements.

7. It should be noted that the availability and utilization of ketones by the fetus is not without risk but may have an adverse effect on neuropsychologic development. Maternal ketonuria, whether secondary to total starvation, a very low carbohydrate diet, or diabetes, has been associated with significant reduction in IQ in such children tested at 4 years of age.

E. Glucose and Insulin

1. In pregnancy the metabolic response to feeding is characterized by hyperinsulinemia, hyperglycemia, hypertriglyceridemia, and a diminished sensitivity to insulin. Thus despite the hyperinsulinemia observed in pregnancy, the blood glucose response to oral or I.V. carbohydrate load is higher than that observed in the nonpregnant state. Because of the greater rise in glucose, specific adjusted norms must be used to evaluate the response to the glucose tolerance test in pregnancy, in order to avoid misdiagnosis as diabetes (see Table 3-5).

2. The increase in blood glucose in the

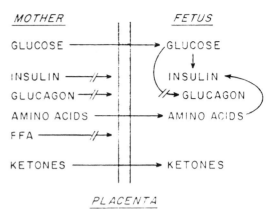

Fig. 3-4. Maternal-fetal fuel and hormone exchange. Glucose, amino acids, and ketones are transferred from mother to fetus while insulin, glucagon, and free fatty acids (F.F.A.) are not. Glucose in the fetal circulation stimulates secretion of insulin and inhibits secretion of glucagon by fetal islet cells. Amino acids are also potent stimuli of fetal insulin secretion. (Felig, P.: Body fuel metabolism and diabetes mellitus in pregnancy. Med. Clin. North Am., *61*:43, 1977)

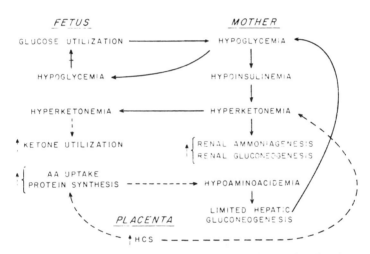

Fig. 3-5. Placental-fetal-maternal fuel-hormone interaction in the fasted stage in pregnancy. Fetal glucose utilization results in maternal hypoglycemia, leading to hypoinsulinemia and hyperketonemia. Maternal hepatic gluconeogenesis cannot keep pace with these augmented demands because of fetal siphoning of gluconeogenic amino acids particularly alanine, resulting in maternal hypoaminoacidemia. Placental secretion of HCS (HPL) may also contribute by enhancing maternal lipolysis (and ketogenesis) and fetal amino-acid uptake. (Felig, P.: Body fuel metabolism and diabetes mellitus in pregnancy. Med. Clin. North Am., *61*:43, 1977)

the pregnant state is due to the failure of the liver to take up glucose, which then escapes into the circulation. This indicates that the liver is resistant to insulin in pregnancy. This resistance is shared by peripheral tissues, notably muscles. Tissue sensitivity is reduced by as much as 80% in normal pregnancy. Nevertheless, the 24-hr blood glucose range does not exceed 45 mg./dl. and is below that of nonpregnant subjects,

a. The diminished tissue responsiveness to insulin in the fed state in pregnant subjects coupled with the effects of pregnancy in unmasking diabetes constitutes the basis for characterizing the effects of pregnancy as "diabetogenic."

    b. The factors that may be responsible for the diabetogenic effects of pregnancy are associated with the variety of hormones secreted by the placenta—human placental lactogen (HPL), progesterone, and estrogen.

    c. HPL, also called chorionic somatomammotropin (HCS) is a polypeptide hormone produced by syncytiotrophoblasts. Chemically and immunologically, it is similar to growth hormone, but the concentration of HPL in the blood is 1000 times that of growth hormone. HPL, has an anbolic effect on protein metabolism, and is both mammotropic and luteotropic. HPL, like growth hormone, alters carbohydrate metabolism by diminishing the effect of insulin. It also shares the lipolytic effect of growth hormone, causing a substantial increase in the mobilization of free fatty acids from peripheral fat depots. The single most important factor in determining the secretion of HPL is the total placental mass, but nutrient availability also influences maternal levels of this hormone.

    d. Despite the known antiinsulin effects of HPL, no constant relationship between maternal HPL levels and insulin requirements during diabetic pregnancy has been demonstrated.

  F. Estrogen and Progesterone

    The placental phase of gestation is characterized by the increasing secretion of these hormones which readily enter the circulation. Estrogen acts as an antagonist of insulin effects rather than as an inhibitor of insulin secretion.

  G. Other Hormones

    1. Increased level of cortisol may affect maternal carbohydrate metabolism in pregnancy. Hypercorticism would contribute to the diabetogenic state by increasing glucose production in the liver, antagonizing the action of insulin in muscle and possibly augmenting glucagon secretion.

    2. In contrast to cortisol, the secretion of pituitary growth hormone, an important

antagonist of insulin in the nongravid state, is inhibited, particularly in late pregnancy.

  H. The effects of maternal and placental hormones on nutrient metabolism during pregnancy are summarized in Table 3-4.

INTRAUTERINE GROWTH RETARDATION

I. Basic Principles

  A. Under normal circumstances there is a linear relationship between gestational age and fetal growth as reflected by the anthropometric parameters of weight, length, and head circumference.

    1. Prematurity or postmaturity as determined by gestational age are causes of increased perinatal morbidity and mortality.

    2. Birth weight is a poor determinant of gestational age.

  B. Babies who are either too large or too small for gestational age are victims of deviant fetal growth.

    1. Examples are:

      a. The newborn (of a diabetic mother) who weighs more than 4000 g. at birth in spite of shortened gestation and

    2. The infant (of the mother suffering from severe preeclampsia) who weighs less than 2000 g. at birth notwithstanding the prolonged gestation.

  C. It is important to differentiate intrauterine growth retardation from shortened gestation because of differences in prognosis, problems, and management.

  D. Within limits, a 37-week pregnancy is expected to yield an infant who weighs about 2500 g.

    1. However, 30% of 37-week pregnancies produce babies with birth weight of less than 2500 g.

    2. These undergrown and often malnourished neonates differ from their "normal" preterm counterparts because their maturation is relatively advanced despite their small size.

  E. Intrauterine growth retardation is second only to prematurity as a cause of perinatal mortality. Newborn infants who have a low birth weight for gestational age because of malnutrition of the mother have a mortality rate of 3 to 5%.

II. Normal Fetal Growth

A. At a cellular level, growth occurs in three sequential stages:

1. A hyperplastic phase in which growth is due primarily to rapid cell proliferation

2. A combined or intermediate phase in which cell proliferation continues but is associated with an increase in cell size and

3. A final hypertrophic phase during which growth is due primarily to an increase in cell size without increase in numbers.

B. If growth were inhibited by malnutrition during the hypertrophic phase, the effect may be temporary, and, with proper intervention, complete recovery may follow. Interference with growth in the cell proliferation phase is not so readily overcome.

III. Regulation of Fetal Growth

A. Fetal growth is determined by:

1. The inherent growth potential of the fetus and

2. The growth support provided by the mother through the placenta.

B. In the first and second trimesters, growth is predominantly determined by the inherent fetal growth potential because growth support far exceeds the needs of the fetus. By the third trimester, the adequacy of the placental growth support becomes the limiting factor.

C. Fetal growth is influenced by genetic, environmental, including nutrient supply, and endocrine factors and, to a lesser extent, the central and autonomic nervous systems.

D. Figure 3-6 demonstrates the regulating mechanisms and the role of nutrients in fetal growth.

IV. Mechanism of Intrauterine Growth Retardation

A. Adequate fetal growth and development depends on a steady supply of nutrients from the mother to the fetus. The availability of nutrients to the fetus will depend upon:

1. The concentration of nutrients in the maternal blood

2. The rate of maternal blood flow through the placenta

3. The rate of transfer of nutrients across the placenta to the fetal circulation

4. The adequacy of fetal circulation.

B. Fetal growth can be impaired by:

1. Deficient dietary intake

2. Inadequate absorption of nutrients from the gut

3. Abnormal metabolism of proteins, lipids, carbohydrates, and micronutrients in the maternal organism

4. Insufficient placental circulation

5. Abnormal utilization of nutrients by the fetus, singly or in combination.

C. Diminished growth support, a form of growth slowing or cessation occurring in a fetus with normal growth potential, represents 60% of instances of clinical growth retardation. The basic defect implies impairment in transplacental nutrient supply. The common denominator of this type of growth retardation probably is fetal hypoxia. Interference with both hyperplastic and hypertrophic growth occurs. Clinically these neonates appear wasted with an increase in head size to body size.

D. Maternal factors can be cited as causes of fetal growth retardation in almost 50% of cases. These include poor nutrition as evidenced by low pre-pregnancy weight and small weight gain during pregnancy. In addition, a number of other factors, some indirectly leading to maternal malnutrition such as socio-economic conditions, smoking, narcotic addiction, alcoholism, teenage pregnancy, ind ill health.

E. Within ethnic groups an overall improvement in social conditions, including the nutrition of the population, is almost

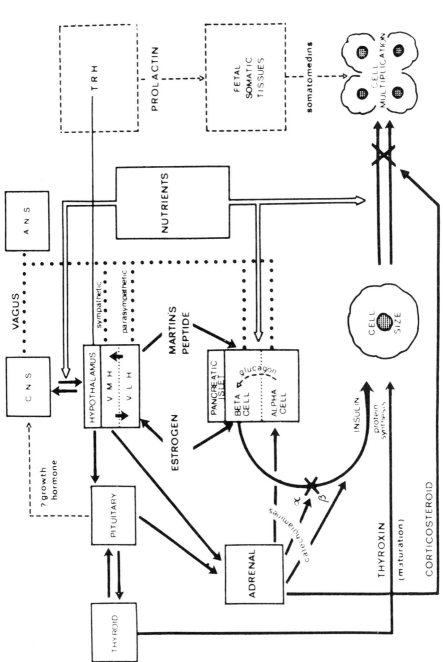

Fig. 3-6. Regulation of fetal growth. (Cheek, D. B., Graystone, J. E., and Niall, M.: Factors controlling fetal growth. Clin. Obstet. Gynecol., *20*:925, 1977)

always reflected by an increase in birth weights, and particularly a decrease in the proportion of low-birth-weight infants. The reverse is also true.

V. Prevention, Diagnosis, and Management of Intrauterine Growth Retardation

A. A comprehensive approach involving early and regular prenatal care—including correction of poor nutritional state—intrauterine monitoring and intensive perinatal surveillance has been shown to be effective in significantly reducing the incidence and complications of intrauterine growth retardation.

B. Prenatal diagnosis of growth retardation involves:

   1. Serial Measurements of the Uterine Fundus, which will detect about 30% of fetal retardation

      a. Fetal growth retardation during the latter half of the pregnancy may be suspected clinically if the mother fails to gain weight appropriately or if the uterus is smaller than expected for the gestational age.

   2. Ultrasound Cephalometry

   3. Measurement of Urinary Estriols

   4. Lecithin/Sphyngomyelin (L/S) Ratio

      a. The L/S ratio remains about 1:1 until the 32nd week of gestation, then it begins to rise.

      b. A ratio of 2:1 is considered mature.

      c. In diabetic pregnancy the rise in L/S ratio is often delayed, which may be associated with fetal hyperinsulinemia.

VI. Long-Range Consequences of Low Birth Weight on Intellectual Development

A. The possible long-term adverse effects of retarded fetal growth on the development of intellectual function can be great.

1. Some recent studies suggest that the effects of impaired fetal growth on mental development are lifelong. This is discussed in Chapter 26.

B. The Collaborative Perinatal Study of the National Institute of Neurological Diseases and Stroke shows that infants of low-birth-weight have a disproportionately increased incidence of perinatal death and later neurologic abnormality.

HIGH-RISK PREGNANCIES

I. Pregnancy in Adolescence

   A. Definition of Population at Risk

      1. Adolescent pregnancy is considered to be a major health problem in the U.S. In 1975, there were approximately 900,000 pregnancies in women younger than 20 years of age.

      2. The reason for this excessive neonatal mortality and low-birth weights is that adolescent growth and pregnancy make competing demands for nutrients and the results are detrimental to both the mother and the infant.

      3. The Working Group on Nutrition and Pregnancy in Adolescence of the National Research Council's Committee on Maternal Nutrition investigated the nature and magnitude of biologic and social problems which accompany pregnancy and childbirth in adolescent girls. Girls who become pregnant before 17 years of age are at great biologic and psychologic risk.

      4. Girls are at biologic risk if pregnancy occurs before cessation of growth. In the U.S., the average age at menarche is 12.5 to 13.0 years. The great majority of girls have completed linear growth and achieved gynecologic maturity by 17 years of age. This conclusion is supported by natality and mortality data indicating that the course and outcome of pregnancies of girls 17 to 20 years of age resemble those of young mature women (20 to 24 years).

      5. Because they are growing, most girls under age 17 have greater nutritional

requirements in relation to body size than adult women. The additional nutrient demands of pregnancy may compromise their growth potential and increase their risk in pregnancy. When growth is completed (usually at age 17), the nutritional requirements become similar to those of mature women. This is reflected in the recommended dietary allowances, which are differentiated for various age groups (see Table 2-1).

6. Adolescent pregnancy is accompanied by an increased morbidity of the child born. About 20% of low-birth-weight babies born alive in the U.S. were born to mothers under 15 years of age. The neonatal mortality rate per 1,000 live births for infants born to white mothers under 15 years of age is 32.1% compared to a rate of 15.9% for mothers 20 to 24 years of age. For nonwhite mothers, the respective figures are 46.5% and 25.3%.

II. Anemia in Pregnancy

A. Pregnancy is in fact associated with enhanced hematologic activity. Plasma volume and red call mass both increase. However, the increase in red cell mass does not equal the expansion in plasma volume and the disproportionate rise of the latter causes a gradual fall in hematocrit, reaching its lowest level in the 32nd week of gestation. As red cell mass tends to increase toward the end of pregnancy, hematocrit rises to near prepregnancy levels. Assuming normal blood loss with delivery and a hematocrit of 38 to 40% at term, the hematocrit will rise to 42 to 43% on the second to third postpartum day as a result of physiologic diuresis and contraction of blood volume.

B. The classic macrocytic anemia of pregnancy diagnosed by the characteristic changes in the peripheral blood represents a combined deficiency of iron and folic acid.

1. Severe iron deficiency may mask megaloblastosis and peripheral macrocytosis.

2. Megaloblastic anemias develop with equal frequency before and after delivery. Appearance before the 30th week of gestation points to unusually high folate requirements (e.g., twin pregnancy) or defective absorption.

3. Treatment should include oral ferrous sulfate, 300 mg., three times daily, and folic acid, 1 mg. orally daily. A reticulocyte response is usual at 4 days, with peak at 7 days.

III. Diabetes in Pregnancy

A. Basic Principles

1. Diabetes in pregnancy is associated with insulin resistance, an increase in insulin requirement, and a greater tendency to ketosis and ketoacidosis.

2. Pregnancy, like obesity, causes an increased resistance to the action of insulin because gestational hormones counteract the action of insulin.

3. Changes in maternal metabolism, especially during the last two trimesters of pregnancy, result in aggravation of the diabetic state.

4. In pregnancy, glycosuria can be found in the presence of normal blood glucose levels.

a. This glycosuria is attributed to the reduced renal threshold for glucose.

b. However, the glucose tolerance test is normal in 75% of pregnant women who have asymptomatic glycosuria.

B. Influence of Pregnancy on Diabetes

1. The effect of gestation on the clinical course of diabetes varies according to the state of pregnancy (see Fig. 3-7).

2. During the first half of pregnancy, the transfer of maternal glucose to the fetus is primarily responsible for the altered carbohydrate homeostasis.

a. The siphoning of glucose by the fetus causes a tendency to fasting hypoglycemia in the mother.

b. This can be symptomatic and may necessitate a reduction in the dose of insulin.

c. Diminished food intake as a con-

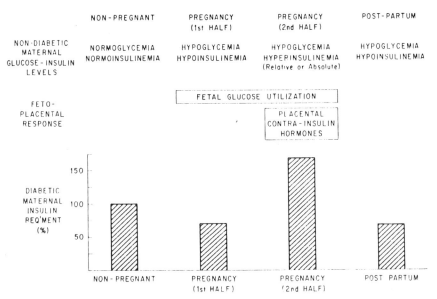

Fig. 3-7. Influence of pregnancy on glucose and insulin levels in nondiabetic subjects and on insulin requirements in diabetic subjects. The prepregnancy insulin dose is shown as 100%. The insulin requirement generally declines in the first half of the pregnancy and in the puerperium and is increased in the second half of pregnancy. (Tyson, J. E., and Felig, P.: Medical aspects of diabetes in pregnancy and the diabetogenic effects of oral contraceptives. Med. Clin. North Am., *55*:947, 1971)

sequence of the nausea and vomiting of early pregnancy may also contribute to the reduced insulin requirement.

3. In the second half of pregnancy, the diabetogenic action of placental hormones outweighs the effect of continual siphoning of maternal glucose by the fetus.

a. This causes an increase in insulin requirement averaging 67%.

4. Coincident with the increased resistance to insulin, there is an increased tendency to ketoacidosis.

a. The recognition of diabetic acidosis in pregnancy is often more difficult than in the nonpregnant diabetic because blood glucose levels are not markedly elevated.

b. Diabetic acidosis must be differentiated from starvation ketosis, which is also associated with ketonuria, but requires administration of glucose rather than insulin.

c. The continuous drain of glucose by the fetus accelerates the normal metabolic response to starvation and is manifested by blood ketone levels two to three times greater than those observed in the non-pregnant state after an overnight fast.

d. In starvation ketosis no hyperglycemia is observed despite the intense ketonuria. Treatment with I.V. glucose solution alleviates the condition.

e. It is essential to promptly diagnose diabetic ketoacidosis for if not treated promptly, fetal mortality may be increased by 50%.

f. Ketoacidosis is treated with rapid acting insulin, a loading dose of 6 units administered intravenously followed by a continuous infusion of 6 units per hour, hypotonic fluids (0.45% saline), and potassium supplements.

(1) Bicarbonate administration is reserved for patients with an arterial *p*H of

7.1 and a bicarbonate concentration of 5 mEq./L.

(2) Blood glucose, blood ketones, and arterial pH should be monitored at frequent intervals, every 2 to 4 hours to determine the need for additional insulin.

5. In the post-partum state, maternal insulin requirements are reduced, frequently to amounts below the prepregnant dose.

a. This is due to the rapid fall in the blood levels of placental hormones, estrogen and progesterone, as well as a continued suppression of growth hormone secretions.

b. Patients have a gradual return to the prepregnancy diabetic state in the ensuing 3 to 6 weeks.

C. *Classification of Diabetes in Pregnancy*

1. Diabetes in pregnancy is classified according to the clinical state and prognostic signs.

a. PREDIABETES

(1) This is suspected in women delivering babies of 10 lb. or more, or who have a history of habitual stillbirths.

(2) Glucose tolerance is normal.

(3) These patients can be expected to develop diabetes sometime in the future.

b. CLASS A—GESTATIONAL OR CHEMICAL DIABETES

(1) These women have asymptomatic chemical diabetes.

(2) Glucose tolerance tests during pregnancy are abnormal.

(3) Fasting blood glucose levels are either normal or minimally elevated.

(4) They do not usually require insulin.

c. CLASS B

(1) These women have overt diabetes.

(2) Onset of diabetes has been after age 20.

(3) Duration of diabetes is less than 10 years.

d. CLASS C

(1) These women have overt diabetes of 10- to 20-years duration.

(2) Onset has usually been before age 20.

e. CLASS D

(1) Overt diabetes has been present for more than 20 years prior to the pregnancy, or

(2) Onset of diabetes was before the age of 10.

(3) Benign retinopathy may be present.

f. CLASS E

(1) This is characterized by calcified pelvic vessels.

(2) This classification is generally no longer employed.

g. CLASS F

(1) This refers to pregnant diabetics who have diabetic nephropathy.

(2) Proteinuria is present, usually with azotemia.

h. CLASS R

(1) These women have malignant (proliferative) retinopathy.

2. The incidence of stillbirths and neonatal deaths, generally increases in proportion to the severity of the diabetes from Class A to Class R.

3. Excessive birth weight (macrosomia) is most common in Classes A through C.

4. Class-F and -R diabetic patients frequently are advised to undergo therapeutic abortion because of persistently high perinatal mortality.

D. *Diagnostic Criteria*

1. In the asymptomatic patient, diagnosis is suspected when a fasting blood sugar of 120 mg. per 100 ml. or greater is found.

2. Gestational diabetes is identified by a glucose tolerance test.

a. The indications for performing a glucose tolerance test in pregnancy are: repetitive glycosuria, strong family history, excessively obese patients, history of previous infant over 10 lb., hydramnios, recurrent stillbirths, neonatal deaths, or congenital anomalies.

    b. The most sensitive screen test for gestational diabetes is a blood glucose over 130 mg./dl. 1 hour after an oral glucose load of 50 g.

    c. If the screen test is positive, a 3-hour standard oral glucose tolerance test using 100 g. of glucose is necessary to establish the diagnosis.

    d. The criteria for the diagnosis of diabetes in pregnancy differ from those in the nonpregnant state.

    e. The accepted values for diagnosis of gestational diabetes with the oral glucose tolerance test (100 g. glucose load orally) are listed in Table 3-5.

       (1) In keeping with the tendency of fasting hypoglycemia and postprandial hyperglycemia characteristic of pregnancy, the fasting blood sugar value is lower, and the 2-hour and 3-hour blood sugar values are higher in the gravid state as compared with the nongravid state.

       (2) Diagnosis of gestational diabetes is established when two or more values exceed the limits shown in Table 3-5.

       (3) Of the subjects showing a positive test, 20 to 30% will develop permanent diabetes within 2 to 8 years.

       (4) A positive test indicates gestational diabetes and possible high-risk pregnancy.

       (5) Glucose tolerance in these patients reverts to normal in the postpartum period.

    3. Random glycosuria is frequently observed in pregnancy

    a. This is attributed to reduced renal threshold for glucose.

    b. Therefore, glycosuria is considered a poor indicator of impaired glucose tolerance.

    c. Two overnight fasting urine specimens should be used for testing.

    d. Glycosuria is said to be associated with abnormal GTT in 85% of pregnant women.

  E. Complications

    1. The most frequent complication of pregnancy in the diabetic are:

    a. Maternal morbidity

       (1) Hydramnios

       (2) Preeclampsia

    b. Fetal mortality (5 to 15%)

       (1) Stillbirths (5 to 10%)

       (2) Neonatal deaths (5 to 10%)

          (a) Respiratory distress syndrome

          (b) Congenital anomalies

    c. Fetal morbidity

       (1) Macrosomia (excessive size for gestational age)

       (2) Hypoglycemia (10 to 25%)

       (3) Congenital anomalies (5 to 10%)

       (4) Respiratory distress syndrome (25 to 30%)

Table 3-5. **Criteria for Diagnosis of Diabetes by Oral Glucose Tolerance Test***

| | *Blood Glucose/Plasma Glucose (mg./dl.)* | |
Time	*Pregnant†*	*Nonpregnant*
Fasting	90/100	110
1 hour	165/180	170
2 hours	145/160	120
3 hours	125/140	110

*The figures apply to whole venous blood in subjects given a 100-g. oral dose of glucose If plasma rather than whole blood is used for analysis, the values should be increased by 15%.
†The diagnosis of diabetes is established if two or more values exceed the limits shown.
(Data from O'Sullivan, J. B., and Mahan, J.: Criteria for the oral glucose tolerance test in pregnancy. Diabetes, *13*: 278–285, 1964)

(5) Hyperbilirubinemia (5 to 40%)

(6) Hypocalcemia (25%)

2. Although perinatal mortality in diabetic pregnancy has declined progressively during the last three decades, fetal deaths are still three to six times higher than in the general population.

3. The Report of the National Commission on Diabetes' Workshop on Pregnancy (1976) indicates that in 1973 as many as 4,500 infants died in the U.S. as a result of perinatal loss associated with undiagnosed or untreated gestational diabetes.

4. Fetal hyperglycemia and hyperinsulinism.

a. The placenta is permeable to glucose but not to insulin. This together with maternal hyperglycemia leads to fetal hyperglycemia and fetal hyperinsulinism.

b. This is believed to be responsible for a large percentage of fetal complications and deaths.

5. The major causes of fetal deaths in diabetic pregnancies are intrauterine stillbirths, congenital malformations and respiratory distress syndrome.

6. The incidence of respiratory distress syndrome (hyaline membrane disease) is two to three times greater in diabetic pregnancies than in the normal population.

a. It has been postulated that delayed pulmonary maturation owing to inhibition of cortisol-induced synthesis of lecithin is responsible for fetal respiratory distress syndrome.

7. Macrosomia (excessive fetal size for gestational age) results from increased fat deposition associated with excessive insulin concentrations in the fetus.

a. A similar sequence of events has been implicated in the pathogenesis of neonatal hypoglycemia.

F. *Management*

1. Adequate control of the diabetes throughout pregnancy

a. Strict control of maternal hyperglycemia purportedly has contributed to an appreciable drop in perinatal mortality and of fetal respiratory distress syndrome. It is responsible for an overall decline of fetal mortality in recent years.

b. However, careful monitoring of maternal blood glucose levels reveals that even under optimal circumstances—hospitalization, individualization of insulin doses, and dietary control—overly rigorous diabetic control can lead to the complications of noctural hypoglycemia.

(1) It was formerly believed that maternal hypoglycemia had no severe consequences, but recent studies in a large series of nondiabetic pregnant women have shown that maternal hypoglycemia may be associated with a two- to threefold increase in fetal mortality.

(2) Further, the incidence of cerebral palsy and seizure disorders are two to three times greater in infants of diabetic mothers than in nondiabetic women and are possibly related to maternal hypoglycemia.

(3) Therefore, although strict control of diabetes during pregnancy is desirable, it is important to avoid hypoglycemia.

c. It is recommended that a single daily dose of intermediate acting insulin (e.g., NPH or lente insulin) to which rapid acting insulin may be added should be used.

d. The goal in treatment is to maintain random blood glucose levels below 150 mg./dl. and the fasting blood glucose below 110 mg./dl.

e. If these goals cannot be achieved, a second evening dose of intermediate or short acting insulin should be added.

2. Timing of the delivery so as to minimize both intrauterine fetal death and neonatal deaths owing to lung immaturity are of crucial importance.

a. In previous years, the optimal time for delivery was empirically determined to be around the 36th or 37th week of gestation because intrauterine deaths rise 25% after this period.

b. Modern techniques, which monitor fetal well-being as well as maturity, have increased the optimal timing of delivery.

3. Ideally, pregnant diabetic women who are insulin-dependent should be hospitalized from weeks 30 to 32 of gestation until after delivery.

a. This is common practice in many European countries.

b. This may not be feasible in the U.S. with currently available health insurance schedules.

G. Dietary Treatment of the Pregnant Diabetic

1. Diet is of vital importance in the management of diabetes in pregnancy.

a. When the goals of diabetic control of the mother and adequate fetal nutrition are in conflict, the needs of the fetus must take precedence.

b. Accordingly, in the dietary management of the insulin-dependent pregnant diabetic, the principles which apply to the nongravid diabetic and those applying to normal pregnancy should be coordinated.

2. A diet containing 30 to 35 Cal./day/kg. of body weight is recommended.

a. The total weight gain allowed is about 24 lbs. (10.4 kg.), but weight gain should not be less than 20 lbs.

b. An increase of about 1 lb. per month is recommended during the first half of gestation and 1 lb. per week during the second half.

c. Calculated on the basis of the usual daily requirement of 30 Cal./kg. of ideal body weight, a sedentary woman requires about 2100 Cal./day during the first trimester, 2200 Cal./day during the second trimester, and 2300 Cal./day during the last trimester. About 600 additional Cal./day are required for physically active pregnant women.

d. If the patient is hospitalized and relatively inactive, the diet can be reduced to 1600 to 1800 Cal./day.

3. Carbohydrates should provide about 45% of the calories with a minimum of 200 g./day.

a. This takes into account the glucose lost to the fetus and moderate glycosuria.

b. In patients with marked glycosuria, an additional 50 g. or more of carbohydrates may have to be given to make up for urinary losses.

c. Concentrated sweets should not be used.

d. Starchy foods are utilized to provide carbohydrates.

(1) These are absorbed relatively slowly, particularly if they are rich in fibers.

(2) Starchy foods are more suited to the diabetic patient's insulin apparatus, which responds slowly.

4. The protein intake should average 2 g./kg./day or about 100 to 120 g. daily.

5. The remainder of the caloric allowance is made up with fat calories.

6. Regularity of food intake and between-meal snacks are important to prevent insulin reactions.

7. For further details on the diabetic diet including exchange lists, see Chapter 16.

IV. Malabsorption Disorders

A. Basic Principles

1. Malabsorption states, including those related to food allergy or intolerance, are most likely to contribute to poor nutritional status of pregnant women owing to depleted reserves on entering pregnancy, inadequate nutrients in the maternal circulation, or both.

2. Malabsorptive states are associated with impaired absorption, excessive loss of nutrients, or maldigestion owing to deficiency of pancreatic or small intestine enzymes.

3. Allergy to milk, often manifested as a protein-losing enteropathy, and lactose intolerance are among the most frequent causes of food-induced malabsorption in pregnant women.

a. Their recognition in view of the

importance of milk as a nutrient source for pregnant women needs no emphasis.

4. Because malabsorption may be either global (involving all nutrients) or more specific (involving only one or more substances, such as calcium or fat-soluble vitamins), clinical symptoms may show wide variations. Incomplete digestion or unabsorbed food residues in the intestine may be toxic and may lead to secondary metabolic alterations.

a. Weight loss, fluid and electrolyte imbalances, or specific vitamin deficiency syndromes generally are manifestations of malabsorption states.

5. Considerable evidence has accumulated demonstrating the interrelationships between nutritional deficiencies, particularly protein-calorie malnutrition and infections on one hand, and impairment of immune defenses on the other.

a. It has been suggested that intrauterine malnutrition may cause impairment of cellular immune function in the small-for-gestational-age fetus.

6. The diagnosis and management of malabsorption disorders are discussed in Chapter 12.

7. Dietary modifications have been demonstrated to be quite effective in correcting a number of malabsorptive states, especially those due to food allergy or intolerance, lack of pancreatic enzymes, and other conditions. The practitioner can obtain the assistance of a dietitian-nutritionist in devising an appropriate diet that will both replenish depleted stores and provide adequate sources of essential nutrients for pregnancy needs.

a. Representative corrective diets for various causes of malabsorption are presented in Chapter 12.

PREECLAMPSIA/ECLAMPSIA

I. Hypertensive states, which complicate some 6 or 7% of pregnancies in the U.S., remain among the leading causes of maternal deaths and also account for a substantial portion of perinatal deaths as well as low-birth-weight infants.

II. Hypertension in pregnancy may represent several diseases. The Committee on Terminology of the American College of Obstetricians and Gynecologists has recommended classification of hypertensive disorders of pregnancy into:

A. Acute preeclampsia

B. Chronic hypertensive disease of pregnancy

C. Acute preeclampsia superimposed on chronic hypertension

III. About 75% of the pregnant women who exhibit hypertension have acute preeclampsia. Of the remaining 25%, one-third have chronic renal disease, and the rest show a transient rise in blood pressure during pregnancy and are likely to develop essential hypertension in subsequent years.

IV. The Working Group of the National Research Council defined preeclampsia as hypertension with proteinuria or edema, or both, appearing after the 20th week of pregnancy. By hypertension is meant a systolic blood pressure of 140 mm. Hg and a diastolic blood pressure of 90 mm. Hg, or both, or alternatively a rise of 30 mm. Hg in systolic or 15 mm. Hg in diastolic pressure observed on at least two occasions 6 or more hours apart.

A. The rise in diastolic or systolic pressure is a more dependable warning sign of preeclampsia than the upper limit of 140/90 mm. Hg, particularly because young women in the 18 to 34-year age group tend to have a normal blood pressure of 120/80 mm. Hg or less, and the normal blood pressure of teenagers, who are at the greatest risk of developing eclampsia, rarely exceeds 90/60 mm. Hg.

B. Diagnosis of hypertension is further complicated by the normal physiologic drop in blood pressure in mid-pregnancy.

V. The precise influence of nutrition on the development of preeclampsia is disputed. It has been stated repeatedly that nutritional deficiencies have an important, although not primary, role in preeclampsia, but convincing evidence of a cause-and-effect relationship is lacking.

A. An unusually high incidence of preeclampsia has been found in epidemiologic surveys in the U.S. among socio-economically deprived groups, and this has variously been interpreted as meaning that the high incidence is related more to the degree of nutritional deficiencies than to any other environmental factors.

B. Some uncontrolled clinical studies purported to show an increased incidence of preeclampsia in poorly or very poorly nourished patients, or that protein-calorie supplementation to such patients reduced the incidence.

VI. Sodium Metabolism and Volume Homeostasis

A. In normal pregnancy, total body water is increased about 6 to 8 L., of which 4 to 6 L. are extracellular. Plasma volume starts to rise in the first trimester, but most of the increase occurs in the latter half of pregnancy. There is also a cumulative retention of sodium (500 to 900 mEq.), part of which is stored in the fetus, while the other part is necessary to maintain the elevated blood volume.

B. The most significant renal adjustment in normal pregnancy is the increase in glomerular filtration rate (G.F.R.; up to 50%), which results in an additional filtered load of sodium amounting to 5,000 to 10,000 mEq./day. Most of the sodium is reabsorbed by the tubules under the influence of aldosterone, the secretion of which is increased.

C. Pregnant women handle sodium load similarly to nonpregnant women, but they adjust more slowly to sodium restriction, and substantial amounts of sodium may be lost in the urine before homeostasis is reestablished.

D. The mechanism of edema in preeclampsia is not completely understood, but it differs from that seen in normotensive pregnancies.

1. In most normal pregnancies there is some retention of sodium, occasionally accompanied by edema. However, there is a rapid appearance of sodium retention and edema in some cases of pre-eclampsia. This gave rise to the belief that fluid retention may be due to excessive salt intake and that sodium restriction and/or diuretics might be beneficial.

2. Prophylactic therapy has been claimed to reduce the incidence of preeclampsia, but the claims have not been substantiated in other studies. After a decade of enthusiastic use diuretics have been abandoned as being of little value and potentially harmful. For despite the elevated blood pressure, some patients with preeclampsia show hypoalbuminemia and a contracted intravascular volume, and the further decrease in blood volume is believed to have a deletrious effect on placental perfusion.

3. While most pregnant women adjust to restricted sodium intake some are said to tolerate it poorly. Thus there is less tendency to routinely restrict salt intake, although some controversy still exists. There is no evidence, however, that mild sodium restriction is harmful.

ENVIRONMENTAL FACTORS

I. Alcoholism and Pregnancy

A. A 1974 report of the National Institute of Alcoholism and Alcohol Abuse (NIAAA) to the Congress of the U.S. stated that the proportion of women alcoholics, especially in the 21 to 29 age group, is increasing steadily. The number of women among 9 million alcoholics is variously estimated between 1.5 and 4.5 million. Teenage drinking is also said to be increasing, and, thus, the number of fetuses being exposed to alcohol can be expected to increase.

B. Heavy maternal drinking causes growth retardation prenatally (affecting body length and head circumference more than body weight) as well as postnatally (owing presumably to continued drinking by the mother and neglect of the child) and may also contribute to physical abnormalities of the child, but whether alcohol is a specific teratogen is questionable. The frequency and spectrum of the so-called fetal alcoholic syndrome remains undefined, and there are no systematic studies of the amount and duration of alcohol consumption before conception and during the various stages of gestation necessary to induce physical abnormalities in the offspring.

C. It is not clear whether alcohol through its metabolites acts as a direct toxin or the presence of associated factors (perhaps amenable to correction) are necessary to induce physical anomalies in the offspring. The quantity and frequency of alcohol consumed at the time of conception and during the various stages of pregnancy may have different effects. It is considered likely that heavy drinking affects mainly fetal development during the first trimester and fetal nutrition and size near term.

D. Malabsorption of vitamins, particularly of vitamin A, thiamine, and folic acid, has been well documented in alcoholics.

E. Alcohol has a direct toxic effect on the pancreas, and acute hypoglycemia may be precipitated by binge drinking. Congenital malformations are increased in diabetic pregnancy, and it has been proposed that hypoglycemia of early pregnancy may be related to congenital anomalies of offspring of alcoholic mothers.

F. Both human- and animal-study data indicate that any effects of alcoholism are dose-related, but safe levels in pregnancy have not been defined. The NIAAA believes that maternal ingestion of the equivalent of 3 oz. of absolute alcohol (approximately six drinks a day) places the fetus at risk. Peak blood alcohol concentration probably is more critical than the frequency (even if only one drink or less per week), therefore, pregnant women should not take more than two drinks a day.

G. Most patients tend to minimize the amount of alcohol consumed daily. However, a reasonable estimate of the daily supply of calories resulting from alcohol intake can be determined by applying the following formula:

$$0.8* \times Proof \times oz. = Cal. (whiskey)$$
$$0.8* \times (2 \times \%) \times oz. = Cal. (beer, wine)$$

H. Although whiskey is stated as "proof" (e.g., 86-proof), wine and beer are specified as "percent of alcohol." Therefore, by doubling the "percent of alcohol," the same formula is applicable for calorie calculations.

II. Caffeine

A. During pregnancy, the woman consumes many foods and other substances which cross the placental barrier, enter the fetal circulation, and may possibly affect fetal development adversely.

B. Of great interest in this regard are the borderline forms of drugs used habitually, which include alcohol, caffeine, and nicotine. Among these, caffeine use in the U.S. appears to have the greatest prevalence,

*0.8 = 0.829 Cal./Proof/oz. (a constant)

Table 3-6. **Caffeine-Containing Beverages**

	Caffeine/cup*	Sodium/cup*	Potassium/cup*
Coffee, brewed	100–150 mg.	0.6 mg.	2.6 mEq.
Coffee, instant	60–80 mg.	1.4 mg.	1.7 mEq.
Sanka, instant	3–5 mg.	0.2 mg.	2.2 mEq.
Sanka, freeze dried	3–5 mg.	0.3 mg.	2.3 mEq.
Sanka, ground roast	3–5 mg.	2.0 mg.	4.0 mEq.
Tea	40–100 mg.	0	2.5 mEq.
Cola beverages	17–55 mg.	15–30 mg.	0

*Six-ounce cup; instant made with 2 g. of coffee.
(Coffee and Cardiovascular Disease. The Medical Letter, *19*[Issue 485]:65, 1977)

principally in coffee, but also in tea, cocoa, and cola. Each year the U.S. uses almost 3 billion lbs. of green coffee beans—a per capita consumption of about 15 lbs.

C. The average cup (200 to 300 ml.) of coffee contains a therapeutic dose (50 to 100 mg.) of caffeine as well as 0.5 mg. niacin, 15 to 20 mg. magnesium, and 45 to 65 mg. potassium.

D. In Table 3-6, the amounts of caffeine, sodium, and potassium are compared in coffee, decaffeinated coffee, tea, and cola.

E. In comparison with other drug dependencies, although caffeine shows no physiologic dependence, it does produce psychologic dependence, is easy to manufacture and use, and is socially acceptable. Although the conclusion of most investigators is that caffeine produces few unfavorable effects in the human fetus, other studies appear to suggest a role of caffeine in reproductive difficulties.

F. Caffeine readily crosses the human placenta and enters the fetal circulation. The neonate, during development and for the first several days after birth, appears to lack the enzyme or enzymes necessary to demethylate caffeine.

G. In one study, 800 households were contacted, and complete data was obtained from 489. The results of evaluating the outcome of pregnancy in relation to caffeine consumption are presented in Table 3-7.

H. Although these data do not establish a cause-and-effect relationship between a high level of caffeine consumption (at least eight cups of coffee daily, more than 600 mg./day of caffeine) and a high risk of fetal loss, the results suggest that women may have reproductive difficulties. However, other behavioral excesses (e.g., alcohol and nicotine), either alone or in combination with a high level of caffeine consumption may have adverse effects on pregnancy outcome.

I. Because of the unique physiologic effects of caffeine, high intakes of caffeine beverages may be an important factor in subfertility, repeated spontaneous abortion, miscarriage, and otherwise unexplainable perinatal mortality. When both men and women in the same households ingest large amounts of caffeine, the possibility exists that the altered patterns of reproductive outcome may be male-mediated.

III. Oral Contraceptives—Effect on Nutrition

A. Oral contraceptives have a definite effect on the nutritional status of patients.

B. The need for many nutrients is increased, and, if supplements are not being administered concurrently, the serum level will be decreased.

C. The nutrients that are principally affected are folic acid, vitamin B_6, vita-

Table 3-7. **Outcome of Pregnancy in Relation to Caffeine Consumption**

Daily Caffeine Consumption (Estimate)	Number of Households (Pregnancies)	Outcome of Pregnancy			
		Spontaneous Abortion	Stillbirth	Premature Birth*	Uncomplicated Delivery
≥ 600 mg. by woman	16	8	5	2	1 (6.3%)
> 600 mg. by man, < 400 mg. by woman	13	4	2	2 (1)	5 (38.5%)
300–450 mg. by man, woman, or both	23				23 (100%)
< 300 mg. by man, woman, or both	81	7	17	5 (3)	52 (64.2%)
None	356	33	38	6 (3)	279 (78.4%)

*Numbers in parentheses indicate deaths within 48 hours after birth.
(Weathersbee, P.S., Olsen, L.K., and Lodge, J.R.: Caffeine and pregnancy. Postgrad. Med., *62*:64, 1977)

min B_{12}, riboflavin, vitamin A, and zinc. On the other hand, the blood levels of vitamin A, iron, and copper are increased, indicating perhaps decreased tissue utilization.

D. The nutrient aberrations attributed to oral contraceptive drugs are listed in Table 3-8.

Table 3-8. **Nutritional Aberrations Attributed to Contraceptive Steroids**

Nutrient	Effect
Folacin	Serum level decreased
	Erythrocyte level decreased
	Megaloblastic anemia (rare)
Vitamin B_{12}	Serum level decreased
Riboflavin	Erythrocyte level decreased
	Glossitis (rare)
Vitamin B_6	Disturbed tryptophan metabolism
	Plasma PLP decreased
	Depression
Ascorbic acid	Leukocyte content decreased
	Platelet level decreased
Vitamin A	Plasma level increased
Iron	Serum level increased
	TIBC increased
Copper	Plasma copper increased
	Ceruloplasmin increased
Zinc	Plasma zinc decreased

(Winick, M. (ed.): Nutritional Disorders of American Women. pp. 37–49. New York, John Wiley & Sons, 1977)

E. The effect of oral contraceptives on nutrition is extremely important because if a supplement was not being administered concurrently, it can be presumed that nutritional deficiency exists.

F. Should a person become pregnant shortly after discontinuing the anovulatory drug, it will be necessary to give additional supplements from the inception of pregnancy to make up this deficiency.

IV. Smoking

A. It is clear that smoking during pregnancy correlates with lowered mean birth weights and apparently also with an increased risk of perinatal mortality. On the average babies of women who are heavy smokers—variously stated as more than 10, 15, or 20 cigarettes per day—weigh 150, 200, or 300 g. less than babies of nonsmoking mothers.

B. The effect of smoking on birth weights seems to be mediated in large part, if not exclusively, through depressed maternal food intake and weight gain during pregnancy.

C. In one series of reports, perinatal mortality was 27% higher in infants of smoking mothers as a group than in those of nonsmokers. Smoking less than one package of cigarettes a day increased the risk of perinatal mortality by 20% and more than one pack a day by 35%. Heavy smoking increased the risk of perinatal mortality 70 to 100% in infants of older mothers, mothers of high parity or of poor nutritional status, or those with less than 11 g./dl. of hemoglobin, whereas the excess risk was only 10% in infants of young mothers of low parity or normal hemoglobin levels.

D. The critical period when smoking would exert its most harmful effect has not been established, although most authors believe the effect is greater during the second half of pregnancy. Babies of women who stopped smoking after the fourth month purportedly showed improved prognosis.

E. Irrespective of the immediate effects of maternal smoking on the fetus, the long-term deleterious effects of smoking are undisputed. From the Massachusetts Department of Public Health comes the recommendation that health professionals involved in prenatal care should take advantage of the unusual opportunity afforded by the concern of pregnant women about the outcome of their pregnancies and their eagerness to heed medical advice aimed at improving their chance of delivering a healthy baby, for educating pregnant women about "the danger of smoking and provide positive reinforcement in helping to eliminate this habit."

V. Drug Addiction

A. Growth retardation of methadone-
and heroin-exposed fetuses is believed to be
multifactorial in origin. The direct effect of
heroin, undernutrition, magnified by the
high carbohydrate level in the diet in periods of low drug supply, intercurrent infections, and episodes of involuntary heroin
withdrawal symptoms all play a role.

ASSESSMENT OF MATERNAL
NUTRITIONAL STATUS

I. Because there is much evidence that
poor nutrition, both on entering pregnancy
and during gestation, is related to the outcome of pregnancy, sophisticated prenatal
care includes evaluation of maternal nutritional status.
II. Gross nutritional deficiency is rarely
found in the U.S., but subclinical or latent
malnutrition is not unusual. The goal in
evaluating the nutritional status of the
pregnant woman in an office-practice set-
ting is not only to recognize obvious nutritional failure but also to detect the factors
which puts the patient in a special category
of nutritional risk and to determine who
may need special testing and more extensive nutritional care.
III. In taking a medical history, it is helpful to keep in mind recognized nutritional
risk categories in pregnancy.
  A. *Categories of Nutritional Risk**
    The presence of any one or a combina-
tion of the following factors is sufficient to
warrant a more intensive nutritional assessment than the routine history, physical, and
laboratory tests:
    1. Poverty: Economic disadvantage,
especially among minority groups, is probably the most readily identifiable risk category.
    2. Adolescence: The nutritional bur-

---

*Aubry, R. H., Roberts, A., and Quencs, V. G.: The
assessment of maternal nutrition. Clinics in
Perinatology, 2:207, 1975.

den of pregnancy, when added to the special metabolic needs at this age, make for
unusually frequent nutritional inadequacy.
    *3. Low Prepregnancy Weight and/or
Weight for Height:* Often a reflection of
lifelong or at least long-term nutritional inadequacy, this risk factor is further magnified if followed by inadequate weight gain
during the pregnancy.
    4. High Parity: Frequently linked
with other risk factors, this is especially a
problem when associated with short inter-
conception interval (less than 1 year).
    5. Chronic Systemic Illness: Among
the more important are: diabetes, chronic
infection, drug abuse or addiction, alcoholism, malabsorption syndromes, and severe
emotional/psychosocial problems.
    6. Unusual Nutritional Patterns:
Food faddists and constant dieters are at
especial risk. Frank pica is also to be
watched for.
    7. History of Anemia or Obesity:
This often indicates long-term inappropriate or unbalanced diet.
    8. Poor Reproductive History: Prior
low birth weight or premature labor with or
without perinatal mortality or morbidity is
an especially important finding.
IV. Fundamental to all nutritional assessment is the evaluation of dietary intake. Detailed information can readily be obtained
by making use of preprinted sample ques-
tionnaire self-administered by the expectant mother. A sample diet history question-
naire based on the 24-hour recall method is
reproduced in Table 3-9.
V. From the clinical point of view, qualitative information about the adequacy of the
diet is more to the point than detailed calculations of nutrient intakes based on food
consumption tables. From data on the intake of major food groups and essential nutrients, consumption of unusual foods, or a
bizarre dietary pattern perhaps, it can be
surmised whether nutritional handicaps
may be a major influence on the patient's
health.
VI. Physical evidences of poor nutrition,

Table 3-9. Dietary History—24-Hour Recall, for Use in Pregnancy

Name _____ Age _____ Weight _____ Height _____ Date _____

Food	Unit	# Units	Prot./Unit	Total Prot.	Cal./Unit	Total Cal.
Morning						
Fruit or juice	½ cup		—		50	
Cereal w/milk	Sm. bowl		6 g.		150	
Bacon	1 slice		—		45	
Egg	1		7 g.		90	
Bread	1 slice		2 g.		60	
Butter/marg.	1 tsp.		—		45	
Other						
Noon						
Soup	1 cup		2 g.		55	
Meat, fish, or chicken	1 serv. (3 oz.)		21 g.		220	
Yogurt, plain	1 carton		8 g.		125	
Egg	1		7 g.		90	
Cheese	1 slice		7 g.		90	
Cottage cheese	¼ cup		7 g.		60	
Cold cuts	1 slice		5 g.		81	
Bread	1 slice		2 g.		60	
Butter/marg.	1 tsp.		1 g.		45	
Veg.—raw	1 cup		1 g.		20	
—cooked	½ cup		1 g.		50	
Salad	½ cup		1 g.		20	
Salad dressing	2 tsp.				45	
Fruit—fresh	½ cup		—		50	
Other						
Night						
Meat, fish, or chicken	1 serv. (3 oz.)		21 g.		220	
Veg.—raw	1 cup		1 g.		20	
—cooked	½ cup		1 g.		50	
Noodles/rice/ potato/spag.	½ cup		2 g.		70	
Bread/roll	1 piece		2 g.		70	
Butter/marg.	1 tsp.		—		45	
Other						
TOTALS						

Food	Unit	# Units	Prot./Unit	Total Prot.	Cal./Unit	Total Cal.
Desserts						
Cake w/icing	1 piece		2 g.		180	
Cookies	1		1 g.		40	
Doughnut/pastry	1		1 g.		125	
Fruit w/syrup	½ cup		—		75	
Gelatin	½ cup		1 g.		65	
Ice cream	½ cup		3 g.		150	
Pie	1 piece		3 g.		375	
Pudding	½ cup		3 g.		50	
Other						
Snacks						
Bread	1 slice		2 g.		60	
Candy—hard	1 small		—		30	
—choc.	1 bar		—		150	
Crackers	1		—		20	
Jam/jelly	1 tsp.		—		15	
Peanuts	Sm. bag		7 g.		120	
Peanut butter	1 tbsp.		5 g.		90	
Popcorn	1 cup		1 g.		80	
Potato chips	Sm. bag		—		150	
Pretzels	1 (Dutch)		—		60	
Other						
Beverages						
Milk—whole	lg. gl.		8 g.		170	
—choc.	lg. gl.		7 g.		208	
—skim	lg. gl.		8 g.		80	
Coffee/tea	1 cup		—		—	
w/sugar	1 tsp.		—		15	
w/milk	1 oz.		1 g.		20	
Soda (non-diet)	lg. gl.		—		100	
Beer	lg. gl.		1 g.		114	
Wine—dry	½ cup		—		95	
—sweet	½ cup		—		160	
Whiskey	1 jigger		—		125	
Other						
TOTALS						

Grand Total Intake: Protein _____ g. per 24 hr. (76 g. recommended); Calories _____ per 24 hr. (2400 recommended).

(Aubry, R.H., Roberts, A., and Quencs, V.G.: The assessment of maternal nutrition. Clinics in Perinatology, 2:207, 1975).

except in gross malnutrition, tend to appear relatively late and, even when present, are often subtle and nonspecific. Also, physical signs may be confounded by changes peculiar to normal pregnancy.

A. With these limitations in mind a list of some common findings may be useful:*

1. *Hair:* dull, dry, thin, color changes, or easily plucked

2. *Face:* depigmentation, excess pigmentation, edema, nasolabial seborrhea, parotid enlargement

3. *Eyes:* pale conjunctivae, Bitot's spots, fissuring at corners of eyelids

4. *Lips:* redness, swelling, angular fissures

5. *Tongue:* swelling, scarlet, smooth, atrophic papillae

6. *Teeth:* loose, missing, erupting abnormally, caries

7. *Gums:* bleed easily, recession, glossitis

8. *Neck:* thyroid enlargement

9. *Skin:* dry, pale, cool, depigmentation, ecchymoses, petechiae, poor subcutaneous fat (skin fold thickness calipers), follicular hyperkeratosis

10. *Nails:* spoon-shaped, brittle, and ridged

11. *Musculoskeletal:* poor strength, frontal bossing, beading of ribs, knock knees or bow legs, short stature, low weight for height

12. *Others:* cardiomegaly, abnormally high or low blood pressure, hepatomegaly, paresthesias, loss of vibratory sense, decreased ankle or knee jerk

B. The relation of these findings to specific nutrient deficiencies in pregnancy is summarized in Table 3-10.

VII. Specific laboratory tests are valuable as they tend to reflect impaired nutrition before clinical signs appear.

A. It is well to remember that laboratory data must be interpreted in the context of

the extensive physiologic adjustments of pregnancy, which also involve metabolic processes. These adjustments may be translated into altered values for hematologic and biochemical tests, which in comparison with standard values obtained in healthy nonpregnant women may appear to be abnormal.

B. Further, these adjustments represent a dynamic process, and laboratory indices may change repeatedly as pregnancy advances. Also lack of established standards for normal pregnant women limits the value of many laboratory tests. Table 3-10 and Table 3-11 presents a succinct summary of basic nutrients, metabolic role, and test values obtained in normal pregnant women and in deficiency states.

DIETARY COUNSELLING

I. Nutritional Guidelines and Diets

A. "Advice on nutrition in pregnancy is an important aspect of health counselling for the mother, the baby, and the future family." This has been recommended by the American College of Obstetricians and Gynecologists and the Committee on Maternal Nutrition of the National Research Council.

B. The Committee on Maternal Nutrition advocates that ideally, to promote successful reproduction, nutritional counselling should begin long before childbearing is undertaken. The U.S. Department of Health, Education and Welfare (HEW) has recommended abandoning the apparent naive approach of depending on prenatal nutrition counselling alone to prepare the woman adequately for successful reproduction.

C. Only with continuous appropriate nutritional support through childhood and adolescence can the mature woman enter pregnancy in optimal nutritional condition to provide for the development of a healthy infant without undue stress to herself.

(Text continues on p. 60.)

---

*Aubry, R. H., Roberts, A., and Quencs, V. G.: The assessment of maternal nutrition. Clinics in Perinatology, 2:207, 1975.

Table 3-10. **Nutritional Assessment in Pregnancy**
Part I

Nutrient	R.D.A. (Adult Female)			Physiologic and/or Biochemical Role	History and Physical Findings in Deficiency States
	Nonpreg.	Preg.	Lact.		
Total calories (Cal.)	2100	+300	+500	Overall nutrition Energy and metabolism	Dieters, lethargy, weakness, faintness, nausea and vomiting, poor weight gain
Protein (g.)	46	+30	+20	Biosynthesis of cell proteins, cellular integrity, growth	Underweight, underheight, lethargy, anemia, edema, fatty liver
Carbohydrate and lipids				Energy metabolism, biosynthesis of polysaccharides, cholesterol, and steroids	Underweight, underheight, lethargy, anemia, edema
Vitamin A (I.U.)	4000	5000	6000	Formation of rhodopsin, epithelial integrity, and rod vision	Growth failure, night blindness, xerophthalmia, follicular hyperkeratosis
Vitamin D (I.U.)	400	400	400	Calcium and phosphate metabolism, bone growth and development	Rickets, stunted growth, osteomalacia or osteoporosis
Vitamin C (mg.)	45	60	60	Integrity of intercellular substances, amino acid metabolism, adrenal function	Scurvy, anemia, hemorrhagic disorders, poor wound healing
Vitamin K				Integrity of clotting factors	Hemorrhages
Thiamine (mg.)	1.1	+0.3	+0.3	Oxidative decarboxylation reactions	Alcoholism, anorexia, beriberi, polyneuropathy, cardiomyopathy
Riboflavin (mg.)	1.4	+0.3	+0.5	H electron transport	Oral lesions, ocular lesion glossitis, dermatitis
Niacin (mg.)	14	+2	+4	H electron transport	Pellagra; dermatitis, diarrhea, contusion, oral lesions, anorexia
Pyridoxine (B_6) (mg.)	2	2.5	2.5	Coenzyme in amino acid metabolism	Anemia, polyneuropathy, seborrheic eczema
Folic acid (μg.)	400	800	600	Biosynthesis of purine bases, histidine, choline, serine	Glossitis, macrocystic, megaloblastic anemia
B_{12} (mg.)	3	4	4	As folic acid, labile methyl groups	Glossitis, peripheral neuropathy, macrocytic anemia
Iron (mg.)	18	+18	18	Oxygen transport, cytochromes	Anemia, glossitis, achlorhydria
Calcium (mg.)	800	1200	1200	Skeletal system bone formation	Osteomalacia
Iodine (μg.)	100	125	150	Thyroid function	Goiter, hypothyroidism

(Aubry, R.H., Roberts, A., and Quencs, V.G.: The assessment of maternal nutrition. Clinics in Perinatology, 2:207, 1975)

Table 3-11. **Nutritional Assessment in Pregnancy**
Part II

Laboratory Tests	Normal Range		Findings in Deficiency States
	Nonpregnant	Pregnant	
Urinary acetone	Negative	Faint positive in A.M.	Positive
Serum protein, total	6.5 to 8.5 g. per 100 ml.	6 to 8	<6*
Serum albumin	3.5 to 5 g. per 100 ml.	3 to 4.5	<3.5*
Blood urea nitrogen	10 to 25 mg. per 100 ml.	5 to 15	<5
Urine urea nitrogen/total nitrogen ratio	>60	>60	<60
FBS	70 to 110 mg. per 100 ml.	65 to 100	<65
2-hr. postprandial blood sugar	<110 mg. per 100 ml.	<120	—
Cholesterol	120 to 290 mg. per 100 ml.	200 to 325	—
Vitamin A, serum	20 to 60 μg. per 100 ml.*	20 to 60	<20
Carotene, serum	50 to 300 μg. per 100 ml.	80 to 325	<80*
Serum calcium	4.6 to 5.5 mEq. per L.	4.2 to 5.2	<4.2 or normal
Serum phosphate	2.5 to 4.8 mg. per 100 ml.	2.3 to 4.6	No change
Alkaline phosphatase	35 to 48 I.U. per L.	35 to 150	No change
Ascorbic acid, serum	0.2 to 2.0 mg. per 100 ml.*	0.2 to 1.5	<0.2
Prothrombin time	12 to 15 seconds	12 to 15	Prolonged
Thiamine, blood	1.6 to 4.0 μg. per 100 ml.	—	Decreased
Thiamine, urinary	>55 μg. per g. creatinine	—	<50
Lactic acid, blood	5 to 20 mg. per 100 ml.	—	Increased
Riboflavin, urine	>80 mg. per g. creatinine	—	<90*
N-methyl nicotinamide	1.6 to 4.3 mg. per g. creatinine	2.5 to 6	<2.5*
Kynurenic acid excretion	3 mg. per 24 hr.	—	Increased
Xanthurenic acid excretion	3 mg. per 24 hr.	—	Increased
Folic acid, serum	5 to 21 ng. per ml.	3 to 15	<3
FIGLU excretion	<3 mg. per 24 hr.	—	Increased
—after 15 g. L-histidine	1 to 4 mg. per 24 hr.	—	Increased
Vitamin B_{12}, serum	330 to 1025 pg. per ml.	Decreased	Decreased
Methylmalonic acid	<10 mg. per 24 hr.	—	Increased
Hgb/Hct	>12/36	>11/33*	<11/33*
Serum Fe/Fe-binding capacity	>50/250 to 400 μg. per 100 ml.	>40/300 to 450	<40/>450
Calcium, serum	4.6 to 5.5 mEq. per L.	4.2 to 5.2	Normal
Serum thyroxine (T_4)	4.6 to 10.7 μg. per 100 ml.	6 to 12.5	Decreased or normal

*Criteria from the "Ten State Nutritional Survey.
(Aubry, R.H., Roberts, A., and Quencs, V.G.: The assessment of maternal nutrition. Clinics in Perinatology, 2:207, 1975)

D. For the nonpregnant, pregnant, and lactating woman, the National Research Council has specified the Recommended Daily Dietary Allowances (see Table 2-1).

E. A food guide for the pregnant and lactating woman is presented in Table 3-12.

F. Nutrient needs during:

1. First Trimester: If the diet has been adequate previously, nutrient requirements parallel those for the normal diet, with increases in folate and iron.

2. Second and Third Trimesters: An increase is needed in calories, protein, minerals (with special emphasis on calcium and iron), and vitamins (especially folate).

3. Lactation: The basic nutritional requirements during pregnancy persist throughout lactation, with the additional need for increasing calories, protein, minerals, vitamins, and fluids.

G. Dietary habits of every pregnant woman are influenced by various aspects of

Table 3-12. **Food Guide For Pregnant and Lactating Women**

Food Group	Amounts	
	Pregnancy	*Lactation*
Protein Foods		
Animal protein: In addition to protein, supplies iron, riboflavin, niacin, B_6, B_{12}, phosphorus, zinc, and iodine	two 3-oz. servings	two 3-oz. servings
Vegetable protein: In addition to protein, supplies iron, thiamine, folacin, B_6, E, phosphorus, magnesium, and zinc	Serving size varies. Plan with nutritionist.	
*Milk and Milk Products**		
Supply calcium, phosphorus, vitamin D, riboflavin, A, E, B_6, B_{12}, magnesium, and zinc, protein	4 servings	4 servings
	Serving equals 8 oz. of milk or its equivalent	
Grain Products		
Supply thiamine, niacin, riboflavin, iron, phosphorus, zinc, magnesium (whole grains provide more magnesium and zinc and should be encouraged). and fiber	3 servings	3 servings
	Serving equals 1 slice of bread or ½ cup of macaroni, rice, or hot cereal	
Vitamin C-Rich Fruits and Vegatables		
Supply ascorbic acid; when fresh supply fiber	1 serving	1 serving
	Serving equals approximately ½ cup fruit or ¾ cup of vegetables	
Leafy Green Vegetables		
Supply folacin, A, E, B_6, riboflavin, iron, magnesium, and fiber	2 servings	2 servings
	Serving equals approximately 1 cup raw or ¾ cup cooked	
Other Fruits and Vegetables		
Include yellow fruits and vegetables, which supply large amounts of vitamin A as well as B complex, E, magnesium, phosphorus, zinc, and fiber	1 serving	1 serving
	Serving equals approximately ½ cup	

*Vitamin D is necessary for the utilization of calcium. Milk is fortified with vitamin D, most other sources of calcium are not. A supplement to ensure an adequate vitamin D intake may be necessary if milk is not consumed.

(Howard, R.B., and Herbert, N.: Nutrition in Clinical Care. pp. 245–267. New York, Copyright © 1978. McGraw-Hill Book Company. Used with permission of McGraw-Hill Book Company. Adapted from Maternal and Child Health Unit: Nutrition During Pregnancy and Lactation. pp. 34–40. California Department of Health, 1975)

her life, which can be considered pyramidal in nature. Initially, the pyramid base represents cultural and family food patterns. Later, individual childhood food-related experiences are added. Finally, the triangle apex reflects the woman's special dietary influences during pregnancy.

H. Many methods and services which are associated with health education can be used to help improve the nutritional status of the population and ultimately its readiness for the reproductive experience.

I. Therefore, to help improve maternal health and fetal well-being, nutritional education and dietary guidance are recommended for both children and adults of both sexes, as well as for special subgroups with unique food habits or economic disadvantages. A sample menu for a nutritionally adequate diet with cultural variations is presented in Table 3-13.

J. The identifiable persons with a special need for nutrition education have significant risk factors in reproduction. These include nonwhite persons, poor persons, uneducated persons, very young or old persons (less than 17 or more than 35 years old), alcoholics, drug addicts, diabetics, women with first pregnancy or high parity, women with pregnancies less than one year apart, women with prior obstetrical complications or fetal wastage, and unwed mothers. Women who are in one or more of these categories are also more likely to have low-birth-weight infants with physical or mental defects, and who will die during the first year of life.

K. A basic daily diet used in diet counselling is described in Table 3-14.

NUTRITIONAL ASPECTS OF LACTATION (DIET FOR NURSING MOTHERS)

I. Recommended Dietary Allowances

A. An optimal diet for lactating women furnishs somewhat more of each nutrient with the exception of vitamin D, than the amounts recommended for the nonpregnant female (see Table 2-1).

II. Major increases are given for energy intake (an additional 500 Cal./day) and protein (an additional 20 g./day). Because approximately 900 Cal. are required for the production of 1 L. of milk, the energy cost to produce 850 ml. of milk per day needed by the infant is approximately 800 Cal., and the fat stored during normal pregnancy (approximately 4 kg.) can be metabolized to provide the additional 200 to 300 Cal./day needed over 100 days of lactation.

III. An additional 500 Cal./day is added during the first 3 months of lactation to permit readjustment of maternal body stores with completion of the reproduction cycle. This allowance is to be increased if lactation continues beyond this period or if maternal weight falls below the ideal weight for height. Allowances are increased further for women nursing more than one infant.

IV. Assessment of Energy Requirements

A. The energy intake of lactating mothers was found to be 2,716 Cal./day as compared with 2,125 cal./day for nursing mothers, a difference of 591 Cal. Adding the energy equivalents assumed to be lost as body weight, the total energy available to the two groups of women was calculated as 2,977 and 2,364 Cal./day, respectively. If it is assumed that the energy requirement for basal metabolism and activity are equivalent for the two groups, the energy for milk production is calculated at 618 Cal.

B. The energy content of daily milk production is considered to be 560 Cal. Therefore, the production efficiency for human milk is 90%. Actually, the 20 g./day of additional protein recommended to cover the requirement for milk production allows for a 70% efficiency of protein utilization.

V. Food Sources

The increased energy and protein needs of lactation can be met by drinking slightly less than 1 quart of milk daily. This

(Text continues on p. 64.)

Table 3-13. Sample Menus*

		Regular	Mexican	Black	Oriental	American Indian	Lacto-Ovo
Breakfast	2 energy foods	1 cup Cream of Wheat 1 tbsp. sugar	2 corn tortillas 2 tbsp. jelly	1 cup grits 1 tbsp. sugar	1 cup rice 1 tsp. sugar (in tea)	1 cup corn mush 1 tbsp. sugar	1 cup brown rice 1 tbsp honey
	1 calcium/protein food	1 cup milk	½ cup evaporated milk in coffee	1 cup milk	1 cup milk	1 cup milk	1 cup milk
Lunch	1 vitamin C food	1 cup orange juice	1 cup orange juice	1 cup orange juice	1 cup orange juice	1 cup orange juice	1 cup orange juice
	1 energy food	1 slice bread	1 tortilla	1-2* square corn bread	½ cup rice	1 slice Indian fried bread	1 slice whole wheat bread
	2 protein foods	2-1 oz. slices cheese	1 cup beans	1 cup pork and beans	3½ oz. tofu 1 egg	1 cup pinto beans	1 cup lentils
	1 calcium/protein food	1 cup milk	½ cup evaporated milk and chocolate	1 cup milk	1 cup milk	1 cup milk	1 cup milk
Dinner	1 vitamin A food	½ cup spinach	½ cup spinach 1 Green pepper	½ cup collard greens	⅓ bok choy	½ cup spinach	½ cup spinach
	1 vitamin/mineral food	1 banana	1 banana	1 banana	1 banana	1 apple	1 banana
	1 energy food	1 small baked potato	½ cup Spanish rice	2 halves candied yams	½ cup rice	½ cup fried potatoes	1 small baked potato
	3 protein foods	3 oz. beef roast	1 cup beans 1 cup caldo	3½ oz. fried pork chops	Okazu (stewing beef 3 oz. and ½ cup broccoli) and 2 oz. tofu	3½ oz. fish	3½ oz. cheese (cheddar)
	1 calcium/protein food	1 cup milk	½ cup evaporated milk and coffee	1 cup milk	1 cup milk	1 cup milk	1 cup milk
	2 vitamin/mineral foods	1 stalk broccoli 1 cup fruited Jello	1 cup fruited Jello	1 cup peas 1 cup fruited Jello	1 cup fruited Jello	1 stalk broccoli 1 cup fruited Jello	1 stalk broccoli ½ cup fruited Jello
Snacks	1 calcium/protein food	1 cup custard	1 cup flan	1 cup custard	1 cup custard	1 cup custard	1 cup custard
	1 vitamin/mineral food	1 pear	1 pear	1 pear	1 pear	1 pear	1 pear
	1 energy food	2 oatmeal-raisin cookies	2 oatmeal-raisin cookies	2 oatmeal-raisin cookies	2 oatmeal-raisin cookies	2 oatmeal-raisin cookies	2 oatmeal-raisin cookies

*These menus show the cultural variations possible when planning a nutritionally adequate prenatal diet. All meet the Recommended Dietary Allowances for calories, provide a minimum of 90 g. protein and exceed the Recommended Dietary Allowances for vitamin A and C and calcium. Only the black and Mexican dietary patterns meet the Recommended Dietary Allowances for iron, providing 21.9 mg. and 23.1 mg. The regular, American-Indian, and the Oriental patterns provide 15.3 mg., 15.8, and 15.3, respectively. The Lacto-Ovo plan provides only 12.0 mg. (Cross, A.T., and Walsh, H.E.: Prenatal diet counseling. J. Reprod. Med. 7:274, 1971)

Table 3-14. Basic Daily Pregnancy Diet

Predominant Nutrient	Foods	Number of Servings*
Protein and iron	Lean meats, fish, poultry, lentils, dried beans and peas, eggs, nuts	3 or more (7 oz.)
Protein and calcium	All milks, cheese, cottage cheese	4 or more
Vitamin C	Citrus fruits and juices, broccoli, brussels sprouts, greens, peppers	1 or more
Vitamin A	Fortified margarine, kidney, dark green and deep yellow vegetables	1 or more
Energy and B vitamins	Whole grain or enriched breads and cereals	5
Other vitamins and minerals	All fruits and vegetables	2 or more
Energy	Fats and sugars	Only as needed for energy

*A 2–3-oz. serving of lean cooked meat, fish, or poultry without bones is:
  ¼ lb hamburger after it is cooked
  ½ cup cooked diced lean meat, fish or poultry
  One medium meat or fish patty
  One slice roast meat or poultry, 5 × 2¼ × ¼ in.
  Two frankfurters
  Two slices of liver
  Two slices meat loaf
  Two medium chicken drumsticks (fryer)
  One chicken leg, including thigh
  One medium-sized fish steak
A substitute for a 2–3-oz. serving of lean cooked meat, fish or poultry without bone is:
  ½ cup cottage cheese   ½ cup shelled peanuts
  3 ounces cheddar or jack cheese   4 tablespoons peanut butter
  1 cup cooked dried peas, beans or lentils   3 eggs
A serving of vegetable or fruit is:
  ½ to ¾ cup or a portion as ordinarily served such as
    1 medium apple   1 medium potato
    1 medium banana   ½ medium grapefruit
    1 medium orange   ½ medium cantaloupe
A serving of whole grain or enriched breads and cereals is:
  1 slice enriched or whole grain bread
  ½ to ¾ cup cooked whole grain cereal such as cracked wheat, oatmeal, brown rice, rolled wheat
  ½ to ¾ cup cooked enriched cereal such as grits, cornmeal
  ½ to ¾ cup enriched noodles, macaroni, spaghetti
  ¾ cup enriched ready-to-eat cereal
  ½ to ¾ cup rice, enriched or converted
  1 large enriched flour tortilla
  2 small corn tortillas
(Cross, A.T., and Walsh, H.E.: Prenatal diet counseling. J. Reprod. Med. 7:273, 1971)

will not, however, provide the increased amounts of ascorbic acid, vitamin D, and folic acid recommended, but this can be taken care of by adding fruits, vegetable oils, and meat to the diet.

VI. Nutritional Supplements

  A. Generally, these are not needed except in situations in which intake of one or more nutrients is deficient. Women who do not drink sufficient milk may need calcium supplements.

  B. Some authorities advise supplements of iron (ferrous sulfate), fluoride, and vitamin D for breast-fed infants. The La-Lache League reportedly does not advocate their administration.

SUGGESTED READINGS

Barsivaia, V. M., and Virkar, K. D.: The effect of oral contraceptives on concentrations of various components of human milk. Contraception, 7:307, 1973.

Bell, W. R.: Hematologic abnormalities in pregnancy. Med. Clin. North Am., 61:165, 1977.

California Department of Public Health, Maternal and Child Health Unit: Nutrition during pregnancy and lactation. Sacramento, California, 1975.

Committee on Nutrition, American Academy of Pediatrics: Commentary on breast-feeding and infant formulas, including proposed standards for formulas. Pediatrics, 57:278, 1976.

Felig, P.: Body fuel metabolism and diabetes mellitus in pregnancy. Med. Clin. North Am. 61:43, 1977.

Filer, L. J., Jr.: Maternal nutrition in lactation. Clinics in Perinatology, 2:353, 1975.

Jacobson, H. N.: Nutrition in pregnancy: a critique. J.A.M.A. 225:634, 1973

Jones, K. L., et al.: Outcome in offspring of chronic alcoholic women. Lancet, 1:1076, 1974.

Kaminetzky, H. A., Langer, A., and Baker, H.: The effect of nutrition in teenage gravidas on pregnancy and the status of the neonate. Part 1. A nutritional profile. Am. J. Obstet. Gynecol. 115:639, 1973.

Kitay, D. Z., and Harbort, R. A.: Iron and folic acid deficiency in pregnancy. Clinics in Perinatology, 2:255, 1975.

Kreutner, A. K., Hollingsworth, D. R.: Adolescent Obstetrics and Gynecology. Chicago, Year Book Medical Publishers, 1978.

McAnarney, E. R.: Adolescent pregnancy: a national priority. Am. J. Dis. Child, 132:125, 1978.

National Research Council, Committee on Maternal Nutrition, Food and Nutrition Board: Maternal Nutrition and the Course of Pregnancy. Washington D.C., National Academy of Sciences, 1970.

O'Sullivan, J. B. et al.: Screening criteria for high-risk gestational diabetic patients. Am. J. Obstet. Gynecol. 116:895, 1973.

Ouellette, E. M. et al.: Adverse effects on offspring of maternal alcohol abuse during pregnancy. N. Engl. J. Med. 297:528, 1977.

Pitkin, R. M.: Nutritional support in obstetrics and gynecology. Clin. Obstet. Gynecol. 19:489, 1976.

Weathersbee, P. S., Olsen, L. K., and Lodge, J. R.: Caffeine and pregnancy. Postgrad. Med., 62:64, 1977.

White, P.: Pregnancy and diabetes. In Marble, A., et al. (eds.): Joslin's Diabetes Mellitus. ed. 11. pp. 581–598. Philadelphia, Lea & Febiger, 1971.

4. NUTRITION IN THE INFANT AND YOUNG CHILD

Frank K. Thorp, M.D., Ph.D.

Paula Peirce, M.S., R.D.

Catherine Schneider, M.S., R.D.

NUTRITIONAL REQUIREMENTS FOR CHILDREN

I. Basic Principles

A. During the 20-year period required for maturation of the human body, there is a remarkable integration and synchronization of a complex series of processes, described collectively as growth and development.

1. Nutrient requirements and body composition vary tremendously during this period and depend on the child's sex and developmental level.

2. Requirements reflect needs for immediate growth as well as storage for such future demands as puberty and pregnancy.

B. The nutritional status of a child can modulate the genetic potential for growth and development.

1. During "critical periods" of cell division, calorie and protein deprivation may lead to cessation of cell division. Under certain conditions, such deprivation may lead to restriction in the number of cells in certain organs and, therefore, a permanent decrease in organ size.

2. Severe protein-calorie malnutrition of a pregnant woman in the last trimester and similar malnutrition of the infant in the first 6 months of life may decrease brain cell count by as much as 20% and may not be reversible with subsequent repletion. (Socio-economic factors are also involved in this process; see also Chapter 26).

3. Overfeeding young children, on the other hand, may trigger overproduction of adipose tissue cells leading to a form of refractory obesity in adult life.

C. Certain types of chronic illness, and probably emotional deprivation as well, may result in growth retardation, which may be reversed with adequate treatment of the disorder.

1. It appears that boys are affected more adversely than girls suffering the same disorder, but boys exhibit more rapid catch-up growth.

2. Reversibility is more rapid and more complete in the younger child.

3. During the recovery process, weight deficit is generally corrected before height deficit. Bone maturation (biological age) is the last of the functions to show acceleration.

NUTRIENT GROUPS

I. Water

A. The body of the infant contains proportionally more water (75 to 80%) than the adult (60 to 65%). The adult value is reached at about 12 months of age.

1. Fifty-four percent of an infant's total body water is in the extracellular space. When the infant is about 9 months old, this drops to 35–40% of the total body water, a level found in most adults.

2. Dehydration is common in infants. Since much of an infant's body water is in the extracellular space, and since body water is more easily lost from the extracellular space, dehydration can occur quickly and be quite serious.

B. Water requirements in the child include four components. Water is required for growth, to replace loss from skin and lungs, to replace fecal loss, and for excretion of renal solutes.

1. Fever increases evaporative losses by about 12% per Celsius degree of temperature elevation.

2. Diarrhea increases fecal loss. Ing-

ested food or fluids, generating solutes, will increase obligatory renal losses.

C. Water requirements are related to metabolic rate, energy requirements, and nutrient composition of food (see Table 4-1).

Table 4-1. **Approximate Daily Fluid Requirements of Normal Children Under Ordinary Conditions**

Age	Maintenance (ml./kg.)
Low birth-weight	
Newborn	50–70
3 days	70–100
Normal infant	
Newborn	60–80
3 days	80–100
Normal Children	
2 weeks–6 months	125–150
6 months–1 year	150–125
1–3 years	125
4–6 years	100
7–12 years	75
Over 13 years	50

II. Calories

A. There is considerable variation in energy needs during childhood. The infant requires two to three times as many calories per unit of body weight as an adult.

1. The infant's greater surface-area-to-weight ratio and higher basal heat production contributes to this increased calorie requirement.

2. Energy needs for growth are greatest in the first 4 months of life. They decelerate rapidly during the rest of the first year and remain relatively low until the second period of rapid growth and development in puberty.

B. Physical activity may consume an average of 15 to 25 Cal./kg./day, and, even in the infant, such activity as crying may double the metabolic rate.

1. Activity level accounts for considerable variation in energy requirements of individual children of the same age and size.

2. The degree of activity as well as the growth pattern must be evaluated in estimating individual needs.

III. Protein

A. Protein requirements are greatest in infancy.

1. Since a high proportion of the protein is used for growth, these requirements are best related to caloric intake in the first year and to weight thereafter.

2. There should be some allowance for irregularities of intake, poor mastication, and reduced biological quality of protein.

3. These intakes range from 1.9 g./100 Cal. (birth to 4 months) to 1.7 g./100 Cal. (4 to 12 months).

B. Human milk is believed to contain an ideal pattern of amino acids and is thus of high biological value. The protein-to-calorie ratio is also optimal in human milk.

C. Protein synthesis cannot occur in the body unless all essential amino acids are present simultaneously in the diet. The absence of one will lead to negative nitrogen balance.

D. In addition to those essential amino acids required by the adult (isoleucine, leucine, lysine, methionine, phenylalanine, threonine, tryptophan, valine), the infant requires histidine and the premature infant requires tyrosine and cystine.

IV. Carbohydrate

A. Breast milk provides 37% of the calories as carbohydrates in contrast to 42% in commercial formulas and about 50% in the diet of the older infant.

B. Hypoglycemia is a common problem in infants and children.

1. The newborn infant has a proportionally smaller liver-glycogen reserve than does the adult.

2. In addition, since some low-birth-weight infants have depleted fat reserves

and ineffective gluconeogenic activity, the newborn infant is dependent on glucose derived from milk lactose to maintain plasma glucose.

3. Preschool children are particularly likely to develop hypoglycemia or ketosis under relatively mild conditions of stress and starvation.

4. Attention must be directed toward adequate dietary intake of carbohydrates in each of the above situations.

V. Fat

A. Metabolically, the term infant appears to be geared to a nutrient mix containing a respectable amount of fat.

1. Early feedings of glucose-water solution are not physiological and may delay normal nutrient utilizations.

B. Human milk contains approximately 40% of the calories as fat.

C. Breast-milk fat is exceptionally well absorbed, and the pattern of constituents appears to facilitate calcium absorption.

D. Skin changes from essential-fatty-acid deficiency do not develop when the diet contains more than 1% of calories as linoleic acid.

E. Skim milk and 2% milk provide high protein intake, but low intake of fat and possibly inadequate intake of essential fatty acids.

F. Cholesterol in the infant's diet may facilitate formation of steroid hormones and bile acids.

G. For the above reasons, it is ill advised to limit fat and cholesterol intakes in children under 2 years of age unless nutrient adequacy can be monitored.

VI. Minerals

A. Sodium and Potassium

1. A large percentage of the sodium stores of infants and small children is located in an exchangeable pool from which salt is easily lost under stress.

2. Minimal dietary sodium and potassium requirements are estimated as approximately 2 to 3 mEq./day, the recommended intake being 6 to 8 mEq./day in infants and young children.

3. More liberal estimates of daily allowance for older children are potassium 1.5 mEq./kg./day and sodium 2.0 mEq./kg./day.

4. For maintenance in parenteral fluid therapy, potassium values of 2 to 3 mEq./kg./day are recommended.

5. There is now concern that excess intake of sodium, which may result from the ingestion of some commercial baby foods, may predispose infants to hypertension in later life.

B. Calcium and Phosphorus

1. Shortly after birth, serum calcium falls transiently and then rises in the first few months to levels that are higher throughout childhood and adolescence than in the adult.

2. Phosphorus levels remain higher in infants than in older children and adults for the first 3 to 4 years.

3. Delayed hypocalcemia in infancy may result from several factors, one of which may be excess intake of dietary phosphorus such as occurs with cow's-milk feeding.

4. During treatment, the calcium-phosphorus ratio in the diet should be raised to 4:1.

5. Phosphorus depletion syndrome occurs under conditions of malnutrition and has been found in children who have diabetic ketoacidosis and in those who require total parenteral nutrition (TPN).

a. In this disorder, serum phosphorus and 2,3-diphosphoglyceric (2,3-DPG) acid levels are low.

b. 2,3-DPG facilitates oxyhemoglobin dissociation, and its absence leads to tissue hypoxia even with a normal P_{O_2}.

c. Rapid delivery of intravenous glucose solutions can accentuate this disturbance leading to muscle weakness, convulsions, and hemolytic anemia.

C. Magnesium

1. Hypomagnesemia in infants and children is often associated with hypocalcemia and with symptoms of tetany and convulsions.

2. Low serum-magnesium levels may be caused by malabsorption accompanying surgical procedures of the intestine, celiac disease, or protein-calorie malnutrition. It may also occur as a familial disorder.

D. Copper

1. Copper deficiency can result in anemia, neutropenia, and scorbutic-like bone changes.

  a. Copper deficiency has been observed during prolonged parenteral feeding and in association with chronic diarrhea, cystic fibrosis, and celiac disease.

  b. It can occur as a congenital metabolic disorder of copper absorption (Menkes' syndrome).

2. Requirements for copper are estimated to be 50 to 110 μg./kg./day in the term infant.

E. Zinc

1. Zinc deficiency has been associated with decreased taste acuity, growth retardation, inhibited sexual maturation, and impaired wound healing.

2. It has been described in children with protein depletion states, such as chronic inflammatory bowel disease.

3. Zinc deficiency can contribute to poor appetite and poor growth rates in apparently healthy children.

VII. Vitamins

A. Vitamin deficiencies are uncommon, although problems with the fat-soluble vitamins are occasionally seen in children with steatorrhea.

B. Many infants, especially those who are breast-fed, develop vitamin K deficiency and hemorrhagic disease of the newborn in the first few days of life.

1. Administration of phytonadione (vitamin K_1) at the time of birth prevents this disorder.

C. Children with steatorrhea (e.g. cystic fibrosis), or low-birth-weight infants, may develop vitamin E deficiency with excess creatinuria and increased erythrocyte hemolysis. This state may be accentuated by administration of iron and by a high diet-intake of polyunsaturated fatty acids.

VIII. Recommended Dietary Allowances

The recommended dietary allowances (RDA) provide guidelines for nutrient intake for the general population but may not be strictly applicable to a given person (see Table 4-2).

IX. Total Parenteral Nutrition

A. For the child requiring multiple surgical procedures or resection of the major portion of the small intestine, and for the child with chronic, intractable diarrhea, total parenteral nutrition (TPN) can be life-saving.

B. Patients must be selected carefully. The catheter or needle site must receive meticulous care, and frequent nutritional monitoring is essential.

C. For the appropriate patient, use of nasojejunal feeding, alone or in combination with parenteral nutrition, may offer nutritional advantages and decreased complication rates. In this technique, it is essential to use an isotonic formula delivered through open-ended silicone rubber tubes.

D. Optimal requirements for nutrients by the intravenous route have not been conclusively established. The following represent typical formulations used at present.

1. Composition of infusate for TPN

  a. Formula for Use With Central Venous Catheter

  (1) Purpose: To provide 110–120 Cal./kg./day in the infant and 50–80 Cal./kg./day in the child over 10 kg. by constant infusion of hyperosmolar solution.

  (2) Composition:

Water: 120–130 ml./kg./day

(Text continues on p. 73)

Glucose: 10–15 g./kg./day initially as 10% glucose going to 25–30 g./kg./day as 20–25% glucose.

Amino acids (crystalline): 1–1.5 g./kg./day initially, going to 2–4 g./kg./day

Electrolytes:

    Na: 2–4 Eq./kg./day

    K: 2–3 mEq./kg./day

    Cl: 3–4 mEq./kg./day

    Ca: 0.5–2 mEq./kg./day

    Mg: 0.25–1 mEq./kg./day

    PO$_4$: 2 mEq./kg./day

Vitamins, multiple vitamin: M.V.I., 1 ml./day in infusate for age 0–12 months, 0.3 ml./kg./day over 1 year of age

(3) B$_{12}$: 5–10 μg.; K$_1$: 250–500 μg.; and Folic acid: 50–75 μg. should be added to the infusate or given intramuscularly.

(4) Iron as iron dextran, 1 mg./kg. every other week should be given by intramuscular injection.

(5) Trace mineral solutions (especially copper and zinc) or infusions of 10–20 ml./kg. fresh-frozen single-donor plasma twice weekly may be given for children on long-term total alimentation (over 4 weeks).

b. Composition of Infusion for Peripheral Veins, With Intralipid

(1) Purpose: To provide 90–100 Cal./kg./day in the infant and 60 Cal./kg./day in the older child over 10 kg., by constant infusion through the peripheral vein. By infusion of large volumes of a less-concentrated solution, the solute concentration may be kept below that level resulting in vein sclerosis.

(2) Composition:

Water: 150 ml./kg./day in the infant and 100 ml./kg./day in the older child over 10 kg.

Glucose: 10% glucose in electrolyte solution at 100 ml./kg./day in the newborn increased to 150 ml./kg./day over a two-day period.

Amino acids (crystalline): 1–2 g. (protein)/kg./day initially (after 50–60

Cal./kg./day being given from glucose) going to 2–3 g./kg./day.

10% Intralipid: 3–4 g./kg./day through separate line with separate infusion pump, mixing with other solutions in "Y" connector just prior to entry at needle site.

(3) Electrolytes, vitamins, and iron should be administered as listed above with the central venous catheter formula.

E. The peripheral route may not be possible and may be dangerous in the adolescent due to the development of thrombophlebitis, especially with more concentrated glucose and amino acid solutions.

F. Incompatibilities

1. Calcium or magnesium may precipitate with NaHCO$_3$, and calcium may precipitate with MgSO$_4$.

a. Sodium acetate or lactate may be substituted for NaHCO$_3$ to prevent this.

2. Infusate levels of 10 to 15 mEq./L. phosphate, 5 mEq./L. calcium, 5 to 10 mEq./L. magnesium are rarely incompatible, if properly mixed in a large volume of solution.

INFANT FEEDING

I. Breast-Feeding

A. Advantages over formula feeding may include:

1. Avoidance of formula-mixing and dilutional errors

2. Bacteriological safety

3. Immunological benefits providing smooth transition to immune independency (colostrum macrophages, secretory IgA, lysozyme, lactoferrin)

4. Decreased stool pH preventing overgrowth of *E. coli* and pathogens

5. Improved iron and calcium absorption

6. Lower renal solute load, optimal Ca-P ratio

7. Decreased incidence of subsequent obesity, allergies, respiratory illness, mortality and, possibly, necrotizing enterocolitis

8. Improved nurturing, sensual closeness and infant stimulation (as compared to bottle-propping)

9. Changing nutrient composition of breast milk during the feed (increasing protein and lipid concentrations) perhaps providing an appetite-control mechanism.

B. Contraindications to breast-feeding include:

1. Drugs being given to the nursing mother that are excreted in human milk and can be toxic to the infant

a. Drugs which are contraindicated when breast-feeding include atropine, anticoagulants, antithyroid drugs, iodides, narcotics, ergot, tetracyclines, and metronidazole.

2. Metabolic abnormalities or prematurity of the newborn which require the use of special therapeutic formulas

3. Lipoprotein lipase secreted in the milk of some women occasionally causes hyperbilirubinemia by inhibiting glucuronide formation. Rarely is this severe enough to warrant termination of breast-feeding.

4. Serious illness in the mother

C. Although breast-feeding is to be encouraged, caution is needed in dealing with mothers who cannot or do not wish to breast-feed.

1. Normal growth and development are possible with the use of available infant formulas.

2. Adequate educational programs for pregnant women, assistance with nursing problems and positive reinforcement from the health care team are important in the encouragement of breast-feeding.

3. Breast-fed infants require vitamin D supplementation of 400 units/day and, if the mother's diet is inadequate, vitamin C supplementation of 35 mg./day.

4. Iron supplementation may be required if the infant is at risk for development of anemia and if solid feedings are delayed.

II. Formula Feeding

A. Special attention should be given in infant formulas to adequate nutrient composition, ease of digestibility, and reasonable distribution of carbohydrate, protein, and fat.

1. Adequacy of nutrient composition should be based on the RDA for infants.

2. Excesses of any nutrients are not desirable.

3. Comparison of human and cow's milk suggests a reasonable distribution of the major nutrients.

	Protein (%)	Carbohydrate (%)	Fat (%)
Formulas	7–16	35–65	30–55
Human Milk	7	38	55
Cow's Milk	20	30	50

B. Calories

1. Standard formulas contain 20 Cal./oz. which is adequate to meet the 117 Cal./kg. requirement of the term infant.

2. The premature infant may require a more concentrated formula to provide as many as 130 Cal./kg. of body weight.

C. Protein

1. Formulas should provide a minimum of 1.8 g. of protein per 100 calories.

2. The biologic value of the formula protein should be at least comparable to that of the milk protein, casein.

D. Carbohydrate

1. Lactose is the carbohydrate in human and cow's milk and is the main source of carbohydrate in milk-based formulas.

2. Other carbohydrates such as sucrose, corn syrup solids, maltose, and dextrins are often used in lactose-free formulas, especially when milk protein (traces of lactose) is to be avoided by allergic infants.

3. Monosaccharides and disaccharides are more easily digested by the infant than complex polysaccharides (starches).

E. Fat

1. Aside from providing an efficient

source of calories, fat is necessary in the diet to provide the essential fatty acids, linoleic and arachidonic acid.

2. These fatty acids are not synthesized by the body and are necessary for optimum caloric utilization and skin composition.

3. In the standard infant formula 2.7% of the calories should be supplied by essential fatty acids.

4. Fat included in the diet enhances absorption of fat-soluble vitamins.

F. Vitamins and Minerals

1. Iron-deficiency anemia is the most common nutritional deficiency in infants today.

2. Thirty-two ounces of an iron-fortified formula will provide the RDA of iron (10 mg.).

3. Hemolytic anemia has been reported in premature infants receiving formulas high in polyunsaturated fatty acid without increased vitamin E levels.

a. To avoid this hemolytic anemia in the premature infant, it is recommended that the ratio of vitamin E to polyunsaturated fatty acid be not less than 0.4 mg. of vitamin E to 1 g. of polyunsaturated fatty acid.

4. High intake of iron has also led to hemolytic anemia, possibly by decreasing vitamin E availability.

a. For this reason the infant should not receive more than the recommended dietary allowance for iron.

5. Supplementation with fluoride is generally considered necessary for good dental health if the water supply provides less than 1.0 mg./L. (Information on fluoride levels is usually available from local officials.)

G. Formula osmolality is important in estimating the potential for diarrhea, food intolerance, and, possibly, necrotizing enterocolitis.

1. This differs entirely from the osmolality of the estimated potential renal solute load generated by the formula (due to dif-fering metabolic clearances of the major nutrients).

2. This renal solute load results from nonmetabolizable compounds of the diet, particularly excess electrolytes and metabolic by-products of protein metabolism.

3. Under conditions of illness, high environmental temperature, or water restriction, the infant may be unable to excrete all of the solute presented to the kidney and may develop hypernatremia, acidosis, and growth failure.

4. In the infant, optimal urine osmolality should range between 300 and 400 mOsm./L.

5. The estimated potential renal solute load, in total milliosmoles per liter, is 79 for human milk, 221 for cow's milk, 308 for boiled skim milk, 139 for SMA, and 166 for Similac (Foman).

H. Frequency of feeding ranges from 3 to 5 hours for the full-term, healthy infant with 60 to 90 ml. of formula offered per feeding.

1. This amount is increased with age to about 180 to 210 ml. per feeding at 3 to 4 months of age.

2. Frequent burping during feeding prevents gaseous distension of the stomach and regurgitation.

3. Formula-feeding is not an excuse for "bottle-propping". The infant should be cradled in the parent's arms during feeding to provide nurturing.

I. Nutrient content of common milks, formulas, and oral solutions is listed in Table 4-3.

III. Feeding the Low-Birth-Weight Infant

A. The low-birth-weight infant requires a high calorie intake to achieve a growth rate comparable to that which would have been present in utero. In addition, absorption of certain fats may be compromised, aspiration of liquids may be a serious problem, and renal-solute loads may be excessive if volume of feeding is low.

B. Breast- or bottle feeding may be employed for infants who weigh over 2,000 g. at birth.

C. For infants weighing 1,500 to 2,000 g., early feedings of 5 to 15 ml. of 10% glucose may be offered in the first 2 to 12 hours at 2- to 3-hour intervals.

1. Gradually, a 100 Cal./100 ml. formula may be offered at 3-hour intervals (initial formula to be diluted equally with glucose water) with an increase in volume of each feeding by 3 to 5 ml./day until urine solute concentration is 300 to 400 mOsm./L.

2. By the fifth or sixth day, and when the volume has been increased to 140 ml./kg./day, the calorie concentration should be decreased to 67 to 80 Cal./100 ml., depending on the rate of weight gain.

3. Expected weight increments for infants of various birth-weights can be projected from published grids.

D. For infants under 1,500 g. or for distressed larger infants, intravenous fluids are necessary at maintenance rates, with a decrease in volume administered as gavage feedings are tolerated and sequentially increased (initial gavage feedings of distilled water, then of diluted formula).

1. Volume of feedings must be individualized. Frequency of feedings is usually every 2 to 3 hours.

2. When 100 ml./kg./day of a 100 Cal./100 ml. formula is tolerated, urine osmolality may be monitored as above.

3. With discontinuance of the intravenous fluids, formula concentration should be reduced to 80 Cal./100 ml.

4. Weight gain may be delayed for 10 to 14 days.

E. For the low-birth-weight infant receiving breast milk, a supplementary formula may be necessary to augment the protein requirement as rapid growth occurs.

F. Vitamin intake should be watched, especially if formula intake is low.

1. Although exact requirements have not been established, needs for vitamin C may be as great as 50 mg./day and for vitamin D as great as 800 to 1,000 units daily.

G. Minerals

1. As the infant gains weight, 5 to 10 mg./day of elemental iron may be given in the form of an easily absorbed iron salt.

2. Calcium requirements are excessive and cannot be met by the usual available formulas.

3. Copper requirements are higher in premature infants, and it has been suggested that their formulas contain a minimum of 90 μg. copper/100 Cal., in order to provide 100 to 500 μg. copper per day.

IV. Adding Solids

A. Solids may be added to the diet at 4 to 6 months of age.

1. Earlier introduction of solids has not been shown to be beneficial and may contribute to obesity and food allergies.

B. Feeding schedules are somewhat arbitrary, however cereals, such as rice, may be initially offered diluted with formula.

C. Fruits, such as applesauce and bananas, are well tolerated at about the same time.

D. Vegetables may be added at 4 months, and meats and egg yolk at 6 months.

E. Formula may be discontinued and whole cow's milk substituted at that time.

F. Crackers and desserts (puddings) may be added at 6 to 8 months.

G. It is best not to introduce more than one new food per day, and it should be presented in a small, dilute feeding.

H. It may be advisable to delay introduction of certain foods (orange juice, egg white) for infants with a strong family history of allergy.

I. Many parents need assistance with practical aspects of infant feeding, otherwise, underfeeding with failure to thrive or overfeeding with obesity can result.

FEEDING OLDER CHILDREN

I. Guidelines and Problems

A. Bite-size pieces of food which can be easily picked up with finger or spoon by the young child should be provided.

1. Such foods as raw carrots and peanuts should be avoided until they can be chewed well, and there is no danger of aspiration.

2. Food should be served in small portions so as not to overwhelm the child.

B. During the second year of life, growth rate decelerates, caloric requirements drop, and children may demonstrate marked disinterest in food.

1. Children should not be forced to eat. If they refuse, the food should be removed without comment, and offered again at the next scheduled meal or snack.

C. A child should be encouraged to feed himself as soon as he is ready to manipulate a cup and spoon. Messy table manners are part of this process and should be tolerated.

D. Milk should be used as a beverage toward the end of the first year with two cups per day.

1. The bottle should not be used as a pacifier or be taken to bed at night.

2. Solids should be offered first during a meal, with milk to follow.

E. It is very helpful to feed children with the rest of the family. Mealtimes should be pleasant and free of dissension and strife.

F. Between-meal snacks may be offered if they do not reduce appetite and if they are not purely carbohydrate without other nutrients. Fruits and nuts are excellent choices.

II. The Handicapped Child

A. Parents of mentally retarded or physically handicapped children must show great care and patience when teaching them to eat.

1. Training in sucking can be facili-

tated by use of sweet or highly flavored liquids and bottles with large, soft nipples with big openings.

2. Children with cleft palate may be able to "chew" formula from a bottle.

3. A plastic straw filled with fluid and slowly emptied into the child's mouth may encourage sucking.

B. Swallowing problems can be circumvented by gently stroking the throat downward and placing food on the back of the tongue.

1. Leisurely feeding of strained foods and small, frequent feedings are also helpful.

2. Exercises for tongue control can be devised during meal time.

C. The child with chewing problems may need to be shown the necessary jaw motions by placing hands on his jaw and moving them up and down.

D. Thickened feedings may help the child who chokes on liquids.

E. Special problems include the long time required for feeding, obesity in an inactive child, and underweight in overactive children or those requiring more energy in muscle action.

F. The handicapped child should be fed with the rest of the family, if possible.

G. Handicapped children should be encouraged to progress in eating skills to the limit of their ability.

NUTRITIONAL STATUS OF U.S. CHILDREN

I. Findings From the Ten-State Nutrition Survey (1968–1970) and the HANES report (1971–73)

A. Children of the poor grow less, and less well than those of the affluent. Quantity of food rather than quality appears to be the major dietary problem.

B. Fatter children are taller and more advanced in bone- and sexual development than leaner children.

Table 4-4. **Assessment of Nutritional Status in Children**

Degree of Investigation	History		Clinical Evaluation	Laboratory Evaluation
	Dietary	Medical and Socio-economic		
Birth to 24 Months				
Routine	Source of iron Vitamin supplement Milk intake (type and amount)	Birth weight Length of gestation Serious or chronic illnesses Use of medicines	Body weight and length Gross defects	Hematocrit Hemoglobin
Mid-Level	Quantitative 24-hr. recall Meat, egg yolks, supplement Energy nutrients Micronutrients— calcium, niacin, riboflavin, vitamin C Protein Food intolerances Baby foods— processed commercially; home cooked	Family history of diabetes, tuberculosis Maternal height Prenatal care Infant immunizations Tuberculin test	Head circumference Skin color, pallor, turgor Subcutaneous tissue paucity, excess	RBC morphology Serum iron and total iron-binding capacity Sickle cell testing, transferrin
Intensive	Quantitative dietary history and nutrient calculation	Prenatal details Complications of delivery Regular health supervision	Cranial bossing Epyphyseal enlargement Costochondral beading Ecchymoses	Above, plus vitamin and appropriate enzyme assays; protein and amino acids; electrolytes, calcium, phosphorus, alkaline phosphatase, magnesium
2 to 5 Years				
	Determine amount of intake	Probe about pica Medications	Add height at all levels Add arm circumference at all levels Add triceps skin folds and bone age at in-depth level	Add serum lead at mid-level Add serum micronutrients (vitamins A, C, folate, etc.) at in-depth level
6 to 12 Years				
	Probe about snack foods Determine whether salt intake is excessive	Ask about medications taken; drug abuse	Add blood pressure at mid-level Add description of changes in tongue, skin, eyes for in-depth level	All of above plus BUN

Table 4-4. **Assessment of Nutritional Status in Children** *(Continued)*

Degree of Investigation	History		Clinical Evaluation	Laboratory Evaluation
	Dietary	*Medical and Socio-economic*		
		Adolescents		
Routine	Frequency of use of food groups Habits, patterns Snacks Socio-economic status	Previous diseases and allergies Brief system review Family history	Height Weight	Urine, protein and sugar Hemoglobin
Mid-Level	Above Qualitative estimate 24-hour recall	Above in detail	Above Arm circumference Skin fold thickness External appearance	Above Blood tests: albumin; iron and TIBC; vitamins A and β -carotene; RBC indices; BUN; cholesterol; zinc
Intensive	Above Quantitative estimate by recall (3–7 days)	Above	Above Radiograph of wrist and bone density	Above Blood tests: Folate and vitamin C; alkaline phosphatase; RBC transketolase; RBC glutathione reductase; lipids; zinc; electrolytes; calcium, phosphorus; alkaline phosphatase; 2, 3–DPG; magnesium Urine: creatinine; nitrogen; zinc; thiamine; riboflavin; loading tests (xanthurenic acid/FIGLU) Hair root: DNA; protein; zinc; other metals Immune status: DNCB

(Modified from Christakis, G. [ed.]: Nutritional assessment in health programs. Am. J. Public Health, [Suppl.] *63*:46, 1973.)

C. Black children tend to be taller, to have greater bone density, and more advanced bone and dental development than white children.

D. Of the nutrients examined, low vitamin-A and -C levels correlated with low income, as did calorie intake level and evidence of calcium-phosphorous imbalance.

E. Iron intake at all age groups is below accepted standards (95% in the 1- to 5-year age group).

CRITERIA FOR ASSESSMENT OF NUTRITIONAL STATUS IN CHILDREN

The criteria to be used in assessing the nutritional status of children are listed in Table 4-4.

NUTRITIONAL DISORDERS AND DISORDERS AMENABLE TO DIET THERAPY

The following examples of disorders with nutritional implications in children include those unique to the pediatric age group and those in which the nutritional approach differs from that used with adults. In many of these disorders, the physician will require the services of a nutritionist/dietitian who can assist in planning the nutritional therapy and can effect an educational program.

I. Diarrheal Diseases and Transient Lactase Deficiency

A. Basic Principles

1. Disorders associated with frequent, watery stools are of concern in children because of the common complications of fluid-electrolyte imbalance and malabsorption-malnutrition.

a. Mild, acute infectious diarrhea of nonbacterial origin is commonly managed by diet change.

b. Because of abnormalities of intestinal mucosal architecture, malabsorption of xylose and fat, and impaired electrolyte and water transport, simple liquid foods are offered during the active phase of these illnesses.

2. Bacterial production of hydroxy fatty acids from dietary long-chain fatty acids may enhance diarrhea in some patients. Poorly absorbed butterfat should be avoided.

3. Impaired digestion of milk lactose is frequently the result of depression or loss of intestinal lactase activity during an acute gastroenteritis.

a. This abnormality may persist for several weeks or longer after the gastroenteritis has disappeared.

b. Occasionally intolerance to other disaccharides also is present.

c. Lactase deficiency may also accompany such conditions as cystic fibrosis and gluten-induced enteropathy and can occur following intestinal surgery.

4. Home diet manipulations may contribute to hypertonic dehydration or hypokalemia if inappropriate amounts of high-solute- or low-potassium feedings are used.

a. Prolonged diarrhea or dehydration may require parenteral fluid therapy (urine osmolality over 400 mOsm./L. in the infant).

B. Therapeutic Approach

1. Eliminate cow's milk and encourage frequent, small feedings of liquids containing simple sugars and electrolytes (see Table 4-3).

a. A variety of foods such as fruit juices, very small amounts of beef broth (excess solute food), liquid gelatin, and soda pop may be used in combination for mild diarrhea.

b. Oral electrolyte solutions of known composition are preferable in providing a safe balance of solutes.

2. By the second day, soft foods may be added with a gradual return to the regular diet.

3. If diarrhea occurs on reintroduction of milk, return for a brief period to a milk-free regimen.

4. If a brief second trial of milk is unsuccessful, institute a lactose-free formula (some require the addition of glucose) and lactose-free diet for 1 to 3 weeks with subsequent return to regular food.

5. Avoid prolonged periods of a liquid diet or of vacillations between liquids and solids.

a. Starvation diarrhea and malnutrition may soon occur with the traditional "bowel rest" regimen.

b. Offer a predigested formula, even though diarrhea continues, in amounts estimated to provide maintenance nutrition above fecal losses.

    c. Despite continuing diarrhea, increased absorption from increase in availability of nutrients will usually occur.

    6. Chronic intractable diarrhea may be treated by TPN instituted soon after recognition of the problem. Prolonged attempts at diagnostic studies usually are fruitless and result in further nutritional depletion.

II. Obesity

A. Basic Principles

    1. It is difficult to give an adequate definition of obesity in children. The actual appearance of the child may be more helpful than data from height and weight tables. In the obese child, there is a generalized excessive accumulation of fat in the subcutaneous and other tissues. In contrast, a stocky child may be in the 97th percentile for weight, but have a larger skeletal frame and more muscle tissue. Another definition of obesity is that of skin fold thickness (triceps and subscapular) greater than two standard deviations above the normal range.

    2. Obesity has come to be known as a serious health hazard. Achievement of ideal weight is both medically desirable and efficacious.

    3. There is evidence that obesity in early childhood is associated with obesity in adult life. Rigorous attempts to halt obesity in children may improve life expectancy.

B. Therapeutic Approach

    1. For a weight reduction plan to be effective, certain changes in life style must be made and maintained. The specifics leading to the individual child's overeating and obesity must be identified and corrected if possible. Understanding of the socio-cultural and familial patterns of obesity in different age groups can be helpful in patient counselling.

    2. It is recommended that the child be seen at specific intervals to assess progress and to offer support. A record of the food intake is a means of determining patient compliance and also nutrient adequacy. Infants and young children should be seen with the mother, whereas adolescents generally require private sessions.

    3. In the moderately obese young child, a weight maintenance program that allows the child to "grow into" his or her weight (the weight remains stable, whereas the height increases) is a desirable goal. In the severely obese child, caloric intake can be restricted to a certain degree and weight loss achieved.

    4. In situations where the entire family is overweight, it is more realistic to approach the family as a unit, rather than the individual child. The family should be brought in for the counselling sessions at which each member is asked to participate. Guidelines for food purchasing, food preparation, and low-calorie snack ideas are helpful.

    5. Restriction of caloric intake can be accomplished by one of several different approaches. It must be emphasized that the plan chosen should be geared to meet the patient's needs. The desired calorie intake should be based on the child's age and ideal body weight. To achieve a 1-lb. weight loss, a calorie deficit of 3,500 calories is needed (500 Cal./day for 7 days).

    a. A meal plan can be written using food lists similar to the diabetic exchange lists (see Appendix 16-A).

    b. The child or parent, with a food calorie booklet, can count the calories in the foods consumed. A specific caloric level is designated, and the foods consumed each day should not exceed this level. This method, if followed, not only restricts the child's total intake but also makes him aware of the caloric density of various foods.

    c. Calories may also be restricted by eliminating one problem food per visit. It must be stressed that if a problem food (such as soda pop) is to be avoided without a concomitant increase in other high-calorie foods, a low-calorie substitute (diet soda) should be offered.

6. Behavior modification may be successful if the patient is well-motivated and able to keep records. The aim is to identify the circumstances and timing of problem eating, set up blocks to the problem behavior, and substitute other behavior patterns. An example might be that of problem eating while watching TV. The child is allowed to watch TV and allowed to eat, but he or she must leave the TV viewing room and sit in another place to eat. If there is a need to do something else while watching TV, puzzles or other games may be substituted for eating.

7. Exercise is a necessary adjunct to any weight-reduction program. A consistent form of fairly strenous exercise of the child's choosing may be encouraged. Inner-city children may have limited access to safe recreation sources.

8. Free access to spending money for after-school snacking should be discouraged, and junk foods should be eliminated from the home.

9. Despite these various approaches to obesity management, successful and permanent weight reduction occurs in less than 10% in the author's experience. (For a more optimistic assessment of the problem, see Chap. 17.)

III. Malnutrition

A. Basic Principles

1. Malnutrition may accompany insufficient food supply, food faddism (such as recent conversion to poorly planned vegetarian diets), anorexia nervosa, prolonged stress or trauma, malabsorptive states (such as regional enteritis), or postoperative conditions (such as ileal bypass surgery).

2. Marasmus refers to protein-calorie deficiency. This has an insidious onset and long duration of illness with loss of muscle and subcutaneous fat, wizened and alert appearance, growth failure, sodium depletion, and gradual decline in vitamin and mineral levels.

3. Kwashiorkor is protein deficiency

with relative caloric adequacy. This is found with increasing frequency in American children. Onset can be rather rapid, with edema of face and extremities, marked muscle loss, poor appetite, and apathetic or irritable affect, mild growth failure, "flaky paint" dermatitis, and diarrhea. Marked electrolyte and water disturbances (including sodium retention, potassium loss and increased body water), serum protein depletion, hypoglycemia, and low levels of vitamins (especially fat-soluble vitamins) partially due to depletion of lipid transport proteins, can occur.

4. Repletion must be slow and gradual. Protein should be of high biological value.

B. Therapeutic Approach

1. Institute a liquid diet with predigested, lactose-free formula. Frequent feedings or glucose supplementation may be necessary to avoid hypoglycemia. Protein intake initially should be 1 to 2 g./kg./day.

2. Solids may be added in the severe case by the second week. The formula can be increased to provide 100 Cal./kg./day. In 1 or 2 weeks, with the small child, over 120 Cal./kg./day and 2 to 5 g. protein/kg./day may be necessary for recovery.

3. Edema should be treated gradually.

   a. Potassium supplements (4 to 5 mEq./kg./day) and sodium restriction (less than 1 mEq./kg./day) may be necessary, particularly in the child with severe anemia.

   b. Magnesium supplements are recommended.

4. Water-miscible vitamin A, 50,000 I.U., may be given initially in the severe case, or daily multi-vitamins may be administered.

5. Recovery is slow. Diuretics and transfusions, aimed at speeding recovery, often do more harm than good.

6. Nutritional repletion may be accomplished in the strict vegetarian patient with vegetable proteins, although nitrogen absorption is less effective than with animal proteins, and mixed vegetable sources may

be necessary to provide complementary amino acid patterns. Supplemental vitamin B_{12} must be provided, as there is no plant source of this vitamin.

IV. Iron Deficiency

A. Basic Principles

1. Iron deficiency is the most prevalent nutritional disorder in American children.

2. Since iron-deficiency anemia leads to increased susceptibility to infection, fatigue, poor attention span, and interference with learning in school, prevention and treatment of this disorder are important.

3. During the early months of life there is a demand for iron as blood volume increases with growth. Low-birth-weight infants with poor iron stores are particularly at risk. After 6 to 9 months of life, iron stores may be exhausted, and the infant diet contains little iron. Anemia may develop gradually from 9 to 24 months of age.

4. Excess ingestion of cow's milk (low in iron) may facilitate anemia by suppressing appetite for iron-containing solids. Occasionally, chronic intestinal blood loss is produced from exposure to a heat-labile protein in the whole milk. Such children are referred to as "milk babies" and are plump and anemic.

B. Therapeutic Approach

1. The severely anemic child may require a slow transfusion of packed red cells to prevent decompensation with congestive heart failure, which can be triggered by stress or infection.

   a. Transfusions should not bring the hemoglobin value to normal in order to avoid hypervolemia, but only to 6 to 7 g./100 ml. The remainder of treatment should be nutritional, to emphasize the nature of the disorder to the family and to prevent recurrence.

2. Milk intake should be decreased to 2 cups daily, and the bottle should not be used as a pacifier. Solids should be offered first and milk should be used only as a bev-

erage toward the end of the meal. Diet content of red meats, egg yolk, and iron-fortified cereal should be increased.

3. Supplemental, therapeutic doses of iron as 6 mg./kg./day of elemental iron should be provided in three divided doses between meals. Ferrous sulfate (20% elemental iron) or ferrous gluconate (10 to 20% iron) may be used. Reticulocytosis should occur promptly.

4. Iron therapy should be continued for 4 to 6 weeks after the hemoglobin level has returned to normal, in order to saturate body stores. If fecal blood loss continues after resolution of the anemia, a cow's milk substitute or heat-treated milk may be used.

5. Prevention may be achieved by use of iron-fortified formulas or iron supplementation of the diet of high-risk infants, no later than age 4 months in term infants and 2 months in pre-term infants.

V. Rickets

A. Basic Principles

1. Nutrition rickets from vitamin D deficiency, in otherwise healthy children, is rare but is still seen occasionally.

2. Causative factors include vitamin D deficiency in the mother, prematurity of the child, breast-feeding without vitamin supplements, dislike of fortified milk, and lack of exposure to sunlight.

3. Children with steatorrhea and malabsorption syndromes may develop secondary rickets.

4. Since the active forms of vitamin D (hydroxylated calciferols) are produced by the liver and kidneys, diseases of these organs (biliary cirrhosis, renal failure, and osteodystrophy) may lead to secondary rickets.

5. Increased turnover of vitamin D as a result of anticonvulsant-induced hepatic enzyme activation may lead to rickets in certain children with seizure disorders.

6. Familial forms of rickets also exist, either as calciferol hydroxylase enzyme deficiency (dependency rickets) or as a pre-

sumed renal tubule disorder (resistant, hypophosphatemic rickets).

B. Therapeutic Approach

1. Administration of 1,500 to 3,000 I.U. daily of calciferol by mouth or 600,000 I.U. in a single oral or intramuscular dose will produce radiological evidence of bone healing in 2 to 4 weeks in nutritional rickets. After healing is complete, maintenance doses may be continued.

2. Large oral doses of calciferol should be given as a concentrated preparation in oil; large amounts of the dilute propylene glycol preparation would produce intoxication and stupor.

3. Hypocalcemic tetany may accompany rickets. This requires immediate treatment with intravenous calcium gluconate followed by oral calcium gluconate or lactate for several days.

    a. Vitamin D in daily doses of 2,000 to 5,000 I.U. should also be administered immediately, to avoid recurrent hypocalcemia.

4. Anticonvulsant-induced rickets requires 10,000 to 15,000 I.U./day of vitamin D to sustain healing and 1,000 to 2,000 I.U./day for maintenance if anticonvulsants are continued. Patients on such drugs should be screened by periodic evaluation of serum calcium, phosphorus, and alkaline phosphatase.

5. In vitamin D-dependent rickets, an inherited disease with an autosmal recessive pattern, rickets will develop despite the usual prophylactic administration of vitamin D. It is necessary to continually administer large doses of vitamin D, to insure adequate intestinal absorption of calcium.

VI. Juvenile Diabetes Mellitus

A. Basic Principles

1. Optimal treatment of this disorder in children requires careful matching of meal plan, insulin dose, and activity pattern.

2. At present insulin management is rather imperfect and artificial in that exogenously administered insulin reaches peak levels at predetermined times, depending on the type of insulin used and the time of injection. This contrasts with the normal physiologic state of insulin levels responding to fluctuating plasma levels of carbohydrate and amino acids.

    a. In addition, despite traditional teaching, a given type of insulin may reach peak levels at quite different times in different children.

    b. It is difficult, therefore, to avoid wide variation in plasma glucose levels and marked postprandial hyperglycemia, unless the caloric and carbohydrate intake of the child is monitored in such a way as to match insulin levels in a consistent fashion from meal to meal and from day to day.

B. Therapeutic Approach (see also Chap. 16)

1. Children with the juvenile type of diabetes do not require caloric limitation or dietetic foods.

    a. This is in contrast to obese diabetic adults or the occasional child with adult type diabetes.

    b. The individual meal plan may be based on the family's customary eating style and pattern, with alteration of the carbohydrate distribution in meals and snacks, and an attempt at consistency of nutrient intake.

    c. Access to refined sugar is restricted, since unrestrained hyperglycemia may result.

2. There are three main approaches to diet: free (generally no monitoring except restriction on foods high in refined sugar); measured or weighted (precise monitoring); and estimated (monitoring using an exchange diet based on simple household portions).

3. A calorie level should be selected that is sufficient to maintain ideal body weight and allow for growth. As there is much individual variation, this must be based on the home diet or observed consumption of a regular hospital diet for the child's age.

4. Protein requirements are 2 to 3 g./kg. or usually about 20% of calories.

The diet should provide 45 to 50% of total calories from carbohydrate and 30 to 35% as fat.

5. In the child with well controlled blood sugar, limitation in dietary cholesterol and saturated fat reduces serum cholesterol and triglyceride and may be advantageous over a long period.

6. To simplify initial nutrition education, qualitative alteration of dietary fat should be delayed until the child can master other aspects of diabetes teaching.

7. It should be determined when peak insulin levels occur (by blood and urine sugar testing) under conditions of usual activity, and carbohydrate should be proportioned through meals and snacks in anticipation.

a. Theoretically, as a guide only to initial planning, with a single morning injection of Lente or NPH insulin, the total carbohydrate may be proportioned roughly in percentages of 20 breakfast, 40 lunch, 20 to 30 supper, 10 to 20 divided between afternoon and bedtime snacks.

b. With a mix of NPH and regular insulin in the morning for example, 10% of carbohydrate calories may be taken from supper and snacks and added to breakfast.

8. The distribution and timing of meals must be individualized and may deviate widely from the theoretical. Some children require mid-morning snacks to avoid hypoglycemia before lunch. The child and family need to be involved in all menu planning. Through use of the exchange system or other teaching strategies, the plan may be translated into actual food units. The usefulness of consistency of nutrient intake and meal timing must be emphasized.

9. Extra food must be planned for extra amounts of exercise. Although individual variation is marked, an appropriate amount is one bread exchange per 30 minutes of moderately strenuous exercise in a young adolescent (an increase of 2 to 3 Cal./kg./hr.).

10. The family may need help in planning exchanges for foods often not listed on exchange lists (i.e., pizza, convenience foods). Food for special occasions such as parties or eating out should be discussed. The limits of diet indiscretion that may be allowed occasionally should be indicated.

11. After initial instruction, the meal plan may be reassessed briefly at each follow-up visit to allow for changing requirements, shifts in activity patterns, or unusual weight changes.

a. Children with good control of blood sugar will gain weight rapidly if they overeat beyond energy needs.

12. In diabetic ketoacidosis, during the transition from intravenous to oral feeding, continuing nutritional deficits may be replenished by imaginative use of natural food sources. Potassium, phosphorous, and B-complex vitamins should be readily available.

VII. Cystic Fibrosis

A. Basic Principles

1. Pancreatic insufficiency is present in approximately 80% of patients.

2. In addition to steatorrhea and fat malabsorption, some patients have lactase deficiency as well. Deficiencies of all fat-soluble vitamins may occur.

3. Anorexia and cachexia may be associated with the severe respiratory difficulties.

B. Therapeutic Approach

1. A high-calorie, high-protein diet (no less than 30 to 35% protein) is recommended with moderate fat (15% or less) at a level such that steatorrhea is under control when pancreatic extract (e.g., Viokase) is given.

2. The dose of pancreatic extract to be used at each meal must be individually adjusted by assessment of nutritional status and stool frequency.

3. Certain patients may require lactose restriction.

4. Infants may benefit from high-protein formulas (see Table 4-3) and have developed hypoprothombinemia and edema when fed breast milk or soy formulas.

5. Supplements of water-miscible vitamins A, D (twice the RDA), and E (1 mg./kg./day) should be provided, and vitamin K_1 should be added if hypoprothrombinemia is present. Infants should receive vitamin K_1 prophylactically on a regular basis.

6. Medium-chain triglyceride replacement of dietary fat may be helpful, if steatorrhea cannot be controlled in other ways, but this adds to the considerable expense of therapy.

7. Diet supplements of beef serum hydrolysate-glucose polymer-medium-chain triglycerides have been shown to reverse growth failure in some patients with moderate respiratory involvement. Monotonous diets, however, may discourage children from following other aspects of respiratory therapy and thus jeopardize their status.

8. Deficiency of essential fatty acids has been suggested to be another problem and oral supplementation may prove beneficial in the future.

VIII. Gastrointestinal Disorders

A. Basic Principles
1. Nutritional therapy has been found to be helpful in several types of gastrointestinal disorders in children.
B. Therapeutic Approach (see also Chap. 12)
1. In gluten-induced enteropathy, chronic malabsorption of malnutrition results from distortion of duodenal architecture. This is triggered in sensitized children by a gluten fraction present in certain grains. Steatorrhea and lactose intolerance are sometimes present. A gluten-free diet, excluding wheat, barley, oats, and rye (oats and barley may be tolerated by some patients) is instituted.
  a. This may need to be followed for the life of the child, but subsequent attempts at a normal diet may be made after improvement of growth has occurred.
  b. In the initial weeks of treatment,

a low-fat and lactose-free diet may also be necessary, if clinical intolerances to these foods are present.

2. In children with chronic inflammatory bowel disease, high-protein diets may be used. In addition, substitution of medium-chain triglycerides for dietary fat may be required in some cases of regional enteritis, and lactose-free diets may be indicated for some children with ulcerative colitis.
  a. Supplements of vitamins and iron may be given to children with severe diarrhea and anemia.
  b. Restricted diets at times may only enhance anorexia and lead to further malnutrition.
  c. Marked growth failure may respond to a trial of TPN or diet supplementation with an elemental liquid diet.

3. Children with biliary atresia may benefit from substitution of long-chain fats in the diet with medium-chain triglycerides and supplementation with fat-soluble vitamins given in a water-miscible form (vitamin K, 5 mg./day; vitamin D, 1,000 units/day).
  a. Phenobarbitol and cholestyramine increase the excretion of bile salts and bilirubin, and both may be used to modify hyperlipidemia in children who survive for long periods with intrahepatic biliary atresia.

4. In management of chylous ascites and intestinal telangiectasia, medium-chain triglyceride replacement of one-quarter to one-third of dietary fat may be beneficial, along with reduction of total fat.
  a. Fat-soluble vitamins and linoleic acid should be added to such modified diets in children if they are to be continued for a long time.

IX. Metabolic Disorders

A. Basic Principles
1. Nutritional therapy may have a dramatic effect upon the course of a number of metabolic disorders of children.
2. Many of these disorders are rare

and require complex nutritional strategies for successful treatment.

3. Modulation of deranged metabolic pathways by supplying vitamin cofactors or missing nutrients and by reducing the concentration of metabolites accumulating from an enzyme deficiency often involves nutrients essential for growth and for life.

4. Because careless or inadequate nutritional monitoring of such complex diets can be dangerous, patients requiring such therapies are best referred to experienced centers with adequate laboratory and nutrition expertise.

B. Therapeutic Approach

The physiologic defect and diet therapy required are listed below for some of the more common congenital metabolic disorders (see Table 4-5).

X. Congestive Heart Failure

A. Therapeutic Approach

1. Treatment of cardiac edema may be facilitated by sodium restriction. In children, oral intake of sodium may be reduced to around 500 mg. (22 mEq.) daily.

2. Low-sodium formulas are available for infants.

a. In the infant, sodium intakes of 7 to 8 mEq./day may be employed.

3. Severe congenital heart disease is often associated with failure of the infant to accept usual volumes of formula and may also be accompanied by a degree of hypermetabolism. A diet of high calorie density (100 Cal./100 ml.) is often necessary, but protein calories need to be restricted in order to avoid a high renal solute load.

4. Formulas, severely restricted in sodium, may lead to sodium depletion and

Table 4-5. **Diet Therapy of Metabolic Disorders**

Disorder	Defect	Diet Therapy
Phenylketonuria (mental retardation, convulsions, eczema)	Phenylalanine hydroxylase or Dihydropteridine reductase	Limit phenylalanine, increase tyrosine
Homocystinuria (Marfan's phenotype, ? mental retardation, thromboembolism)	Cystathionine synthetase	Limit methionine, increase cystine; pyridoxine in some types
Pyridoxine dependency (infantile convulsions)	Glutaminc acid decarboxylase	Pyridoxine
Hypoglycemia— undifferentiated		
Hyperinsulinemia	(β–cell hyperplasia, ?functional hyperinsulinism)	Frequent feedings: high protein, avoid concentrated carbohydrate
Leucine sensitive	?(Abnormal insulin release)	Low protein, sucrose after meals
Ketotic	?(Deficient muscle alanine efflux)	Carbohydrate during fasting periods; frequent feedings: high protein-high carbohydrate
Glycogen storage disease Type I (massive hepatomegaly, growth failure, hypoglycemia, ketoacidosis)	Glucose–6–phosphatase	Frequent feeding: decrease fructose (sucrose), galactose (lactose), purines, protein, saturated fats; increase glucose, starch, polyunsaturates
Galactosemia (cataracts, growth failure, mental retardation, liver disease)	Galactose–1–phosphate uridyl transferase	Eliminate galactose (lactose)

growth failure. Preferred formulas manufactured from demineralized whey contain a low solute load and optimal protein levels for heart failure management.

PREVENTATIVE NUTRITION

I. Obesity

A. Prevention of obesity in the adult should begin with the establishment of sound feeding and exercise habits in the child.

B. A current theory states that obesity may result from an increase in either number or size of adipose cells, or both.

1. There are periods of active hyperplasia of adipocytes in the fetus during the last trimester of pregnancy, in the first 2 years of life, and from age 10 to 14.

2. After adolescence, the number of adipose cells is generally fixed throughout life, although cell hypertrophy may occur at any age.

3. During the active period of cell hyperplasia, an overfed child may become obese because of stimulation of cell hyperplasia.

4. In obesity resulting from cell hyperplasia, the number of fat cells will not decrease with any later attempts at weight reduction. There will only be a decrease in individual cell size.

5. Thus it is important that ideal body-weight be maintained during the critical period of cell hyperplasia, for weight gained during this period may lead to obesity more resistant to treatment than obesity resulting from cell hypertrophy alone.

C. Bottle-fed babies tend to gain more weight per unit length than breast-fed babies.

1. Such overfeeding may contribute to later obesity, either because of increased fat cell number or establishment of the habit of overeating.

2. Addition of solid foods to the diet of the infant before 3 months of age contributes to an unnecessary intake of calories.

D. Another common practice is the indiscriminate offering of a bottle to a fretful or crying infant. This may lead to a pattern or life style in which the frustrated child seeks, or is given, food as a means of consolement.

II. Atherosclerosis

A. Because of the finding of cholesterol deposits in the coronary arteries of children and young adults, efforts at prevention of atherosclerosis may be necessary in childhood.

B. It is hoped that some consistent restriction of saturated fats in the diets of children over 2 years, as well as a regular program of exercise, may prove to be beneficial.

C. Children at high risk for adult atherosclerosis, such as those with diabetes or familial hypercholesterolemia, may well be advised to moderate fat intake under close nutrition supervision.

III. Hypertension

A. It is possible that the excess sodium content of the American infant's diet may contribute to subsequent hypertension.

B. Since salt intakes of infants are clearly well above requirements and since added salt does not increase palatability of food for infants, salt intake should be limited.

IV. Dental Medicine

A. Prevention of dental caries can occur at any age, if a few sound nutritional principles are consistently followed.

1. There are several factors in prevention of tooth decay. Improved oral hygiene is perhaps the most important, followed by decreased sucrose content of the diet, decreased frequency of snacking, and modification of the texture of food eaten.

B. Streptococci in the mouth metabolize sucrose to glucose and fructose, which then form long polymers of glucose (dextrans) or

Table 4-6. **Possible Nutritional Effects of Drugs in Pediatric Practice**

Class	Agent	Nutritional Effect
Pharmacologically active substance in food	Oxalate in spinach, rhubarb Phytates in soy and oat flour Iodate additive to bread	Hypocalcemia Decreased absorption of calcium Hidden dietary source of iodine
Antibacterial	Ampicillin Chloramphenicol Kanamycin Nalidixic acid Neomycin Penicillin G Sulfonamides	Diarrhea Decreased protein synthesis; lactose malabsorption Generalized malabsorption Decreased glucose tolerance Generalized malabsorption, vitamin B_{12} malabsorption Diarrhea; hyperkalemia (potassium salt) Decreased intestinal synthesis of vitamins K and folic acid
Antifungal	Griseofulvin Trimethoprim	Increased absorption and toxicity with fatty meals; hypogeusia Decreased folate utilization
Antitubercular	INH PAS Ethambutol	Antipyridoxine Vitamin B_{12} malabsorption Increased urinary zinc excretion
Ion Exchange Resin	Cholestyramine	Steatorrhea; decreased absorption of fat-soluble vitamins (especially D and K) and of calcium and potassium
Antipyretic	Acetylsalicylic acid	Hypoglycemia; decreased protein synthesis; amino aciduria
Anticonvulsants	Barbiturates Phenytoin	Increased vitamin D turnover; folate deficiency Folate deficiency; increased vitamin D turnover and rickets; decreased glucose tolerance
Antiinflammatory	Prednisone, Triamcinolone	Decreased glucose tolerance; decreased muscle protein; increased potassium excretion; sodium retention; decreased calcium, iron, amino acid and protein absorption; aminoaciduria
Diuretic	Thiazides Furosemide	Increased excretion of Na^+, Cl^-, K^+; decreased glucose tolerance; decreased calcium excretion Increased excretion of Na^+, Cl^-, K^+; decreased glucose tolerance
Antineoplastic	Methotrexate 6–Mercaptopurine	Folate antagonist; mucous membrane ulceration; malabsorption Purine antagonist; nausea; stomatitis; diarrhea
Antacid	Aluminum hydroxide gel Magnesium trisilicate	Decreased phosphorus absorption Decreased iron absorption

(Continued on overleaf)

Table 4-6. **Possible Nutritional Effects of Drugs in Pediatric Practice**

Class	Agent	Nutritonal Effect
Psychotherapeutic	Phenothiazines	Decreased glucose tolerance; hypocholesterolemia
Vitamins	Vitamin A	Increased intracranial pressure; fatigue; anorexia; pyrexia; anemia; hepatomegaly
	Vitamin K analog menadione	Hyperbilirubinemia; mild hemolytic anemia
	Vitamin D	Growth retardation; mental retardation; hypercalcemia; calcification of soft tissue; nausea; diarrhea; polyuria

fructose (levans). These substances contribute to the formation of dental plaque. Fructose also leads to the formation of lactic acid which causes demineralization of the enamel. The plaques prevent salivary neutralization of the acid.

C. Children should be encouraged to brush their teeth after eating, but especially after eating sweets. Their overall intake of foods containing sugar should be limited.

D. There is also evidence that sweets consumed at mealtime are less harmful than sweets consumed continuously throughout the day. For this same reason, the common practice of putting children to bed with a bottle of sweetened juice or milk should be discouraged. Modification of the texture of the food is important in the prevention of dental caries. Foods with a sticky texture (such as caramel) are probably more likely to result in caries.

DRUGS AND NUTRITION IN PEDIATRICS

Certain drugs commonly administered to children may have adverse nutritional effects. These are listed in Table 4-6.

NUTRITION EDUCATION OF CHILDREN

I. Basic Principles

A. Improved compliance in following a new meal plan for a child can result if some effort is directed toward nutrition education of both the child and the family.

B. Nutrition teaching must take into account the child's socio-economic and cultural background, as well as his/her maturation level.

C. The physician can often benefit greatly from the help of a skilled clinical nutritionist/dietician possessing the virtues of patience, enthusiasm, and a sense of humor.

II. Approach

A. Young children prefer to learn from direct involvement in the project, acting out, touching, smelling, tasting.

1. By 5 to 7 years of age, visual representation of subject matter may be employed.

2. Ability to learn from symbolic sources (the spoken or printed word) is not fully developed until 11 to 13 years of age.

3. For these reasons, it is best to avoid lengthy discussions or printed handouts and instead employ the use of specially developed teaching tools or games.

B. Supervised use of "street experience," such as buying food in a cafeteria line or cooking a meal or sharing a brown-bag lunch, contributes to improved communication.

5. NUTRITION IN THE ADOLESCENT

Edward Wasserman, M.D.

Leonard J. Newman, M.D.

Adolescence is the period of life between childhood and adulthood, characterized by a rapid increase in the rate of physical growth and changes involving physiologic development. The age at onset ranges from 9.5 to 13.5 years with an average of 11.5 years for males and 1 to 2 years earlier for females.

Adequate nutrition is necessary to provide the energy and essential nutrients required for increased linear growth, increased body-cell mass and maturation. Because of increased demands on nutrition due to accelerated growth and development, dietary deficiencies are more apt to occur during this period than during other stages, when these processes are progressing at a slower rate.

Finally, the effect of dietary fads or chronic and debilitating illnesses, compromising food-intake or limiting physical activity, is significant because a life style is being developed for the future.

I. Growth, Sexual Maturation and Development

A. Changes which occur during adolescence include an increase in the size of every organ except lymphoid tissue.

1. Muscle mass increases in both sexes, but the increase is much greater in males.

2. Fat tissue increases steadily in females during the entire period, but in males, after an initial increase, there is a marked decrease after 16 years of age.

B. The chronology of sexual development varies significantly, but the sequence is constant.

1. Girls

a. Breast-budding and widening of the hips are the first signs of development and are followed by growth of pubic hair.

b. Menarche occurs after the peak of the growth spurt and can occur from 1 to 6 years after the first signs of adolescence appear, the average age of onset being 13 years.

c. Breast development is usually completed 3 years after onset of budding.

d. In general, weight increase and height spurt occur concomitantly.

2. Boys

a. Testicular enlargement, reddening and rugosity of the scrotum, and growth of pubic hair are the first signs of puberty.

b. The enlargement of the penis occurs concomitantly with the height spurt (peak growth), usually about 1 year after first signs of adolescence.

c. These changes occur over a 2- to 4-year period.

d. Peak increases in height and weight usually occur at about the same time.

II. Nutritional Requirements

A. Basic Nutrients

1. The requirements for calories, proteins, carbohydrates, and fats are best expressed in terms of growth rate and state of physiologic development, particularly of the genitals, which parallel physiologic maturation better than chronologic age.

2. To estimate caloric needs, variables such as physical activity and gender also must be considered.

a. Healthy males, aged 11 to 14 years, in general require 400 calories more per day than do females of this age group, due to a greater spurt of growth and increased activity.

b. Girls have a peak caloric need at menarche of 2400 calories, followed by a slow decline to 2100 by age 16.

c. Males consume 2400 calories at age 10, followed by increases paralleling physiologic development to 3000 calories by age 16.

3. Protein intake is in direct proportion to needs for other nutrients and should provide approximately 12 to 15% of the total caloric intake.

4. Carbohydrates should supply 40 to 50% of caloric intake.

5. Fats should constitute 30 to 45% of caloric intake.

B. Calcium Requirements

1. The importance of calcium lies in its key role in bone formation.

2. Only 10 to 33% of dietary calcium is absorbed. It is carried bound to albumin or in a free ionized form in the blood. It moves from the blood, in and out of bone tissue.

3. Vitamin D and parathormone directly influence calcium needs and utilization.

4. In adolescents with marked bone growth, calcium needs increase dramatically paralleling increased caloric intake.

5. In both males and females, the RDA for calcium increases from 800 mg. at age 10 to 1200 mg. during the growth spurt.

6. The primary source of calcium is dairy products.

C. Iron Requirements

1. The need for iron is markedly increased during adolescence in both males and females.

2. This increased need is due primarily to increase in muscle mass and increase in blood volume in males and, to a lesser degree, in females.

3. In females, menstruation and pregnancy also threaten iron balance.

a. A menstruating female loses 15 to 30 mg. of iron per cycle.

b. A normal pregnancy results in loss of about 3000 mg. of iron.

4. Iron exists in both ionic form (70%) which is loosely bound (i.e., hemoglobin, myoglobin and intracellular iron-containing enzymes), and non-ionic form (30%; i.e., hemosiderin and ferritin as stored iron).

5. In females, the amount of stored iron is about half that found in males.

6. Iron absorption is a complex process that can occur along the entire alimentary tract but is greatest in the duodenum.

7. Absorption is influenced by the form of iron (ferrous, ferric) as well as by other constituents (e.g., phosphates, calcium, acids) in the diet.

a. Some elements cause an increase and others, a decrease in absorption.

b. Iron cooking utensils result in a marked increase in iron content of food.

c. Iron absorption is enhanced by iron deficiency, decreased iron stores, or decelerated erythropoiesis.

d. In general, the mean iron absorption from animal sources is twice that from vegetable foods (see also Chap. 14).

8. Data gathered from the Ten-State Nutrition Survey of 1968–1970* indicates that boys of high-income families, ages 12 to 16 usually met iron needs, but 20% of poverty-level adolescent males were deficient. In contrast, 20% of females were deficient regardless of income level.

9. Data regarding the requirements for adolescents are limited. Standards are needed for adolescents that are based on both age and developmental level.

III. Environmental and Psychological Influences on Diet

A. During the teenage period, there is a strong need for acceptance from peer groups.

B. Our society places great emphasis on body awareness for the teenager. In females especially, the need to be slim often comes into direct conflict with good nutrition.

---

*Ten-State Nutrition Survey, 1968–1970. U.S. Department of Health, Education, and Welfare, Publication (HSM) 72–8133.

1. This has led to poor eating habits and fad diets which invariably result in nutritional deficiencies, particularly of vitamins.

C. Because of the need to participate in after-school activities and athletics, less time is spent having meals.

D. There are fewer "family meals"; meals are wolfed down and carbohydrate-rich, empty-calorie foods are eaten to relieve hunger quickly.

1. The decline of family meals, eaten together, leisurely, in a formal dining-room, has been an adverse factor in adolescent nutrition.

E. The teenager tends to buy inexpensive foods, which usually means high carbohydrate content.

F. Those teenagers who are more athletically inclined and body-conscious may maintain their slimness at the expense of nutritional needs.

1. On the other hand, the less active teenager who snacks frequently on high-carbohydrate foods (e.g., soda, candies and cookies) may become overweight and still have nutritional deficiencies.

G. The ideal nutritional situation, including balanced meals rich in fruits, vegetables and milk, with a few snacks in between, and plenty of time to dine with family or friends, frequently seems impossible for the busy teenager.

H. Between-meal snacks are appropriate for the physically active adolescent because carbohydrates are poorly stored in the body. The adolescent starved for a 6-hour period may deplete this energy source.

IV. Assessing Nutrition

A. History

1. The patient's medical and dietary history is of prime importance in evaluating nutritional status.

2. Ethnic background of the patient should be explored for particular dietary habits.

3. Chronic illnesses (e.g., allergy in childhood resulting in restricted nutritional intake) should be determined.

4. The adolescent's attitude toward correct nutrition and balanced meals should be ascertained, as well as insight into his eating habits.

5. A 24-hour dietary recall, in which the patient is asked to list quantities of food consumed in the past 24 hours, is important.

a. Although this technique for evaluating nutrition is very subjective and open to considerable error, the experienced nutritionist can obtain valuable data for analysis if good rapport is established and if the adolescent is questioned carefully.

b. Results obtained from such data are most valuable when compared to norms. Unfortunately reliable norms are not yet established for adolescents.

c. This method, therefore, gives insight only into gross inappropriateness in diet.

B. Physical Examination

1. Anthropomorphic Measurements

a. Height and weight of the individual and their incremental increases as they compare to standards are perhaps the best measure of satisfied nutritional needs.

(1) These, however, do not give an indication of body composition, isolated deficiencies, or borderline nutritional states.

(2) On the other hand, a cessation of growth may be noted by obtaining these measurements and may indicate onset of nutritional disease, inadequate intake or chronic illness.

b. Skin fold thickness can be measured using a Lange caliper.

(1) Most commonly the triceps or subscapular folds are used, and the values for thickness obtained are compared to norms.

(2) These measurements are indicative of body fat content and are a useful screening device.

(3) When correlated with mid-

arm circumference, they yield information regarding lean body mass.

2. Dentition

a. The condition of the teeth (i.e., number of decayed, missing or filled teeth [DMF index]) has been shown to be influenced by consumption of refined carbohydrates, especially those eaten between meals. Refined carbohydrates include snack foods such as pastries, candies and soft drinks with high quantities of sugar.

b. In addition, poor dentition is more prevalent in low socio-economic groups, where the cost of dental care is prohibitive.

c. The adolescent who devotes little time and effort to dental hygiene generally receives little counselling in this area. He does not plan meals well or devote time to other health care needs.

C. Clinical Assessment

1. There are specific physical findings that indicate a severely compromised nutritional state.

a. Foremost is a delay in onset of secondary characteristics which normally are present in the older adolescent. The lack of development indicates a delayed onset of puberty.

b. The physician must distinguish delay due to organic disease from familial or constitutional delay.

2. The presence of chronic conditions of the gastrointestinal tract (ulcerative colitis, Crohn's disease, celiac disease), urinary tract (infection, nephritis), or endocrine system (hypothyroidism), or infections (tuberculosis) should be ascertained.

a. Other clinical findings may be helpful in this regard (e.g., glossitis, presence of a goiter, clubbing, easy pluckability of the hair, skeletal deformities and muscle wasting).

b. In the Ten-State Survey, hepatosplenomegaly was found in a small but significant percentage of the population, equally among low- and high-income groups. Hepatosplenomegaly probably indicates underlying illness.

D. Biochemical Evaluation

1. The simple, available tests generally detect extreme deficiencies only and ignore the borderline state.

2. More-expensive, less-available tests vary in reproducability, and results vary according to the method used. Most have not been standardized for the adolescent.

a. Norms vary according to the state of development.

b. They also may differ with diets and state of activity.

3. Simple tests include urine protein and sugar, blood smear, hemoglobin, hematocrit and serum total protein.

4. Moderately complex tests include serum Fe, vitamin A, serum carotene, BUN, cholesterol, alkaline phosphatase, folate, B_{12}, lipids, calcium, magnesium, and total iron-binding capacity.

5. Research tests are occasionally helpful but normally are not readily available to the clinician. They are usually performed where nutritional research is being conducted and are listed for informational purposes.

a. Blood and serum levels—namely vitamin C, red blood cell transketolase (thiamine), red blood cell glutathione reductase, zinc, selenium, copper, ionized calcium

b. Urine tests—urine nitrogen: creatinine ratios, urinary riboflavin and thiamine

c. Examination for DNA, protein, zinc and other metals

V. Counselling the Adolescent

A. Nutritional counselling for the teenager is a difficult task. An appeal should be made to the adolescent's need for social acceptance based on a healthy physical appearance.

B. Generally, nutritional planning should take into account the cultural aspects of the family diet and attitudes of peers toward food.

C. The nutritionist should not attempt

to impose an eating schedule but rather should impart information about nutrition and, together with the adolescent, develop a regimen which demonstrates a respect for his independence and his contribution.

D. One should not ascribe a nutritional disorder where none exists.

E. There are many adolescents who have appropriate eating habits and for them prolonged counselling sessions may not be indicated.

VI. Sports and Nutritional Requirements

A. The adolescent athlete is particularly vulnerable to deficiency states because of increased caloric demands created during training periods and athletic events.

B. The markedly increased need for calories should be supplied in the form of a balanced diet rather than by fast foods which satisfy hunger but are carbohydrate-rich.

C. The increased protein need is directly proportional to demands for other nutrients. High-protein diets, more than required, are expensive, of little benefit, and may result in retention of excess body water.

D. The athlete should avoid a diet with carbohydrates as a sole energy source, since sugars are stored in the body for short periods, measured in terms of hours, and will not provide energy during prolonged training.

E. The athlete's need for a balanced diet, with enough calories, protein, fat, carbohydrates, and minerals, should not be taken lightly.

F. Inappropriate weight reduction during training is to be avoided.

G. Athletes desiring to gain weight must realize that training may produce anorexia.

H. Generally, water retention, resulting from excess salt intake as well as food residues, is to be avoided.

I. Caffeine and alcohol deplete body water and are to be avoided.

J. The athlete should lose no more than 2 lbs. after a training period, as he may become water- and salt-deficient.

1. There must be acclimatization; that is, the athlete should train in an environment which approximates that of the particular event for which he is training.

2. For these reasons, it is suggested that the athlete be weighed before and after training.

K. Anabolic steroids, used by some athletes for weight gain and increase of strength, are medically unsafe, as they may decrease bone growth and testicular function.

L. A good intake of iron is particularly important for the female adolescent athlete because of the marked need for this mineral in muscle tissue as well as the excessive demands prevalent in adolescent females.

1. Requirements range from 12 to 28 mg./day at this time.

2. Since the average daily American diet contains 9 to 18 mg. of iron (6 to 8.5 mg./1000 cal.), many adolescents may be borderline or deficient in their intake.

VII. Obesity

A. Obesity is the major nutritional disorder affecting the American adolescent.

1. Obesity does not spare any class; there is little correlation between obesity and income level in the Ten-State Survey.

2. There is a higher mortality rate for obese persons with concomitant cardiovascular, gastrointestinal, and renal diseases and diabetes mellitus.

3. Several studies have shown that the obese teenager becomes the obese, at-risk adult.

B. An obesity problem affects the psyche and self-image to a greater extent in adolescents than in other age groups.

1. During this period of increasing self-awareness, the adolescent with poor body-image may withdraw from social contact or may overcompensate (e.g., aggressive behavior), and still may not make friends easily.

2. Furthermore, the obese person is less apt to participate in athletics because of weak performance as a result of poor form or not enough strength.

3. There is thus a tendency to lead a sedentary life, which initiates a vicious cycle and perpetuates the obesity.

C. There are two principal types of obesity in adolescents.

1. Obesity present from early life is associated with both increased number and size of fat cells.

2. Obesity with its onset in early adolescence, is associated more with an increase in cell size than number.

a. This type is more frequently associated with psychological stress.

D. Obesity is generally characterized by hyperinsulinism which generally is a result of and not the cause of obesity.

1. The enlarged fat cell is less sensitive to the actions of insulin. Thus there is an increased need for insulin to maintain the steady state in carbohydrate and fat metabolism.

2. Related to this is resistance to ketosis that develops. It is thought that ketosis may have an appetite-depressing effect.

3. If the result is increased lipogenesis when "gorging" occurs, other hormonal alterations can occur which are also secondary to the obesity.

E. It is important to consider that prolonged weight reduction is catabolic and may cause cessation of growth.

F. The extra psychological burden of dieting may be compounding an already stressful period.

1. The dietary habits of the entire family should be evaluated.

2. A program of weight loss should not be attempted without the full cooperation of the subject and his family, and a critical approach should be avoided.

G. Weight control should be emphasized with gradual institution of proper dietary habits rather than rapid weight loss (see Chap. 17).

1. At first, reduced portion size should be the only restriction, because even moderate caloric reduction results in negative nitrogen balance.

2. If the patient is in an active growth phase, dieting may result in severe loss of lean body mass.

H. Obesity in itself is not an indication for psychotherapy.

1. When associated with other significant problems (e.g., school or social problems) psychotherapy may be indicated.

2. Those with a poor self-image are best suited to this approach.

VIII. Alcoholism

A. This social disease has not been considered a major nutritional disorder when it occurs in adolescents.

1. New statistics, however, indicate that 5% of teenagers have taken alcohol to relieve social stress; 10% have been intoxicated at least once.

2. In many, chronic alcoholism has resulted in severe nutritional deprivation, liver disease, and central nervous system sequelae.

B. The effect of alcohol on the growth and hormone balance can be quite profound and may result in permanent damage.

C. An intensive program is needed to treat the addicted teenager and to provide proper nutrition and psychological counselling (see Chap. 27).

IX. Anorexia Nervosa

A. This disease is characterized by a disturbed psyche resulting in gradual weight loss due to inadequate caloric intake.

B. Anorexia nervosa must be differentiated from chronic illness of other causes (e.g., neoplasm, Crohn's disease, and hypopituitarism).

C. There is secondary amenorrhea in most cases, with low gonadotropin levels but normal thyroid levels.

1. There appears to be a critical

weight loss level above which hormone function can return to normal.

D. Observations suggest a defect in hypothalmic function which may explain vegetative symptoms.

E. Proper nutrition is mandatory and the patient may even require prolonged periods of nasogastric feedings to reach the critical level in which hormonal improvement occurs.

F. Psychotherapy would appear to be more effective when the patient is not starved and malnourished.

G. Treatment—nutritional and psychotherapeutic—should be begun as soon as it is recognized that the patient has this disorder.

X. Pregnancy

A. Pregnancy during adolescence presents a unique nutritional problem by increasing the demands for proper and adequate nutrition during a period of growth in which the demands are already high.

B. The high incidence of pregnancy in adolescents in lower socio-economic groups with inadequate nutrition is another reason for the higher mortality and morbidity of adolescent pregnancy.

C. Of special note is the increased demand for iron which may result in severe anemia during pregnancy. (The subject of nutrition in pregnancy is covered in depth in Chap. 3.)

XI. Inflammatory Bowel Disease

A. In Crohn's disease and ulcerative colitis, which frequently commences in adolescence, inflammation of the large and small intestine result in increased nutritional requirements due to the excess enteric loss and the catabolic state of the patient.

1. These nutritional requirements may be difficult to meet because of the anorexia and abdominal pain common in this condition.

2. It is especially important to attempt to maintain an adequate calorie and protein intake.

B. Complications of these diseases such as fistulas and strictures require specific nutritional therapies.

1. In fistula formation, there may be excess loss of fluid, protein, fat, potassium, and other minerals requiring parenteral replacement.

2. With strictures, there may be a need for a diet consisting of elemental nutrients with low residue formation or for intravenous hyperalimentation (see Chap. 20).

C. The site of the disease may affect needs. For example, ileal involvement may result in anemia secondary to poor absorption of vitamin B_{12}, and steatorrhea secondary to poor bile acid absorption.

D. Extensive bowel disease can result in an enteric loss of protein with secondary edema and a failure to absorb iron, together with an excess loss from bleeding. This situation often requires parenteral replacement.

E. These patients frequently have delayed onset of puberty and poor growth because of poor nutrition secondary to the decreased ingestion and intestinal absorption. Maintenance of adequate protein-calorie intake can avert this untoward situation (see also Chap. 13).

6. GERIATRIC NUTRITION

Denham Harman, M.D., Ph.D.

BASIC PRINCIPLES

I. Persons aged 65 and over now comprise over 10% of the U.S. population.

A. Of the approximately 20 million persons aged 65 and over, there are about 12 million aged 65 to 74, some 6.5 million aged 75 to 84, and about 1 million aged 85 and over.

B. The ratio of women to men increases with age: from 120 to 100 at ages 65 to 69 to around 160 to 100 at ages 85 and over.

II. Approximately 4% (about 800,000 persons) of the 65+ age group are in nursing homes. Conversely, over 95% of the older population are on their own, living mostly in smaller family units.

III. Along with the increase in the size of the geriatric group, from 4% of the population in 1900 to over 10% today, there has been an increasing interest in geriatric nutrition directed at improving the health of older persons.

A. This 10% of the population uses about 30% of the total health-care dollars. More attention and better care, with especial attention to nutrition, might correct this situation.

IV. The unique role of nutrition in the maintenance of an optimal state of physical, mental, and emotional health is most apparent at the extremes of life when the consequences of aging are most obviously manifest.

A. The nutritional intake of elderly individuals should be no more dependent upon fortuitous factors than is that of infants and children.

B. Prevention of chronic disorders through good nutrition from youth to late maturity promises the greatest rewards in terms of a healthy, active old age.

NUTRITIONAL REQUIREMENTS

I. The nutritional requirements of elderly persons are essentially the same as the requirements of young and middle-aged persons to maintain good health and prevent disease.

A. General Considerations

1. People of all ages require an appropriate intake of proteins, carbohydrates, fats, minerals, vitamins, and water. The recommendations made in Chapter 2, with certain variations, apply to all age groups.

2. Although the absolute amounts of nutrient intake by healthy older persons decreases with age, it was found that the relative amount remains the same (see Table 6-1).

a. In this survey of healthy persons living in households, all the nutrient intakes were above or near the recommended allowances except for a somewhat low calcium intake at the older ages.

b. About one-third of elderly people, however, are not consuming a satisfactory diet.

(1) This group consumes less than 75% of the National Research Council recommended dietary allowance for various essential nutrients (see Table 2-1).

(2) The nutrients most frequently lacking in the diet are calcium, iron, ascorbic acid, vitamin A, and riboflavin and, among the very elderly, total calories and thiamine.

(3) The most neglected food groups are milk and milk products and the green leafy and yellow vegetables.

Table 6-1. **Mean Nutrient Intake Per Day**

	Age in Years			
	35–54	*55–64*	*65–74*	*75+*
Calories (Cal.)	2,643	2,465	2,051	1,866
Protein (g.)	107	99	82	72
Fat (g.)	133	124	100	90
Carbohydrate (g.)	244	228	204	191
Calcium (g.)	0.77	0.70	0.67	0.60
Iron (mg.)	16.9	16.2	13.4	11.3
Vitamin A (I.U.)	6,560	9,740	5,640	4,720
Thiamine (mg.)	1.4	1.4	1.2	1.1
Ascorbic Acid (mg.)	75	78	67	54

(Data from U.S. Department of Agriculture: Household Food Consumption Survey, 1965–1966. Report 11, 1972)

B. Calories

1. The caloric requirements gradually decrease with age because of reduction in the mass of metabolically active cells. This in itself would require a 5% reduction in calorie intake per decade from age 25.

2. There are large variations according to age, sex, size, occupation, environment, physical activity habits, and the presence or absence of chronic illness.

   a. There is obviously a great difference between the needs of a bedridden, immobilized person and those of a vital, active older person.

3. The average 75-year-old woman requires approximately 1900 calories, and a man of that age requires approximately 2100 calories.

   a. These figures would be less if the person was very inactive or confined to a wheelchair or to bed.

   b. These figures would be increased if the person was a spry, active, youthful 75-year-old.

C. Protein

1. Protein requirements must be met in order to maintain tissue health.

2. One gram of protein per kilogram of body weight is sufficient for the average person.

3. Increased intake is not normally advantageous and may be harmful in renal or liver disease.

4. Ten to twelve per cent of the average daily diet should be derived from high quality animal protein foods, such as meat, fish, eggs, poultry, milk, and cheese. This, together with whatever other protein foods are in the diet, should meet the requirements of all elderly persons.

D. Carbohydrates

1. Adequate intake should be maintained, otherwise tissue proteins would be broken down to maintain normal levels of blood glucose for the central nervous system and to make up calorie deficit.

2. Elderly people may have a relatively high intake of carbohydrates because they are less expensive and frequently are available in forms that require little preparation.

E. Fats

1. Fat intake should generally comprise about 25 to 30% of total calories.

2. The current consensus is that the percentage of fat derived from polyunsaturated fats should be increased while that coming from saturated (animal) fats should be decreased.

F. Minerals

1. The two mineral elements that are most frequently lacking in the diets of older people are calcium and iron.

2. The thin, brittle, osteoporotic bones and the increased incidence of fractures among older people may be related to the meager supply of calcium in their diet.

   a. Bone is actively metabolizing

throughout life and needs to replace its calcium content.

b. Though the need for calcium in elderly adults is not as great as in children, it is greater than in young adults.

c. Required intake of calcium is 0.8 to 1.0 g. daily.

d. The inclusion of two glasses of milk or milk substitutes in the daily diet would satisfy the calcium needs of geriatric patients.

3. Iron is necessary at all ages.

a. A superimposed iron deficiency anemia can be a serious handicap in an elderly person with an already impaired atherosclerotic circulation.

b. The need for iron at times may be increased in older people because of a loss of iron from the body secondary to mild bleeding from hemorrhoids or other gastrointestinal lesion (e.g., diverticular disease).

c. Sufficient iron-containing foods, such as green leafy vegetables, meat, and egg yolks, should be incorporated into the daily diet.

G. *Vitamins*

1. Vitamin requirements remain substantially the same throughout adult life.

2. Elderly persons who are unable to consume a sufficient quantity of protective foods (see Chap. 2) for any reason may require a multivitamin supplement to their diet.

3. Taking quantities in excess of recommended amounts is of no value, and excessive dosages (e.g., megavitamins) may actually be harmful.

H. *Water*

1. Although water is often not thought of as a food, it probably is the single most important compound required by the body.

2. A person can survive for many weeks without food, but death can occur within a few days if a person is totally deprived of water.

3. Enough fluids should be consumed

each day to provide for a 24-hour urine volume of about 1½ quarts.

4. Under ordinary circumstances, the sensation of thirst will insure a sufficient intake of liquids. This is not always true, however, among elderly and chronically ill persons.

5. Six to eight glasses of fluid per day will generally satisfy water requirements.

NUTRITIONAL PROBLEMS

I. Overnutrition

A. Obesity is common even among those over 65.

B. It is almost invariably due to overeating.

C. Weight reduction is desirable because of the association of obesity with many chronic diseases (see Chap. 17).

D. Life-long eating habits are very difficult to change, and developing new eating habits may be a slow process.

E. Weight reduction of institutionalized obese patients will reduce the incidence of decubitus ulcers as well as the strain on members of the nursing staff who may have to lift or move the patient.

II. Undernutrition

A. Problems of undernutrition and medically related nutrient problems increase significantly with age.

B. Frequency

1. Overt nutritional deficiencies are rare and comprise no more than about 2 to 3% of the 65+ age group.

2. Subclinical deficiencies manifested by vague feelings of weakness, lethargy, and ill-health are probably higher than overt but are difficult to document.

3. As total food intake goes down, the danger of not getting an adequate intake of vitamins and minerals increases because essential substances may be lost to a variable degree in food processing, storage, and cooking.

4. It is probably desirable in cases of suspected deficiencies to supplement the daily diet with a multivitamin plus minerals preparation.

C. Causes of Malnutrition in the Elderly

1. A combination of socio-economic, psychological, and biomedical troubles that interfere with acquiring and assimilating a balanced diet are responsible for nutritional deficiencies in older people.

2. Socio-economic factors

a. Income: This decreases sharply with age. The income of persons 55 to 64 years old is about twice that of the corresponding 65+ age group.

(1) As their income becomes progressively lower, people buy less meat and more carbohydrates, and later the caloric content may be insufficient to maintain weight.

(2) At times, a home visit may be more useful than diet inquiry in evaluating a patient's ability to purchase a balanced diet.

(3) Some older people are too proud to admit they are destitute and would rather starve than seek help. Their homes may be neat and clean, but the cupboards will be bare. A discussion of food cost, nutritive value, cooking, and use of leftovers may be helpful in improving nutrition at the same or an even lower cost.

(4) Participants in "Meals on Wheels" or in hot meal programs at their church or elsewhere may become malnourished because they may not take enough total meals and may eat little more than the sponsored meal.

(5) Economic factors are not the major cause of substandard nutrition in the elderly, rather lack of knowledge about nutrition or other social and medical problems.

3. Medical problems

a. Ability to get out to purchase food or to cook and prepare meals may be impaired due to arthritis, poor vision, encroaching senility, and other physical problems.

b. Chronic illness may cause difficulty in ingesting, digesting, absorbing, or utilizing nutrients.

4. Social problems

a. Eating is a social event. People generally do not like to eat alone. Cooking and eating alone becomes monotonous. This may result in reduced appetite and decreased motivation for cooking and for planning well-balanced diets.

b. Toast, jelly, and coffee or some other inadequate meal may become the daily fare for people who have to cook for themselves and who are confined indoors.

(1) This type of diet is a prime cause of iron deficiency anemia in the elderly.

5. Effects of age

a. Food intake in older persons can be decreased across the board, or selectively, so as to produce clinically evident deficiencies through a combination of age-associated changes.

(1) Depression, common in older persons, has an adverse effect on appetite.

(2) Poor vision can interfere with eating.

(3) The sense of taste and smell declines with age. This is frequently compounded, particularly in institutional settings, by unappetizingly prepared foods served in unpleasant surroundings.

(4) Edentulous patients or those with poorly fitted plates may limit themselves to easily chewed food. In addition to permitting a person to eat a normal variety of foods, good dentures can have a beneficial psychological effect by making the patient appear younger.

b. Fat clearance from the blood becomes slower with age. This may interfere with sleep in some cases and may indirectly depress food intake. Such persons should be encouraged to eat their main meal at noon.

c. Activity decreases with age. Moderate exercise will not only stimulate appetite and food intake but will also give an increased sense of well-being.

NUTRITION-RELATED PROBLEMS
IN THE AGED

I. Constipation

A. This is a common complaint in older patients.

B. It generally can be treated satisfactorily by increasing intake of fruits, vegetables, prunes, bran, and fluids.

C. A high-fiber diet, when there are no medical contraindications, can prevent the development of constipation (see Table 13-1).

II. Dehydration

A. This is seen usually only in institutionalized patients.

B. Lethargy and a semi-comatose state can be produced by inadequate fluid intake.

C. Treatment is to force fluid intake. Occasionally it may be necessary to give fluid by tube or I.V.

III. Low Serum Potassium Levels

A. This is frequently observed in older persons who are taking diuretics.

B. It can cause weakness and cardiac arrhythmias.

C. Increasing intake of bananas, oranges, and other high-potassium foods may prevent its development.

D. Some persons may require supplemental potassium. This can be given as 20 mEq. of KCl in orange juice once or twice a day.

IV. Tube Feedings

A. This may be necessary at times to maintain an adequate intake of fluid and nutrients in hospital or nursing home patients.

B. A number of commercial liquid products are available (see Table 12-1, 12-3, and 12-5).

C. Tube feedings can also be conveniently prepared with the aid of a blender to liquefy a diet of bread, milk, fruit juice, vegetables, and meat.

D. Patients tolerate tube feedings well, aside from occasional diarrhea; diarrhea can be prevented by small frequent feedings and proper refrigeration.

V. Decubitus Ulcers

A. Unfortunately, this is a common problem in institutionalized older patients.

B. Poor nutritional state, especially protein-calorie malnutrition, is a common etiological factor.

C. Healing may be enhanced by increasing the daily protein intake to around 100 g.

D. Insuring an adequate vitamin intake will also promote wound healing.

SUGGESTED READINGS

Agate, J.: Digestion and assimilation of food. *In* The Practice of Geriatrics. ed. 2. Springfield, Charles C Thomas, 1970.

———: Food and nutrition. *In* The Practice of Geriatrics. ed. 2. Springfield, Charles C Thomas, 1970.

Alexander, M. M., and Stare, F. J.: Nutritional management of geriatric patients. *In* Rudd, J. L., and Margolin, R. J. (eds.): Maintenance Therapy for the Geriatric Patient. Springfield, Charles C Thomas, 1968.

Bonner, C. D.: Homburger and Bonner's Medical Care and Rehabilitation of the Aged and Chronically Ill. ed. 3. Boston, Little, Brown & Company, 1974.

Brocklehurst, J. C.: Textbook of Geriatric Medicine and Gerontology. London, Churchill Livingston, 1973.

Judge, T. G.: Nutrition in the elderly. *In* Anderson, W. F., and Judge, T. G. (eds.): Geriatric Medicine, Academic Press, 1974.

Schroeder, H. A.: Nutrition. *In* Cowdry, E. V., and Steinberg, F. W. (eds.): The Care of the Geriatric Patient. ed. 2. St. Louis, C. V. Mosby, 1971.

Watkin, D. M.: A year of development in nutrition and aging. Med. Clin. North Am., *54:*1589, 1970.

7. PRINCIPLES OF THERAPEUTIC NUTRITION

Seymour L. Halpern, M.D.

BASIC PRINCIPLES

I. Therapeutic nutrition refers to the use of diet as a therapeutic tool in the management of patients.

A. The science of medicine from its founding has been inseparable from that of nutrition. Hippocrates noted, "The art of medicine would not have been invented at first, nor would it have been made a subject of investigation . . . if when men are indisposed, the same food and other articles of regimen which they eat and drink when in good health were proper for them, and if no others were preferable to these."

B. The major effort of all therapeutic nutritional programs is to insure total adequacy of the diet.

1. Good nutrition, when present, must be maintained.

2. The development of deficiencies must be prevented.

3. Abnormal nutritional states should be corrected as rapidly as possible.

C. In constructing a diet for a patient, it is necessary to take into account the following three factors:

1. The normal daily needs of the patient

2. Previous nutritional depletions

3. Increased requirements resulting from current losses as by vomiting and diarrhea

II. The composition of a patient's diet should not be based solely upon the recommended daily dietary allowances for healthy people because this does not take into account the additional demands for specific nutrients engendered by illness, injury, or surgery.

A. The caloric content of a diet, for example, is determined by calculating:

1. The total number of calories normally required by the patient.

2. The amount of calories lost from the system by vomiting and diarrhea or from the skin in burns

3. Extra needs produced by fever and other metabolic causes

4. The amount needed to compensate for previous weight loss

5. The patient's caloric status as determined by height and weight (e.g., obesity or underweight) also should be ascertained in assessing caloric needs.

a. The presence of edema should be taken into account when evaluating weight-to-height status.

B. Similar appraisals are necessary for determining the protein-, mineral-, and vitamin content of a therapeutic diet. The methodology for these assessments will be found in the succeeding chapters.

III. The attention of the physician in a therapeutic program must never be so narrowly focused on drug, surgical, or other specific therapy that the nutritional status of the patient is overlooked.

A. Modern advances in surgical technique and the development of effective medications has brought these modalities of therapy to the foreground.

B. Nutrition, however, should be concurrently utilized in all therapeutic programs to assure the maximum success from drugs and surgery.

1. Closer attention to diet treatment would help assure the ultimate success of surgical procedures, would shorten the period of convalescence, and would improve the quality of wound healing.

2. Proper diet therapy, prescribed at the time medications are ordered, would contribute to successful drug treatment.

C. Close attention to nutrition therapy might obviate the necessity for some surgical procedures (e.g., in peptic ulcer or ulcerative colitis patients).

    1. In certain instances it can preclude the need for medications.

IV. It is virtually impossible to deliver optimal medical care if therapeutic nutrition is not an integral part of the total health care program because nutrition is the most important environmental factor that continuously influences the total state of health.

FACTORS AFFECTING NUTRITION REQUIREMENTS

The diet prescription is affected by any physiologic or pathologic state that accelerates or inhibits nutrient excretion or degradation, as well as by any situation that interferes with digestion, absorption, or utilization of nutrients or that in any other manner affects nutritional requirements.

I. Two types of malnutrition are encountered by the physician.

A. Primary Malnutrition. This refers to an inadequate intake of nutrients to meet the body's demands. This category includes:

    1. Poor selection of foods, which frequently leads to single or multiple deficiencies of vitamins, minerals, protein, or total calories. The inadequate intake may be due to:

        a. Defective knowledge of nutrition

        b. Economic factors

        c. Food shortage

        d. Fad diets

    2. Inability to eat because of anorexia, poor dentition, anxiety, and injuries, such as fractured jaws

    3. Obesity secondary to excess intake of calories is a form of primary malnutrition frequently encountered in highly developed countries (see Chap. 17).

    4. Fad diets, especially those that emphasize a specific category of foods, frequently lead to malnutrition.

B. Conditioned or Secondary Malnutrition. This occurs when the ingested diet would normally be adequate for the person. Included in this category are:

    1. Physiologically increased requirements, as in pregnancy, lactation, or sustained heavy work

    2. Pathologically increased requirements, as in hyperthyroidism or high fever

    3. Decreased absorption, excessive losses, or decreased utilization of nutrients

        a. Burns, uncontrollable diabetes, vomiting, diarrhea, liver disease, ascites, and drug therapy are among the clinical situations that can lead to defective absorption, abberant utilization, or excessive loss of essential nutrients.

II. The extent of the nutritional deficiency will determine not only the makeup of the diet, but the mode of administration. Influencing this are:

A. The total duration of each specific nutrient deficiency

B. The presence of biochemical aberrations and tissue pathology that may have developed

III. In many illnesses, the stage of a disease has a strong influence on dietary requirements.

A. Kidney Disease

    1. In acute or chronic kidney disease in which there are high blood urea nitrogen-, creatinine-, and potassium levels, it will be necessary to reduce the levels of protein and potassium in the diet.

        a. Potassium-containing medications and salt subistutes should not be used.

        b. In addition, drugs associated with potassium retention must be avoided, while drugs that promote potassium excretion can be utilized.

    2. On the otherhand, in kidney diseases associated with marked proteinuria, normal blood urea nitrogens, and low- or normal potassium blood levels, a diet which takes these into account should be prescribed.

    3. When there are significant sodium losses owing to the kidney's inability to

conserve sodium (sodium-losing nephritis), the use of a sodium-restricted diet or of diuretics that promote sodium loss can produce a fatal low-sodium syndrome. Sodium intake will have to be adjusted in accordance with the clinical state (e.g., sodium retention as compared with sodium loss).

B. Liver Disease

1. With most disorders of the liver, a high-protein diet is advantageous.

2. On the otherhand, with severe liver failure a high-protein diet can precipitate hepatic coma.

C. The above demonstrate why the physician must carefully ascertain the nutritional status of his patient and the nature and stage of the pathological disorder when deciding upon diet and drug therapy. Diet and drug therapy must always be correlated.

ANOREXIA

I. A major obstacle to successful nutrition therapy of sick persons is the presence of anorexia.

A. Vigorous endeavors must be made to induce the patient to eat.

1. Anorexia with decreased intake frequently is an etiological agent in producing malnutrition.

2. Contrariwise, loss of appetite frequently is induced by a poor nutritional state.

3. It is often sufficient to explain to the patient that his failure to eat can induce a vicious cycle from which the only escape is the ingestion of more and better food.

4. Appetite training can be a tedious process.

5. As nutrition improves, the appetite will usually improve.

B. The cause of anorexia is not always known.

1. In many cases it appears to be due to a loss of the sense of taste. Zinc deficiency has been implicated in this process.

2. Taste and olfactory sensations frequently are improved by supplying a totally nutritious diet.

C. Cultural and personal food habits, likes and dislikes, and individual idiosyncrasies must be taken into account. Menus should be appetizing and presented in an appetizing fashion.

II. Anorexia is commonly associated with the therapeutic regimen.

A. Medications being administered should be checked to make sure they are not causing anorexia.

B. Extensive exposure to radiation therapy often causes anorexia.

C. Depression and other abnormal emotional states resulting from therapy may induce anorexia.

D. Physical abnormalities, such as radiation esophagitis, produced by therapeutic maneuvers, may increase anorexia.

E. In all of the above cases, the anorexia will be exacerbated if nutritional depletion is allowed to continue.

III. It is rarely necessary to resort to insulin, anabolic drugs, or corticosteroids in an attempt to stimulate the appetite.

A. These have been used with irregular results and have the potential for adverse side effects.

B. Attention to individualization of diet and all factors involved in the anorexia will often be successful in inducing the patient to consume the prescribed diet.

IV. The severely anorexic patient may be content to ingest liquid feedings.

A. Nutritious liquid mixtures can be prepared or commercial preparations utilized that will supply all requirements for calories, proteins, vitamins, and minerals. These types of preparations are described in Tables 12-1, 12-3, 12-5, and 12-7.

B. Occasionally tube feeding may become an unavoidable temporary expedient in severely deteriorated anorexic patients. The liquid preparations described in the preceding paragraph usually can be utilized for this purpose.

C. Because the adverse psychological effects of tube feeding may produce anorexia, oral feeding should always be resumed as soon as possible.

NUTRITION-MEDICATION INTERACTIONS

The relationship of nutrition and medication must be of special concern to all physicians.

I. The composition of a patient's diet may strongly influence the action of many commonly used drugs.

A. It can enhance a drug's action.

B. The effect of a drug may be inhibited because of the patient's nutritional status or the composition of the diet being ingested.

C. The dose requirements or even the necessity for medication may be affected.

D. Diet may determine the development of untoward side effects. For example, sodium depletion enhances lithium toxicity. Thus a severe sodium-restricted diet should be prescribed with caution to a patient receiving lithium carbonate therapy for emotional disturbances. If a sodium-restricted diet is a medical necessity, lithium should be discontinued.

E. Many of the undesirable effects of medication can be prevented by dietary manipulation. Prescribing a diet containing high-potassium foods can prevent the hypokalemia frequently seen with diuretics such as furosemide, ethacrynic acid, and the thiazide drugs.

II. Medications frequently influence a patient's nutritional state.

A. Nutritional disorders may be caused by drugs.

B. The situation may become complicated because a patient's therapy frequently involves more than one drug.

C. It may be difficult at times for the physician to determine whether he is dealing with the disease itself, a drug side effect, or a nutritional deficiency induced by treatment.

D. Some nutritional complications of drug use may come only after long-term use of a medication. Disorders such as osteoporosis produced by corticosteroids may be difficult to detect in its early stages.

E. Metabolic disorders may be influenced by drugs necessitating a change in therapy. Diuretics, especially the thiazides, furosemide, and ethacrynic acid, can cause glucose intolerance aggravating hyperglycemia in overt or prediabetic patients. In overt diabetics, increased dietary restrictions and a change in insulin dosage may be required. Similarly, the diuretics can raise serum uric acid levels and precipitate an attack of gout requiring a change in therapy.

III. Nutritional depletion is a frequent accompaniment of drug therapy.

A. It may produce anorexia, which decreases the intake of many essential nutrients.

B. Many medications induce nausea and vomiting, which cause increased loss of nutrients.

C. They may affect metabolic processes causing an increased need for certain nutrients.

1. For example, anovulatory drugs (oral contraceptives) have been shown to increase the need for certain vitamins, especially folic acid, pyridoxine and to a lesser extent vitamin C.

2. Isoniazid (INH) used in the treatment of tuberculosis can produce pyridoxine deficiency with neuropathy to the extent that most experts now recommend that vitamin B_6 (pyridoxine) supplements should be administered routinely to all patients receiving INH therapy.

3. Contrariwise, pyridoxine can decrease the effects of levodopa that is prescribed for the treatment of Parkinson's disease. When multivitamins are required for patients receiving levodopa, a supplement that does not contain B_6 is preferred.

4. The bile acid sequestrants used in the treatment of hyperlipoproteinemias, cholestyramine, and colestipol can interfere with the absorption of the fat-soluble vitamins A, D, and K. Supplements of these

vitamins in a water-miscible form will be required when the bile acid sequestrants are used over a long period of time. At times, parenteral vitamin K may be necessary.

5. Anticonvulsant-, antimalarial-, and antibiotic drugs also increase the need for vitamins and can induce specific vitamin deficiencies if the increased needs are not met.

6. Many other drugs have the capability of effecting the metabolism, especially in malnourished persons. Before prescribing any drug the physician should familiarize himself with the information on precautions, warnings, adverse reactions, and contradictions contained in the package literature supplied by the manufacturer. Many of these are related to the patient's diet and nutritional state.

D. Some drugs given to pregnant women may alter metabolic processes and nutritional requirement and may lead to fetal malnutrition and birth malformations.

E. Drugs may affect intestinal absorption, storage, utilization, and excretion of many foodstuffs.

IV. Drugs should never be used as a substitute for careful and intelligent diet planning.

A. Diuretics should not be used in place of a low-sodium diet to control congestive heart failure and hypertension.

1. Low-sodium diets may obviate the need for diuretics in some patients.

2. In the case of antihypertensive drugs, the concurrent use of a low-sodium diet can reduce dosage requirements and thus lessen the possibility of side effects. It may also enhance the drug's actions.

3. Using diuretics to eliminate sodium from the body may not produce identical beneficial effects as a low-sodium diet.

B. Carefully controlled clinical research has indicated that patients who have adult-onset diabetes have fewer vascular complications when treated with diet alone than those who are treated with oral hypoglycemic drugs and a more liberal diet.

V. Flavor Substitutes

A. It is necessary to be cautious when using flavoring products.

1. Many salt substitutes contain principally potassium chloride (see Table 9–1). In a patient with chronic renal disease with potassium retention or when a potassium-sparing diuretic is being used, it is possible that use of this type of salt substitute may help induce a dangerous hyperkalemia.

2. Contrariwise, one cannot depend upon the amount of potassium in a salt substitute to correct low-potassium blood levels induced by the injudicious use of diuretic preparations.

B. The safety of many sugar substitutes has been questioned.

1. Although large amounts of sugar in the diet are undesirable for reasons outlined in Chapter 17 and Chapter 22, it is equally undesirable to use large amounts of sugar substitutes.

2. Fruit juices and other nutritious foodstuffs can be used to help sweeten foods rather than sugar calories, which are devoid of any nutritional benefit, or sugar substitutes with their potential hazards to health.

C. It is preferable to gradually alter the diet so that the amount of sugar and salt in the diet is decreased. Appetite retraining can be accomplished with judicious diet prescriptions.

VI. Antacid Medication

A. The milk-alkali syndrome is frequently seen among peptic ulcer patients but is less common since the introduction of non-absorbable alkalizing agents.

1. The excessive administration of calcium, principally in the form of milk, and of absorbable alkalis is responsible for the onset of the milk-alkali syndrome.

a. It is characterized by hypercalcemia, hypercalciuria with possible metastatic calcification, nephrocalcinosis, and renal calculi. These can produce renal insufficiency and azotemia.

2. By altering the diet, so as to lower the milk and total calcium intake,

and substituting non-absorbable alkalis, the hypercalcemia and azotemia are corrected.

B. The non-absorbable antacids can bind various minerals and cause nutrient depletion of these elements.

1. For example, hypophosphatemia secondary to phosphate binding with failure to absorb this element can lead to bone demineralization.

IATROGENIC MALNUTRITION

An inappropriate diet regimen can lead to nutritional insufficiency and metabolic disturbances. This situation has been referred to as iatrogenic malnutrition.

I. Iatrogenic malnutrition is as common a cause of malnutrition in hospitalized patients as are the diseases for which the patients are hospitalized.

A. Many of the symptoms produced by malnutrition are mistakingly attributed to the primary illness.

B. The symptoms of malnutrition frequently go unrecognized because many physicians, as well as other members of the health care team, are not well informed about the rapidity with which nutritional disturbances can occur.

1. This is especially true of surgical patients (see Chap. 11).

C. New dietary restrictions may be imposed upon the patient because the developing symptoms of malnutrition go unrecognized, compounding both medical and nutritional problems.

II. Iatrogenic malnutrition can develop, especially among hospitalized patients, when diets which would be appropriate for the person if he was in an ideal state of health are prescribed, but increased calorie needs are not satisfied, increased requirements for protein are not met, and augmented demands for vitamins and minerals have not been fulfilled.

A. While one aspect of increased needs may be noted, such as losses from vomiting and diarrhea, other causes of changed nutritional requirements, which result from an altered metabolism or from drug therapy and which are less obvious, may not be recognized and taken into account.

III. Iatrogenic malnutrition is a principle cause of tissue depletion of essential amino acids, vitamins, minerals, and calories.

A. This results in a needless delay in convalescence and healing.

MINERAL MALNUTRITION

I. The role of trace metals and minerals in therapeutic nutrition has become increasingly evident (see Chap. 19).

A. Magnesium, zinc, and other minerals apparently have an important role in tissue healing.

B. Maximum nutritional support is not possible unless mineral nutrition is taken into account.

C. The failure of parenteral alimentation and hyperalimentation in treating several disease processes has been attributed to the lack of a mineral, even though all other aspects of nutritional support were carefully observed (see Chap. 20).

II. Increased mineral malnutrition can be expected to occur as a result of iatrogenically-induced depletion, especially secondary to drug therapy.

A. Many diuretics, for example, cause excessive losses of minerals, principally calcium, magnesium, and zinc, as well as of the electrolytes, sodium, chlorides, and potassium.

B. A substance which is being used more frequently in the treatment of rheumatoid arthritis, D-penicillamine, has caused zincurea and zinc depletion with its associated loss of taste and anorexia.

III. The use of minerals in treating specific organ pathology is now being elucidated.

A. For example, the administration of magnesium following an acute myocardial infarction may prevent extensive tissue necrosis and various potentially fatal complications.

B. Zinc has been found to be an important factor in the treatment of many liver disorders.

C. The function of minerals in health and disease, the diagnosis and treatment of excesses and deficiencies, and their evolving role in therapeutics is reviewed in Chapter 19.

OUTLINING THE DIET TO THE PATIENT

I. It is essential to instruct both the patient and his family what foods can be eaten.

A. This is exceedingly important for office patients, as well as for patients who are being discharged from the hospital where their menus invariably were prepared for them.

B. It is not sufficient to enumerate to the patient only the foods that must be avoided.

1. Unwarranted fears of certain foods and food groups which actually are not contraindicated may produce both nutritional imbalance and dietary invalidism.

2. It is necessary to spend sufficient time and to answer all questions posed by the patients and their families so they understand how to assure that a diet that is optimal for the disease is also nutritionally balanced.

C. The need for individualization is as important with diet therapy as with potent pharmaceuticals.

D. The most frequent cause of resorting to quacks, food faddists, health food stores, and faddist books is the patient's lack of understanding of the details of his diet.

E. If the physician does not have the time to explain the diet to his patient, he should designate a member of his staff (e.g., dietician, physician's associate, or medical assistant) who has had training in therapeutic nutrition to review the diet prescription with the patient.

F. The patient should be encouraged to avoid worry, rushing, fatigue, and emotional upsets when eating. Controversial and unpleasant subjects should not be discussed during meals.

II. A diet regimen can be imposed with too much zeal.

A. This has led at times to serious psychogenic disturbances, as well as disruptions of family patterns and of life-style.

B. This situation can lead to dietary invalidism.

1. Dietary regimens should be made as simple as possible.

2. An undue fear regarding the consequence of dietary deviations should be avoided.

C. Rigid dietary restrictions probably are imposed on patients far more often than is actually necessary.

III. Simplified nomenclature should be used.

A. Titles of diets should be specific and should indicate the nature of the nutritional therapy being prescribed.

1. For example, "bland diet" can be used when prescribing for digestive disorders that respond to diets that are chemically- and mechanically nonirritating.

2. Naming diets after a pathological condition or after a particular person increases the total number of diets available to physicians and can be confusing.

a. Furthermore, the basic principles and characteristics of a diet become obscured when pathologic or personal names are attached to a diet.

b. The number of diets in some hospital diet manuals has been decreased by as much as 60 to 70% by eliminating specifically named diets, such as ulcer diet, gall bladder diet, diarrhea diet, Sippy diet, and modified Sippy diet.

c. Designating a diet by the person's medical disorder (e.g., ulcer diet) can be psychologically traumatic to the patient whose medical problems receive emphasis whenever food is thought of.

FAD DIETS

Food faddism has become a major problem encountered by physicians.

I. Vegetarianism.

This is probably the most common fad diet.

A. A vegetarian diet, especially a lacto-ovo-vegetarian diet in which dairy products and plant foods but no meat, poultry, or fish are used, can be a completely nutritious diet.

B. The extreme vegetarian diet that contains no foods from animals frequently leads to an inadequate intake of high quality protein and essential minerals and vitamins.

C. Macrobiotic diets that rely on tea, brown rice, beans, and nuts can produce severe protein-calorie malnutrition and can result in death.

1. Infants raised on this type of diet may develop mental retardation.

D. Vitamin B_{12} is frequently lacking in vegetarian diets because the principle sources of this vitamin are foods of animal origin.

E. There are no special attributes, even of a well-balanced vegetarian diet, that render it superior to a normal diet that includes animal protein foods.

II. Fad Diets Used in the Treatment of Obesity

A. Fad diets invariably are promulgated for the treatment of obesity.

1. The type of diet varies from year to year, if not from month to month.

2. They promise rapid weight loss, frequently without caloric restriction—an impossible feat.

B. Severe restriction of carbohydrates has been the most common form of eccentric diet. It has been presented under many different guises over the last hundred years, often with a physician's name attributed to it.

1. These diets are hazardous in that they produce ketonemia.

2. If there is no restriction of total fat, hypercholesterolemia, hyperlipedemia, and/or hypertriglyceridemia may ensue.

a. This can result in aggrava-tion or precipitation of coronary artery disease.

3. They frequently are deficient in total nutrition content.

4. The initial large weight loss is mostly fluid because the absence of carbohydrate leads to naturesis and diuresis. Small amounts of carbohydrate curtail the sodium wasting. When a normal diet is resumed, the sodium and water diuresis is reversed.

a. This explanation also applies to the initial large weight loss in total fasting or with the protein-sparing modified fast.

C. Some fad diets may result in a decrease of weight as a result of loss of lean body mass, not just fat.

D. The protein-sparing modified fast is a diet that contains approximately 300 cal. and is composed of purified amino acids.

1. This diet is nutritionally deficient and has resulted in sudden and unexpected cardiac deaths from cardiac arrhythmias.

2. This diet should only be used on in-hospital patients who are under careful medical supervision.

E. None of these fad diets for obesity are satisfactory because lost weight is rapidly regained owing to a failure to develop new correct dietary habits.

F. For further discussion of diet treatment of obesity see Chapter 17.

III. Organic or Natural Foods

A. These foods have become very popular in the U.S. and some countries in western Europe.

B. There is no evidence that foods grown with organic fertilizer have more nutritious value than foods grown with an inorganic fertilizer.

1. These foods are more expensive.

2. Organically grown foods are much more perishable and thus have a shorter shelf life.

3. There are many abuses. Because of limited availability, foods sold as organic

foods frequently are mixtures of ordinary foodstuffs and organically grown foodstuffs.

C. Some natural and organic food products are very high in calories and relatively high in fat content. Natural and organic foods are not dietetic foods.

D. Natural foods should be distinguished from organic foods.

1. Natural applies to any food in its natural, unprocessed state. Their use should be encouraged because salt-, sugar- and fat intake will then be decreased.

2. Organic foods apply to foods grown only with organic fertilizer. No artificial fertilizers are used.

IV. Dietetic Foods

A. The label "dietetic food" can be very misleading.

1. Many so-called diet foods may be sugar-free, but are high in total fat and calories.

B. Many different foodstuffs have been called dietetic.

1. The term, therefore, has little practical significance.

2. Patients should learn to read in detail and evaluate nutrition labeling.

CONTROVERSIES IN NUTRITION

I. Hyperlipidemia and Atherosclerosis

Although there is some difference of opinion, most medical experts agree that there is an association between diet, plasma-lipoprotein concentrations, plasma-cholesterol concentrations, and the development of coronary heart disease.

A. For this reason, most nutrition and cardiac specialists have recommended that if the risk of coronary heart disease is to be reduced, a person should ingest less total fat, especially saturated fat, and consume more polyunsaturated fat.

1. High-cholesterol foods also should be reduced in the diet.

B. The controversy revolves around the question of when saturated fat and cholesterol should be reduced or omitted from the diet.

1. There are some physicians who feel that cholesterol and fat restriction should commence in infancy.

2. Because lipids are necessary for the development of many tissues, restriction of cholesterol and fat in the diet should probably not begin before the age of 2. Others feel that limitation should not begin until adolescent growth has ceased.

3. Probably no purpose is served by severely restricting the diet of an elderly person. They should be encouraged to have as much variety as possible in their diet.

C. There is universal agreement that the average adult consumes too much fat and too many calories. Reduction of total fat intake, along with reduction of sugar, will help correct the excess amount of obesity found today.

D. Further details will be found in Chapter 9 and Chapter 10.

II. Salt

A. Most persons consume too much salt.

1. All physicians and nutritionists agree on this.

2. The average salt consumption in the U.S. is 4.8 lbs. to 14.5 lbs./person/year.

B. There is a correlation between salt intake and hypertension.

C. A sharply decreased salt intake is desirable for most persons.

1. This is especially true for patients who have an inherited susceptibility to high blood pressure.

D. Some controversy exists concerning the necessity for all persons to reduce salt consumption.

1. It is the consensus of nutrition specialists and other physicians that:

a. The average American would benefit by limiting his salt intake to 3 to 5 g./day.

b. Salt, as well as sugar, should be eliminated from baby and infant foods.

III. Megavitamins

A. The use of megadoses of vitamins has received much publicity.

B. At the present time there is no evidence that massive doses of vitamins have any role in preventive or therapeutic medicine.

1. On the contrary, massive doses of vitamins may be deleterious to the health.

2. Toxicity from large doses has been proven for vitamins A and D.

3. There is new evidence that megadoses of even the water-soluble vitamins may be harmful. For example, excessive doses of vitamin C can accelerate uric acid excretion, can produce uric acid stones, and may also cause destruction of vitamin B_{12}.

4. Large doses of vitamin E have been associated with the development of hypertension. It also has an adverse effect on anticoagulants.

C. The rational use of vitamins in medical practice is discussed in Chapter 8.

IV. The Role of Nutrition in Clinical Practice

A. Although some controversy may have existed until recently, there is no longer any dispute concerning this subject.

B. The correct application of the principles of therapeutic nutrition, as enunciated in this and the following chapters, will facilitate the treatment of virtually all medical and surgical disorders.

PLANNING FOR ALTERING EATING HABITS
Corinne Mamo Montandon, M.P.H., R.D.

I. Food is eaten for a variety of reasons.

A. Seldom, however, is food chosen for nutrient value alone.

B. Eating habits are habitual and complex.

C. They evolve from various aspects: familial, cultural, social, educational, economical, and environmental.

D. They originate from the first encounter with foods and all subsequent food and eating experiences.

II. Any dietary alterations designed for long-term patient cooperation must consider how the patient perceives and uses foods during health and illness.

III. Therapeutic diet lists do allow the physician an opportunity to view a broad perspective of foods allowed or excluded from the diet.

A. For long-term cooperation, all efforts should be made to individualize the diet plan.

IV. The physician can be assisted by a registered dietitian (R.D.) who is a member of the American Dietetic Association (A.D.A.).

A. During the nutritional counselling session, the dietitian can evaluate food habits, life-style, and value systems as applied to food during health and illness and then design a diet to meet the patient's needs.

B. Further, the dietitian can provide information on the purchase and use of specialty dietary products.

C. Dietary analysis, a component of nutritional assessment, provides an insight into individual food habits.

D. Reasons for evaluating a person's food intake include:

1. To determine the adequacy of a person's food intake

2. To establish a baseline of food habits before recommending modifications

3. To provide an opportunity to evaluate in what area of the person's eating pattern the diet needs improving

4. To approximate the intake of specific nutrients such as calcium, iron, and calories

5. To provide a base to assist in identifying food attitudes, beliefs, and values during health and illness

6. To motivate a person to accept dietary alterations

Name ―――――――――

Date ―――――――――

24-HOUR FOOD DIARY

Please list everything you eat or drink during the next 24 hours. Record the amount of each food or beverage item after it has been consumed. Record each 24-hour period on a separate page, beginning with when you awaken to begin your day until the next day at the same time.

Awake at: ―――――――   To Bed at: ―――――――

Time food or beverage was consumed, where, with whom, emotional atmosphere	Type of food or beverage consumed, amount consumed, and method of preparation		When appropriate, list any specific related items (i.e. physical activity, symptoms)
	Type of food or beverage	Amount consumed	Method of preparation (include all ingredients)	

Fig. 7-1. Twenty-four-hour food diary for evaluating food intake, dietary compliance, and information useful in the clinical care of the patient.

7. To determine the knowledge of food, nutrient values, food safety, and storage

8. To identify availability of resources for purchasing foods

9. In infancy, to identify the baby's stage in development relative to feeding

V. Various techniques have been developed to obtain meaningful information on food intake.

A. The use of one or more of the techniques listed below can be valuable in determining food intake and dietary compliance.

1. Food Diary

a. All foods and beverages consumed in a specified period are recorded, separating each 24-hour period.

b. Amounts consumed are important for quantifying results.

c. Further specific information relating to method of food preparation, such as ingredients in a meat loaf, thickening agent for sauces and gravies, and type of sweetener used on cereal, are essential for defining constituents of the diet (see Fig. 7-1).

d. Included in the diary should be information on symptoms that would be appropriate for the clinical care of the patient.

2. Food Recall

a. The patient is asked to recall foods and beverages consumed during the previous 24-hour period.

b. An attempt is made to quantify amounts consumed and method of preparation.

3. Diet History

a. Patterns of food intake, relationship to various foods and beverages, and food likes and dislikes are elicited from the person.

b. No attempt is made to quantify the intake of foods or beverages.

c. The diet history technique can be relevant when probing for particular reactions to foods or when determining the reliability of other techniques.

4. Frequency of Food Intake

a. The patient is requested to indicate, from a predetermined list, how often a specific food item is consumed (daily, weekly, monthly, yearly, or never).

b. Usually foods of therapeutic interest are included in the list.

B. The above techniques can assist in better understanding of the patient. When the diet is designed to meet the patient's existing eating pattern, he will be likely to adhere to the therapeutic plan.

8. RATIONAL USE OF VITAMINS IN PRACTICE

Richard M. Freeman, M.D.

When considering vitamins from a medical standpoint, one should make clear the distinction between the treatment or prevention of specific deficiency diseases and the uses of vitamins as pharmacologic agents. While the value of vitamins in the vitamin deficiency states has been well documented, use of vitamins as therapeutic agents in pharmacologic doses is often more controversial.

I. Potential Causes for Multivitamin Deficiencies

A. The most obvious cause is that of inadequate intake of vitamin-containing foods.

1. Poor appetite is a common cause.

a. Anorexia may occur in elderly persons, especially those who are mentally depressed.

2. The development of vitamin deficiencies in patients with acute and chronic alcoholism is widely known. Vitamin replacement in such patients, at least while they are hospitalized, is thus a widespread practice.

3. Perhaps more difficult to discern is the vitamin deficiency which develops as a consequence of eccentric diets.

a. Many physicians do not routinely question patients regarding the quality of their diets.

b. Such information is likely to come from nurses, other paramedical personnel, members of a patient's family, or friends.

4. Unusual diets may be present in patients with mild, as well as severe, psychiatric disturbances.

5. Religious beliefs are rarely a cause of vitamin deficiency itself. More frequently they may complicate the otherwise standard treatment of some disease entity.

6. The number of food fads which have proliferated in the United States in the past 10 to 15 years is substantial. Many of these diets are nutritionally unsound but few people stick to them for prolonged periods of time.

7. Obese persons will often try a variety of diets in an attempt to control their weight.

a. The number of popular books written on this subject is astounding.

b. Some of these diets contain inadequate vitamins on a daily basis and are potentially dangerous if utilized for prolonged periods of time.

8. Several diets prescribed by physicians may, under certain circumstances, have inadequate nutrients.

a. For example, the 10 g. protein diet, occasionally advised for patients with uremia, may have inadequate amounts of iron for hematopoietic purposes, as well as inadequate vitamins.

II. Recommended Daily Dietary Allowances of Vitamins

A. A healthy person's diet should provide the recommended daily allowances of vitamins listed below:

Fat-Soluble Vitamins	
Vitamin A	5000 I.U.
Vitamin D	400 I.U.
Vitamin E	12–15 I.U.
Water-Soluble Vitamins	
Ascorbic acid	45 mg.
Folic acid (Folacin)	400 μg.
Niacin	12–20 mg.
Riboflavin	1.1–1.8 mg.

Thiamine	1.0–1.5 mg.
Vitamin B$_6$	1.6–2.0 mg.
Vitamin B$_{12}$	3.0 µg.

Recommended Daily Dietary Allowances. ed. 8. Food and Nutrition Board, National Research Council, National Academy of Sciences, 1974.

III. Increased Tissue Requirements in Health

A. While growth increases the tissue requirements of vitamins in healthy persons, in general this is more a question of reaching adult requirements than clearly exceeding them.

    1. The increased needs for calcium and phosphorus are more definitive in the growing stage.

B. Pregnancy is also known to increase the requirements for calcium and phosphorus more than for vitamins, although the recommended daily allowances for vitamin A, ascorbic acid, folic acid, and the other water-soluble vitamins increase slightly.

C. Lactating women also have slightly increased vitamin needs.

D. Menstruating women require more iron than non-menstruating women, but their vitamin needs are not substantially changed.

IV. Therapeutic Indications for Vitamins

A. There are many circumstances in which specific vitamins may be indicated. Some of them are listed below.

Potential Indications for Certain Vitamins

Fat-Soluble Vitamins

Vitamin A
  Night blindness
Vitamin D
  Rickets
  Hypoparathyroidism
  Renal osteodystrophy
  Vitamin D-resistant rickets
  Malabsorption syndrome
Vitamin E
  Acanthocytosis
  Protein-calorie malnutrition
  Premature infants
  Malabsorption syndromes

Fat-Soluble Vitamins (Continued)

Vitamin K
  Hypoprothrombinemia of newborn
  Inadequate absorption
    Biliary obstruction
    Malabsorption syndromes
    Antibiotics
Inadequate utilization due to severe hepatocellular
  injury
  Drugs
    Dicoumarol and its congeners
    Salicylates
    Excessive vitamin A

Water-Soluble Vitamins

Ascorbic acid
  Scurvy
  Methemoglobinemia
  Hypertyrosinemia of infants
  Common cold (?)
Thiamine
  Alcoholism
    Alcoholic neuritis
    Wernicke's reaction syndrome
    Korsakoff's psychosis
  Neuritis of pregnancy
  Subacute necrotizing encephalomyelopathy
    (Leigh's disease)
  Beriberi heart disease
Nicotinic acid
  Pellagra
  Schizophrenia (?)
  Peripheral vascular disease with or without
    hypercholesterolemia (?)
Riboflavin
  Anemia of protein-calorie malnutrition
  Glutathione reductase deficiency
Pyridoxine
  Isoniazid administration
  Hydralazine-induced neuropathy
  Pyridoxine-responsive hypochromic microcytic
    anemia
  Dialysis patients
Vitamin B$_{12}$
  Pernicious anemia
  Strict vegetarians
  Disorders of stomach
    Neoplastic involvement
    Subtotal and total gastrectomy
  Ileal disease
  Pancreatic disease
  Fish tapeworm
  Blind loop syndrome
    Surgical
    Small bowel diverticula
Folic acid
  Pregnancy
    Oral contraceptive agent
  Alcoholism
  Malabsorption syndromes

Water-Soluble Vitamins (Continued)
Hemolytic anemias
Dialysis patients
Malnutrition
Drugs
   Anticonvulsants
   Pyrimethamine
   Trimethoprim
   Triamterene
Pantothenic acid
   No specific indications
Biotin
   No specific indications

B. There is no evidence that moderate amounts of water-soluble vitamins in excess of the daily requirements have adverse effects.

C. The long-term effects of megadose vitamins of the water-soluble class have not been vigorously studied, but there are now some indications that there may be adverse effects.

V. Vitamin A

A. Clinical evidence of vitamin A deficiency is largely ocular.

1. Night blindness as a consequence of rod dysfunction is the first functional evidence of vitamin A deficiency.

2. Night blindness has been associated with deficiencies in riboflavin and vitamin C and is therefore not pathognomonic of vitamin A deficiency.

3. Not all patients with documented vitamin A deficiency develop clinical night blindness.

4. Evidence of conjunctival involvement includes dryness, wrinkling, loss of luster, and "nonwetability". Corneal involvement may lead to blindness

B. While the serum vitamin A level of 20 to 50 μg./100 ml. is generally considered acceptable, the serum vitamin A level is not an ideal reflection of body stores of vitamin A.

1. The serum level of carotene also is not a reliable index of vitamin A status.

C. Excessive intake of vitamin A can also lead to toxic effects.

1. On an acute basis the symptoms include headaches, vomiting, dizziness, drowsiness, irritability, and, occasionally, desquamation of the skin.

2. Symptoms of chronic vitamin A toxicity include anorexia, pruritus, alopecia, coarse hair, fissures at the angle of the mouth, occasional hepatomegaly, tender swelling of the bones, hypoprothrombinemia, increased alkaline phosphatase, and, occasionally, hypercalcemia.

VI. Vitamin D

A. Rickets in the pediatric age group has largely disappeared in the U.S., although it still occurs in both Canada and Great Britain.

B. Presumably, the decreased incidence is a result of the regular fortification of milk with vitamin D in the U.S.

C. Vitamin D supplementation in normal, healthy children should not be necessary unless milk and milk products cannot be ingested.

D. Vitamin D deficiency is also distinctly rare in adults unless the individuals have diseases which interfere with vitamin D absorption or utilization.

1. Vitamin D requirements may be increased by malabsorption due to steatorrhea, small intestinal disease, prolonged biliary obstruction, and pancreatic insufficiency, all of which interfere with absorption, and by uremia, in which metabolism is abnormal (see Chap. 25).

E. Vitamin D intoxication is a serious consequence of excess vitamin D because metastatic calcification of the kidney often leads to renal failure which is frequently irreversible.

1. Vitamin D excess is likely to be observed in patients who have been treated with vitamin D (often together with a calcium supplement) for the correction of hypoparathyroidism, vitamin D-resistant rickets, renal osteodystrophy, and osteoporosis.

F. Dangers of hypercalcemia should be

discussed with patients. Potential symptoms should be mentioned to patients even though these are admittedly nonspecific—nausea, vomiting, anorexia, constipation, fatigue, and malaise.

1. Serum calcium should be measured at regular intervals, at least three or four times a year. It should be done more often in the patient with renal failure.

2. Hypercalcemia may appear suddenly despite these precautions.

3. Hypertension also may be a manifestation of vitamin D intoxication when hypercalcemia is present.

G. In mild cases of vitamin D intoxication without renal involvement, discontinuing vitamin D in itself may be sufficient.

1. Corticosteroids occasionally are necessary to facilitate correction of hypercalcemia in more severe cases.

VII. Vitamin E

A. Although the importance of vitamin E for fertility in subprimate species, especially rats, has been well documented, the value of vitamin E in human metabolism is far from established.

1. In humans, months of a diet deficient in vitamin E are required before the plasma concentration of vitamin E decreases.

2. No clinical symptoms appeared in these Vitamin E deprivation studies, which did help, however, to generate data regarding normal daily requirements.

B. Although, in the past, it was a popular treatment of habitual abortion in women and sterility in men, there is no conclusive evidence that vitamin E is of any value in these conditions.

C. It is conceivable that vitamin E may occasionally be responsible for anemia in humans.

1. Red blood cells from vitamin E-deficient animals are more susceptible to hemolysis by oxidizing agents than non-deficient erythrocytes.

2. It is presumed that tocopherol protects the lipid in the red blood cell membrane from peroxidation, thereby avoiding membrane destruction and hemolysis.

D. Prolonged excessive intake of vitamin E can produce hypertension and conceivably other adverse effects. Therefore, it should not be ingested for unproved indications.

E. Vitamin E has proved to be of no value in the prevention or treatment of coronary artery disease. There is some suggestive evidence, however, that it may be of some value in peripheral vascular disease.

VIII. Vitamin K

A. Vitamin K is required for the maintenance of normal prothrombin time through its effect on prothrombin and several factors essential in blood coagulation.

B. Daily vitamin K supplements are not needed by the healthy person.

1. The average diet satisfies the vitamin K needs, which appear to be extremely small.

2. The vitamin K which is synthesized by intestinal bacteria is also available to the host.

C. The bleeding manifestations of vitamin K deficiency include ecchymosis, epistaxis, hematuria, gastrointestinal bleeding, and postoperative hemorrhage.

1. While intracranial hemorrhage may occur, hemoptysis is rather rare.

D. In the absence of bile, the fat-soluble vitamin K is poorly absorbed. Either intrahepatic or extrahepatic biliary obstruction may lead to hypoprothrombinemia.

1. When hypoprothrombinemia is a consequence of biliary obstruction, vitamin K therapy, either orally or parenterally, is generally effective in returning prothrombin activity of the blood to normal.

2. The hypoprothrombinemia which occurs with severe hepatocellular damage, however, is less likely to respond favorably to vitamin K administration.

3. The liver cells under these circumstances are presumably unable to

produce the vitamin K-dependent clotting factors which are necessary to promote clotting.

4. In the past, the therapeutic response to parenteral vitamin K administration has been used in an attempt to distinguish jaundice due to obstructive disease, from that due to hepatocellular damage.

5. While the adverse effects of Coumadin and salicylates on the prothrombin time are well known, hypoprothrombinemia as a consequence of vitamin A toxicity is less well appreciated.

IX. Ascorbic Acid

A. Interest in the relationship between vitamin C and the common cold has been with us since World War II, but Pauling's popular book *Vitamin C and the Common Cold* has rejuvenated intellectual curiosity.

1. Clinical trials from 1942 to 1974 have recently been evaluated in an excellent review of this subject.*

2. Of 14 clinical trials, five were poorly controlled by present standards because double-blinding and randomization were not employed.

3. The remaining nine studies were analyzed according to the number of colds per year as well as mean duration of colds in days.

4. In six of the nine studies, the mean number of colds was less in vitamin C treated subjects than in placebo subjects.

5. The overall decrement in colds per year averaged only 0.1, a figure neither statistically significant nor presumably clinically important.

6. Of interest regarding the incidence of colds are studies which demonstrated that vitamin C, 3 g./day given prophylactically 3 to 14 days before inoculation with a

number of different viruses, did not influence the incidence of colds.

B. Although the incidence of colds does not appear to be affected, there is somewhat more evidence to suggest that vitamin C may have a slight beneficial effect on the duration and severity of the common cold.

1. The mean decreased duration of a cold, however, averages only a tenth of a day.

2. The evaluation of severity of a cold is even more difficult because bias may have been introduced by patients who tasted their tablets and therefore correctly identified whether they were in treated or placebo groups.

3. The beneficial effects of vitamin C on the common cold appear to be clinically minor, even if in certain studies they appear to be statistically significant.

4. The recommended prophylactic-therapeutic dose of vitamin C, 1000 to 3000 g./day, exceeds the normal needs of the body.

5. The ethics of advising a pharmacologic dose of an agent of unknown long-term toxicity to treat a disease of minimal mortality is open to question.

C. Approximately 10 mg. of vitamin C are necessary to prevent scurvy.

D. The recommended daily allowance of 45 mg. is four to five times the anti-scorbutic amount.

1. Most U.S. citizens exceed this recommended allowance from normal fruit stuffs without taking supplemental vitamins.

E. Toxicity

1. The effect of prolonged excessive ingestion of ascorbic acid on renal acidification and the urinary excretion of calcium is known and most often postulated as potential adverse side effects from the long-term use of pharmacologic amounts of vitamin C.

2. Other problems may conceivably exist.

---

*Chalmers, T. C.: Effects of ascorbic acid on the common cold. Am. J. Med., *58:*532, 1975.

X. Thiamine (Vitamin B₁) Deficiency Disease

A. Thiamine deficiency as a consequence of starvation is now rather rare in the U.S.

B. It is more likely observed in patients with chronic alcoholism in whom certain of the manifestations may be quite dramatic.

C. The earliest symptom of vitamin B₁ deficiency neuropathy may be heaviness of the legs.

1. Symptoms indistinguishable from intermittent claudication may appear.

2. Burning of the feet is often followed by progressive weakness of the toes, feet, legs, and thighs.

3. Knee and ankle jerks are generally absent if the neuropathy is severe.

D. Patients with nystagmus, paralysis of the extraoccular muscles, ataxia, and mental confusion are said to suffer from Wernicke's encephalopathy.

1. This syndrome may be rapidly fatal if not properly treated with thiamine.

E. Korsakoff's psychosis is a combination of peripheral neuropathy, memory defects, and confabulation.

F. While the manifestations of thiamine deficiency in the alcoholic may be most striking, other vitamin deficiencies are usually present.

1. Multivitamin supplements, in addition to thiamine, should be administered to such patients.

G. It appears that thiamine requirements increase during pregnancy and lactation.

1. The neuritis of pregnancy occurs in patients with inadequate diets or persistent vomiting.

H. Leigh's syndrome (subacute necrotizing encephalomyelopathy) is a potentially fatal genetic disease of children in which extracts of spinal fluid inhibit the enzyme in the brain (phosphoryl transferase) which catalyzes the synthesis of thiamine triphosphate from thiamine pyrophosphate. Many patients respond favorably to high doses of thiamine.

I. Thiamine requirements are related to caloric intake. The recommended dietary allowances are 0.4 mg./1000 Cal. or about 1.0 to 1.5 mg. daily (minimum of 0.8 mg./day).

XI. Nicotinic Acid

A. Nicotinic acid has a mild vasodilatory effect, especially in the cutaneous vessels of the blush area.

B. A dose of 100 to 150 mg. orally may produce warmth and tingling as well as a flush appearance.

C. Evidence that the drug is effective in the management of peripheral vascular disease, for which it has often been prescribed, has not been confirmed.

D. Larger doses of nicotinic acid (3 g. daily) are effective in lowering both plasma cholesterol and triglycerides.

1. The side effects of the drug, however, are substantial. They include intense cutaneous flushing, itching, vomiting, diarrhea, abnormal liver function tests, hyperglycemia, and hyperuricemia.

2. Patients' compliance is understandably poor.

E. There is no clear-cut evidence that nicotinic acid is of value in schizophrenic disorders.

F. The recommended daily allowance for nicotinic acid is about 6.6 mg./1000 Cal., or about 12 to 20 mg. daily.

1. Because the amino acid, tryptophan, is converted to nicotinic acid in the body, if dietary tryptophan is low, the need for nicotinic acid is increased.

XII. Riboflavin

A. Riboflavin deficiency rarely occurs as an isolated deficiency.

B. The requirements for riboflavin are related to energy expenditure. About 0.3

mg./1000 Cal. are necessary to avoid symptoms.

C. The minimal daily allowance of 1.1 to 1.8 mg. takes into account variations in caloric intake and needs.

D. Riboflavin deficiency may be one factor in the development of anemia in patients with protein-calorie malnutrition.

E. Riboflavin is also reported to correct some instances of glutathione reductase deficiency.

XIII. Pyridoxine

A. It has become rather standard practice to give vitamin B_6 to patients receiving long-term isoniazid therapy.

1. Isoniazid is a potent inhibitor of pyridoxal kinase, an enzyme which catalyzes the reaction of pyridoxal to pyridoxal phosphate.

2. The peripheral neuropathy which can develop after isoniazid is a consequence of this chemical inhibition.

3. Hydralazine-hydrochloride-induced neuropathy presumably has a similar pathogenesis, although the prophylactic use of pyridoxine in patients treated with hydralazine hydrochloride is not so widespread.

B. Pyridoxine-responsive hypochromic microcytic sideroblastic anemia is a rare disorder. Megaloblastic anemia due to pyridoxine deficiency is even more uncommon.

C. There is some evidence that certain patients with renal failure receiving long-term maintenance hemodialysis may have biochemical evidence for pyridoxine deficiency.

1. Most dialysis patients receive daily multivitamins.

2. Vitamins are administered because of the anticipated losses of water-soluble vitamins into the dialysate during treatment with the artificial kidney.

3. Dietary restrictions may contribute to increased vitamin needs.

4. For example, in an attempt to reduce the potassium intake, prolonged boiling of vegetables is suggested so that potassium is leached into the boiling water. While this may effectively lead to decreased potassium intake, decreased vitamin intake is also insured.

5. Appetite may also vary because of medical complications.

D. Recommended daily allowance is 1.6 to 2.0 mg. daily.

E. The requirements for pyridoxine may be somewhat increased when oral contraceptive agents are used.

XIV. Vitamin B_{12}

A. Pernicious anemia as a consequence of vitamin B_{12} deficiency is known to most practicing physicians.

1. The diagnosis may not be clinically obvious.

2. It is especially difficult to diagnose in the patient who, for one reason or another, has ample supply of folic acid. Since ample folic acid prevents or corrects the hematological findings of megaloblastic anemia, these may be absent at the time neurological symptoms of B_{12} deficiency begin.

B. Vitamin B_{12} deficiency can develop in strict vegetarians in whom anemia may be minimal.

1. Folic acid levels in vegetarians, however, may be higher than normal.

2. In vegetarians in whom intrinsic factor secretion and the ileum are both normal, an active enterohepatic circulation may maintain small body stores of B_{12}, and evidence of an overt deficiency may develop very slowly.

C. Recommended dietary allowance is 3.0 μg. daily, which is usually met by almost any diet.

XV. Folic Acid

A. Although severe megaloblastic anemia in the pregnant female is no longer commonplace, laboratory evidence of folic acid deficiency is by no means rare. The prophylactic administration of folic acid is generally recommended.

B. The relationship between folic acid and oral contraceptive agents is also of some interest.

1. In several studies, the use of oral contraceptive agents has led to statistically decreased levels of folic acid in the serum as well as in the red blood cells.

2. Oral contraceptive agents have been listed (see p. 116) as a potential indication for folic acid supplementation.

3. Despite the statistical evidence of decreased serum and red blood cell folate, both hemoglobin and hematocrit in oral contraceptive agent users are not necessarily reduced.

4. An occasional patient with megaloblastic anemia, presumably secondary to oral contraceptive agent use, has been described.

5. It has also been suggested that women who discontinue oral contraceptive agents in order to become pregnant are more prone to folic acid deficiency during the subsequent pregnancy.

XVI. Gastrointestinal Disease

A. Patients with disturbances of gastrointestinal absorption are particularly likely to require vitamin supplementation.

1. The necessity of vitamin K in patients with severe diseases of the liver and biliary tract is well established.

B. Prolonged diarrhea may lead to vitamin deficiencies as well as the need for other supplemental elements.

C. The need for vitamin B_{12} therapy in patients with pernicious anemia is well known. The disease, however, may be difficult to diagnose, especially in the elderly.

D. Although sprue is primarily associated with abnormalities in the absorption of fat-soluble vitamins, water-soluble vitamin deficiencies may also develop.

E. Antimicrobial therapy may occasionally induce vitamin deficiencies by modifying the bacterial content of the gastrointestinal tract.

9. NUTRITION AND CARDIOVASCULAR DISEASE

Roger G. Mazlen, M.D.

ARTERIOSCLEROSIS AND CORONARY HEART DISEASE

I. Definitions

A. Arteriosclerosis is a condition in which there is loss of elasticity and thickening and hardening of the arteries.

Atherosclerosis is a lesion of large and medium arteries characterized by yellowish plaques of cholesterol, lipoid or fatlike material, and lipophages or fat-ingesting cells in the intimal layer of the arteries.

B. Coronary Artery Disease (including fatty streak, fibrous plaque, and complicated lesion) is atherosclerotic disease of the coronary arterial wall, involving the intimal layer and occasionally the media, characterized by three types of lesions.

1. Fatty Streak is a yellow, sessile lesion featuring accumulation of intimal smooth muscle cells, containing and surrounded by deposits of lipid.

2. Fibrous Plaque is a whitish, elevated lesion consisting of foci of lipid-laden, intimal smooth muscle cells surrounded by lipid, collagen, elastic fibers, and proteoglycans, which act as a fibrous cover for a larger, underlying deposit of free extracellular lipid and cellular debris.

3. Complicated Lesion is a fibrous plaque altered as a result of hemorrhage, cell necrosis, and mural thrombosis, which contains calcification.

C. Risk Factors is a term used to describe those characteristics, found in so-called healthy persons, that are correlated with the subsequent appearance of coronary artery disease (CAD).

D. Obesity is a condition in which body weight exceeds the skeletal limitation and physical requirement of the body, resulting from excessive accumulated fat.

E. Hypervitaminosis is a condition resulting from excessive ingestion of one or more of the vitamins.

F. High-, Low-, and Very Low-Density Lipoproteins

1. Lipoproteins are a combination of lipids and proteins, which possess the solubility of proteins.

2. Very Low-Density Lipoproteins are those in which hydrated density is less than 1.006 and in which electrophoretic mobility is that of a pre-β-lipoprotein.

3. Low-Density Lipoproteins are those in which hydrated density ranges from 1.006 to 1.063 and in which electrophoretic mobility is that of a β-lipoprotein.

4. High-Density Lipoproteins are those in which hydrated density ranges from 1.060 to 1.210 and in which electrophoretic mobility is that of an α-lipoprotein.

II. Basic Principles

A. Cardiovascular deaths are still the number one killer in the U.S. today. Acute myocardial infarction, hypertension, stroke, myocardial diseases, arteriosclerosis, other arterial diseases, rheumatic fever, and rheumatic heart disease are included in this category.

B. Arteriosclerosis and atherosclerosis are becoming more prevalent as our longevity increases.

C. It appears that the sequence of events leading to the human atherosclerotic plaque begins with injury of some type to the arterial endothelium and the other segments of the intimal lining. A chronic elevation of blood cholesterol may be adequate to produce such intimal injury.

D. The fatty streak is the earliest lesion involved in atherosclerosis and is commonly found in young persons.

1. Lipid droplets have been found accumulating in the arterial wall smooth muscle cell's lysosomes of American preteen children.

2. It is thought that the fibromuscular lesion of the intima is the antecedent lesion to the fibrous plaque.

3. Abnormal proliferation of the smooth muscle cells plays the major role in the formation of the fibrous or atherosclerotic plaque. The lipid in these plaques is primarily cholesterol and cholesterol ester.

4. The complicated lesion, which is believed to be a fibrous plaque altered as a result of calcification, cellular necrosis, local hemorrhage, or mural thrombosis, is often associated with occlusive vascular disease.

E. LDL, or low-density lipoproteins, appear to carry cholesterol to the peripheral tissues for utilization, whereas HDL or high-density lipoproteins appear to transport cholesterol from the peripheral tissues to the liver, where it may be excreted into the gastrointestinal tract for removal or recycled to the blood.

1. The LDL deliver cholesterol/cholesterol esters to the peripheral cells where they bind to a receptor and are then taken into the cell by pinocytosis and split into free cholesterol from cholesterol esters by lysosomal enzyme activity.

2. LDL receptors in animals are saturated at relatively low serum cholesterol levels while in humans this level appears to be about 50 mg./100 ml. indicating that our high-fat American diet has strained the cellular control mechanisms that ordinarily prevent the development of atherosclerosis.

3. Data from the Framingham Study* indicate that the risk of having a heart attack increases as the concentration of plasma LDL increases. Contrariwise, persons with high HDL concentrations appear to have a decreased risk of heart attacks.

---

*Kannel, W. B., and Gordon T. (ed.): The Framingham Study, An Epidemiological Investigation of Cardiovascular Disease. Washington, D.C., U.S. Government Printing Office, 1971.

F. Preliminary evidence indicates that established athcrosclerosis can be made to regress in humans.

1. The cholesterol turn-over time in human atherosclerosis appears to be very slow, being in the range of 442 to 934 days.

2. Although cholesterol in atherosclerotic plaques exchanges very slowly with the plasma, at least partial regression of the atherosclerotic lesion appears to be possible.

3. A rise in HDL levels may possibly induce this regression, as HDL is the major determinant of the pool size of cholesterol.

4. Confirmation of the regression of coronary atherosclerosis in patients with documented coronary artery disease is the crucial evidence now required.

G. Dietary risk factors may contribute in either a major or a minor way to the development and progression of atherosclerotic cardiovascular disease.

1. Serum cholesterol level is one of the major risk factors for coronary artery disease. There is evidence that even within the so-called normal range of serum cholesterol, the higher the cholesterol, the higher the risk.

2. Although a second or recurrent myocardial infarction may not necessarily be prevented by reduction of the serum cholesterol, once a person has had a myocardial infarction, an attempt should be made to reduce plasma LDL levels.

3. The increased risk of developing coronary heart disease conferred by hypercholesterolemia is considerably enhanced by the concomitant presence of hypertension, cigarette smoking, or diabetes mellitus.

a. Cigarette gases include carbon monoxide, hydrogen cyanide, and nitrogen oxides. Of these, carbon monoxide appears to contribute to atherosclerotic plaque formation through increased accumulation of LDL and formation of lipid-laden cells as seen in the arteriosclerotic plaques.

H. Obesity. A moderate or minor risk factor per se, obesity is usually associated with or productive of other risk factors such as glucose intolerance or diabetes mellitus, hypertension, physical inactivity, and increased plasma cholesterol, triglycerides, and uric acid.

I. Diabetes and Glucose Intolerance. In Western nations, diabetic men have two to three times more CHD and diabetic women have five to six times more CHD than do non-diabetics.

    1. Diabetics are especially predisposed to peripheral occlusive vascular disease due to microangiopathic changes and their sequelae.

    2. A myocardial lesion of diabetes mellitus has been described.

J. Triglycerides. An elevation of endogenous triglycerides reflected in a fasting plasma level is a weaker risk factor than the elevated plasma cholesterol level. Studies of lipid levels in angiographically documented coronary artery disease reveal a significantly greater frequence of CAD in patients with levels in the upper two quartiles, defined, respectively, as 151 to 207 mg./100 ml. and over 207 mg./100 ml. (fasting overnight, 10 to 12 hours), as compared to those with levels below 151 mg./100 ml. There was more of a risk for men than for women at any level of triglycerides studied.

K. Diet and Nutritional Status. Certain aspects of our nutritional status and our long-term dietary intake significantly influence the development and progression of CHD.

    1. Dietary fiber alone will not offset the deleterious effects of a high-cholesterol diet. The addition of fiber such as wheat bran to the diet does not lower the plasma cholesterol. There is preliminary evidence, however, that in animals alfafa-derived dietary fiber can significantly lower serum cholesterol. This has yet to be tested in humans in adequately controlled studies.

    2. Sugar has been suggested as a possible risk factor for the development of CHD, but this is open to question.

    3. Coffee. This was once thought to contribute to the occurrence of myocardial infarction, but this has not been proven. Persons who have a tendency to develop premature contractions, however, should restrict their coffee intake to the decaffeinated variety.

    4. Alcohol. There is no firm evidence to suggest alcohol consumption per se as a cause of CHD.

        a. Daily consumption of alcohol in socially acceptable amounts, however, can cause a significant increase in the endogencous triglycerides in hypertriglyceridemic persons (but not in healthy persons).

        b. After a meal, alcohol ingestion causes much higher levels of triglycerides in both healthy and hypertriglyceridemic persons. Too, ingestion of a fatty meal soon after consumption of alcohol has been reported to cause much higher levels of VLDL, which persist at least 12 hours.

        c. Persons with preexisting hyperlipemia respond to moderate amounts of alcohol with marked increases in serum cholesterol levels.

        d. Alcohol, however, is believed to preferentially increase HDL cholesterol and thus alter the HDL:LDL ratio.

        e. Chronic heavy ingestion of alcohol can lead to the development of alcoholic cardiomyopathy, and even well-nourished alcoholics may develop a variety of ethanol-induced cardiac arrhythmias.

    5. Minerals. The level of certain minerals in the diet may influence the development of cardiovascular diseases.

        a. Minerals may be divided arbitrarily into macrometals and trace metals.

        b. Among the macrometals, calcium and magnesium deficiencies in particular have been implicated in both the etiology of CHD and sudden death from cardiovascular causes, but a direct relationship has not been demonstrated. For example, recent studies have linked local magnesium deficiencies in the soil/water axis to an increased incidence of sudden death from cardiovascular disease.

        c. U.S. cardiovascular disease death rates have been reported to be lower in areas where the soil is rich in selenium. In fact, one of the pathologic features of selenium-responsive dietary deficiency disease in experimental animals is heart muscle degeneration.

d. Cadmium, chromium, and lead are among the trace elements that are now under investigation for their possible involvement in the etiology of CHD.

e. Lack of the trace element silicon may be an etiological factor in the development of CHD, for very high amounts of bound silicon are found in the arterial wall, and in the intima in particular. An inverse relationship between the degree of atherosclerosis in the arterial wall and its silicon content has been claimed. Silicon content is high in the food contents of Oriental societies in which CHD is markedly lower than in Western societies.

III. Criteria for Diagnosis

A. Accurate History

1. The history should carefully review the cardiovascular system, and a complete family history should be obtained in which the presence or absence of familial hypercholesterolemia (FH), hypertriglyceridemia, diabetes mellitus, hypertension, obesity is ascertained as well as that of heart disease.

B. Physical Examination

1. The presence of xanthoma, arcus senilis, and psoriasis should be determined.

2. A comprehensive physical examination for signs of atherosclerotic disease should be made.

C. Clinical Testing

1. A complete blood count, 12-lead electrocardiogram, chest radiograph, and urinalysis should be routine.

2. In addition, laboratory determinations of the blood cholesterol, HDL cholesterol triglycerides, fasting or postprandial blood sugar, blood urea nitrogen, creatinine, blood calcium and -phosphorous, and the blood uric acid are indicated.

a. The absolute value of HDL cho-

lesterol as well as the ratio of HDL cholesterol to total cholesterol are said to be of prognostic value in coronary artery disease and myocardial infarction. The higher the value and the greater the ratio of HDL cholesterol to total cholesterol, the more the protection against developing coronary artery disease.

b. It is noteworthy that women during their menstrual years have higher HDL cholesterol values than do men.

3. In special cases in which clinical hypertension is present in a severe or malignant form, a peripheral plasma renin activity and 24-hour urinalysis for sodium excretion are desirable to determine the renin classification. A high plasma renin activity may have an acceleratory effect on atherosclerotic cardiovascular disease through its role in producing angiotensin II and aldosterone.

IV. Management

A. Abnormally elevated plasma cholesterol, if present, should be reduced. Hyperlipidemia, in general, requires treatment that should be directed toward returning and maintaining the elevated lipids near to or within their respective normal ranges.

1. Dietary intervention should have a high priority before CHD becomes clinically evident, and a diet low in saturated fat and cholesterol and high in polyunsaturated fat should be employed for at least 1 year as a therapeutic measure for hyperlipidemia.

2. Although it has not been conclusively proven that reduction of plasma cholesterol reduces the risk of a second heart attack, it is the consensus that treatment of elevated cholesterol in these patients is indicated.

3. If hyperlipidemia persists after reasonable efforts have been made to normalize body weight by altering the makeup of the diet as indicated above, to moderate alcoholic intake, and to promote physical

fitness, a therapeutic trial with drugs then may be instituted (see also Chap. 10).

    a. If not contraindicated, clofibrate may be utilized. This may have the added benefit of raising the HDL level.

    b. Similarly, cholestyramine resin and nicotinic acid have been used to treat hyperlipidemia.

  B. Obesity should be treated simultaneously (see Chap. 17).

  C. Hypertension, cigarette smoking, and other risk factors should be treated concurrently.

  D. There is a significant difference in the incidence of CHD in physically active as opposed to inactive workers.

    1. The exercises that are employed are brisk walking, bicycling, jogging, running, swimming, calisthenics, and heavy work in the house or garden or on the farm.

  E. Strict dietary measures are recommended for patients with diabetes mellitus, even though the evidence that the degree of metabolic control of diabetes influences the risk of developing CHD is not conclusive. An appropriate reduction of carbohydrates and replacement with protein and fats is recommended. Although complete normalization of the blood sugar level is difficult to maintain, it appears that fewer glycoproteins, which are involved in producing diabetic microangiopathy and renal damage through basement membrane deposits, are produced with a strict diet. Good control of diabetes may also prevent the diabetes-induced lesions of the myocardium itself.

  F. Abnormally elevated plasma triglycerides should be reduced. In cases in which hypertriglyceridemia is the predominant lipid abnormality, a reduction of total daily caloric intake to lower and maintain the body weight near its ideal level for the age, height, and body frame of the patient, is the most crucial dietary measure.

    1. The additional dietary measures necessary to correct hypertriglyceridemia are a strict restriction of carbohydrate intake, sugar in particular, to about 40% of

the diet and the limitation of alcoholic intake to two small drinks a day (approximately 45 ml. each).

    2. The hyperlipidemia induced by ethanol is not corrected by hypolipemic agents such as clofibrate, dextrothyroxine, and nicotinic acid.

    3. For the Type-IV hyperlipoproteinemia patient (in whom triglycerides and cholesterol are both elevated), daily cholesterol intake should be maintained in the range of 300 to 500 mg.

    4. With rigorous dietary management, the triglycerides may decrease from 15% to 200% or more, whereas in mixed hyperlipidemia both lipids will decrease at least 30%, with the triglycerides decreasing as much as 300%.

  G. Mineral Factors

    1. In healthy children and adults, it is advisable to insure an adequate daily intake of calcium and magnesium. Both of these macrometals have been established as necessary for cardiovascular health maintenance.

    a. If local water supplies are low in these minerals, they should be supplemented.

    b. Recommendations for magnesium vary, but an intake above 6 mg./kg./day is recommended for adults.

    c. Principal dietary sources of magnesium are grains, fish, some meats, nuts, soybeans, blackstrap molasses, and green vegetables.

    d. Females have an increased magnesium requirement during pregnancy and lactation and when they are using oral contraceptives.

    e. Chronic diuretic therapy of cardiovascular diseases, such as hypertension and congestive heart failure, depletes the body of magnesium, and this may lead to serious cardiac arrhythmias.

    2. Preliminary data suggest that an adequate daily intake of the essential trace element silicon, a component of dietary fiber (from some sources) is essential for the maintenance of healthy arteries.

a. The principal natural sources of dietary silicon are sugarbeet pulp, oat hulls, rice straw, rice hulls, and, to a lesser degree, alfalfa and wheat straw.

b. Wheat brans are a relatively poor source of silicon, although some brands have a higher content than others.

H. Vitamins

1. Vitamin E. There are no conclusive studies showing any role for Vitamin E in preventing the development of CHD.

a. Some forms of vitamin E may prolong the plasma clotting time at a dosage of 300 to 400 mg./day.

b. There is some evidence that vitamin E supplementation may play a role in the treatment of peripheral vascular disease.

2. Vitamin D. Excessive vitamin D ingestion, over 1200 I.U./day, has been reported to abnormally elevate the plasma cholesterol. There also appears to be a positive correlation between the intake of over 1200 I.U./day of vitamin D and an increased incidence of myocardial infarction.

a. It is recommended that, for now, both young adults and middle-aged adults have their daily vitamin D intake from all exogenous sources restricted to less than 1200 I.U.

b. In patients with proven CHD, the daily intake of vitamin D should not exceed the recommended daily allowance of 400 I.U.

HYPERTENSION AND HYPERTENSIVE CARDIOVASCULAR DISEASE

I. Definitions

A. Essential Hypertension. A diagnosis made by the exclusion of any secondary cause of labile or fixed (sustained) hypertension. Essential hypertension encompasses a spectrum of severity ranging from labile or borderline to malignant or accelerated. It also includes various subpopulations that can be categorized by plasma renin activity and for which therapy may be variable.

B. Renovascular Hypertension is hypertension associated with or due to kidney damage or defective renal function.

C. Sympathetic Overdrive. A disease state in which there is an inappropriately increased level of sympathetic nervous activity as reflected by cardiodynamic parameters such as pulse, blood pressure, and cardiac output

D. Azotemia. An abnormal elevation of the blood urea nitrogen and creatinine caused by decreased glomerular filtration rate from hypertensive renal damage

E. Cadmium Toxicity. Pathologic changes, resulting from excessive cadmium deposition in the adrenals, kidneys, and lungs, that can produce hypertension

II. Basic Principles

A. Hypertension is the most prevalent cardiovascular disease in the U.S. today and is the major independent risk factor for the subsequent development of CHD.

B. Hypertension afflicts over 23 million people in this country who run a significantly high risk of developing target organ damage manifested as congestive heart failure, renal failure, and stroke unless their blood pressures are reduced by appropriate therapy. Hypertension is here defined as an accurately measured blood pressure reading in excess of 160 systolic/95 diastolic mm. Hg.

C. An arterial blood pressure fluctuating above and below 140/90 mm. Hg. characterizes the state of labile or borderline hypertension

1. The prevalence of labile hypertension in the U.S. appears to exceed 10%.

2. This is an important population of younger people because it is estimated that as many as 25% of these will progress to fixed hypertension.

D. There are a variety of pathophysiologic changes associated with benign essential hypertension. Specific pathologic changes observed in the arteries when hypertension is present include increased collagen in the arterial wall, increased elastic fibrils and acid mucopolysaccharides in the arterial wall, increased sodium and calcium in the arterial wall, and a proliferation of smooth muscle cells in the arterial wall. All of these lead to an increased arterial thickness and a narrowing of the lumen.

E. Endocrine and metabolic abnormalities are associated with benign essential hypertension. The most well-known are those related to the renin-angiotensin-aldosterone system.

1. Renin, a proteolytic enzyme that converts a precursor glycoprotein to angiotensin I, which later is converted to angiotensin II, is abnormally elevated in about 16% of patients with benign essential hypertension.

2. Renin levels are normal in about 57% of the patients and abnormally low in the remaining 27% of those with benign essential hypertension.

3. Aldosterone plasma levels generally parallel those of renin. Renin is measured as the plasma renin activity (PRA).

4. High plasma renin activity is a frequent occurrence in cases of secondary hypertension due to renovascular disorders.

5. In benign essential hypertension, plasma catecholamines are frequently elevated.

6. Overactivity of the sympathetic nervous system has also been described in benign essential hypertension.

F. Sodium plays a very important role in the causation of clinical essential hypertension. However, once this is established, the restriction of sodium, although essential, may not be adequate in itself to control the blood pressure.

1. In the patient with fixed essential hypertension, the sodium content of the arterial wall is significantly increased. Part of this sodium is readily exchangeable; the other part is fixed in the acid mucopolysaccharide matrix.

2. The average American diet supplies 10 to 15 g. daily of sodium chloride and other sodium salts. Because the necessary daily allowance is less than 1 g., the body is occupied daily with getting rid of the excess sodium, to prevent it from accumulating as it does in the disease state of essential hypertension.

3. The hypertensive person apparently treats a sodium load differently than does the normotensive person. When hypertension progresses to the severe or malignant stages, handling a sodium load is made more difficult due to consistently increased aldosterone secretion.

4. Even early in the course of essential hypertension, in many persons there appears to be a defect in the hepatic inactivation of aldosterone. This decreased metabolic clearance does not appear to be related to sodium balance. When this state of relative and inappropriate hyperaldosteronism is concomitant with a high sodium intake it may call into play other inappropriate responses thus upsetting the regulation of blood pressure.

5. Once hypertensive disease progresses to the point where sodium significantly accumulates in the arterial wall, this sodium potentiates the action of most known vasopressors, especially angiotensin II, thus making natural regulation of the blood pressure more a conflict of opposing forces than a successful homeostatic cascade.

G. In many hypertensives, especially those in the low renin category, there has been shown to be an excessive secretion of one or more mineralocorticoids.

1. In labile and low-renin forms of benign essential hypertension, increased secretion of 18 hydroxy DOC (which is regulated by ACTH production) has been shown.

2. Another adrenal steroid, progesterone, has been found to be increased in the plasma of nearly 50% of patients with benign essential hypertension. Because progesterone blocks the sodium-retaining

effects of aldosterone at the renal tubules, it seems logical to infer that increased plasma progesterone levels reflect an effort to counteract the sodium-retaining effects of an inappropriate aldosterone secretion or of other less potent mineralocorticoids.

H. Finally, some trace elements have been implicated as the possible causes of various forms of hypertension.

   1. The most likely candidate for a role in the etiology of benign essential hypertension is cadmium.

      a. In humans, cadmium has a predisposition to collect in the kidneys, and, in fact, about 33% of the total body cadmium burden in the average American is found in the kidneys.

      b. It is thought to be a possible etiology of human hypertension, although not enough is known yet about the sequelae of such exposure.

      c. Most of our body cadmium load comes from ingestion of food and water. The biologic half-life of much of such ingested cadmium is thought to be between 20 and 40 years.

      d. In smokers, a significant amount of inhaled cadmium may be added to the body burden, especially in the lungs.

III. Criteria for Diagnosis

A. Accurate History

   1. History may provide valuable information related to both primary or essential and secondary hypertension.

   2. A renal history is a key component of the hypertensive evaluation. A history of childhood acute or chronic glomerulonephritis or nephritis would be suggestive evidence for renal hypertension.

   3. As part of the occupational and social history of the patient, he should be questioned about any possible exposure to toxic metals, such as cadmium, lead, or mercury.

   4. The social history should elicit the patient's use of alcohol and the number of cigarettes he smokes each day. Alcoholism

may complicate the hypertensive state because of nutritional deprivation, liver disease, and cardiac disease. It is generally more difficult to obtain an alcoholic's compliance with diet or drug therapy.

   5. A detailed diet history should be obtained, including salt (sodium) intake.

   6. A drug history should be obtained. Use of corticosteroids, which are sodium-retaining, may cause iatrogenic hypertension and may decrease the efficacy of diet or drug therapy.

   7. Prior diet and drug therapy for the hypertension and the outcome should be noted.

      a. A dietary history of sodium (salt) intake or restriction should be established.

      b. Too, the patient's general pattern of potassium intake should be determined.

      c. Concomitant drug usage should be established because this may well affect the success or failure of a therapeutic dietary regimen. For example, some prescription, patent, and over-the-counter medications may have a high sodium content.

      d. Attention should be given to any prior antihypertensive drug side effects or adverse drug experiences including orthostatic hypotension.

B. Physical Examination

   1. This examination should include a bilateral funduscopic examination looking for disc changes, retinal hemorrhages and exudates, arteriolar narrowing, and retinal detachment.

   2. All peripheral pulses should be palpated, and auscultation for bruits over the carotid, brachial, femoral, and radial arteries should be performed.

   3. The measurement of blood pressure should be made initially on both arms using an appropriately sized cuff and bladder.

   4. Examination of the heart for arrhythmias, thrusts, heaves, cardiac enlargement, friction rubs, murmurs, gallops, and clicks is necessary in order to tailor a safe and effective therapy in which adverse drug-drug or diet-drug interactions can be avoided or minimized.

C. Clinical Tests

1. As part of the further work-up of the hypertensive patient, the following clinical tests should be performed: a resting 12-lead electrocardiogram, chest radiograph, complete blood count, urinalysis, blood urea nitrogen, sodium, chlorides and potassium, serum creatinine, serum cholesterol and triglycerides, serum uric acid, serum fasting blood sugar and 2-hour postprandial blood sugar, serum calcium and phosphorous and urinary catecholamine metabolites.

2. Selectively, the following may be performed as clinically required for diagnostic purposes: plasma renin activity, plasma catecholamines, plasma cortisol, plasma T4 iodine, rapid-sequence timed I.V.P. and renal scan.

IV. Management

A. Careful instructions on a diet should emphasize sodium restriction below 100 mEq. (2.3 g.) per day if no diuretics are employed concomitantly.

1. Because normal diets without added salt contain about 2.5 to 4.5 g. salt, it is fairly difficult on an outpatient basis to sustain a sodium-restricted diet of less than 2 g./day.

2. Rigorous sodium restriction is probably of the greatest benefit early in the natural history of essential hypertension.

3. It is reasonable to consider whether excessive sodium in a person's diet may not at some point push the pathophysiologic process of hypertensive disease into an irreversible phase.

a. For this reason, it is recommended that a no-added-salt diet should be prescribed (beginning in young adulthood) for normotensive persons who have a history of essential hypertension in the immediate family.

b. In the hypertensive patient, it is important to continue salt restriction even when diuretics are being employed in order to conserve the dosage of drug used, to min-imize the amount of sodium fixed into the arterial wall, and to reduce the strain on other homeostatic mechanisms called into play when plasma sodium is transiently increased.

B. An adequate ratio of dietary potassium intake to sodium intake should be maintained.

1. Even without any diuretic therapy, potassium intake should be in the approximate ratio of 1.5:1 to sodium intake.

2. Good dietary sources of potassium are citrus fruits, apricots, bananas, dried dates and figs, raisins, artichokes, brussel sprouts, cauliflower, dried lentils, parsley, dried and fresh soybeans, spinach, sweet potatoes, nuts, wheat germ, dried brewer's yeast, cheeses, non-fat dried milk, poultry, and some fish and meats.

3. Potassium supplements may be necessary if diuretic depletion of body potassium stores occurs, as reflected in a lowered serum potassium.

a. When this is the case, it is safer to start with a liquid potassium supplement, such as potassium chloride solution, than with enteric-coated tablets.

b. Even with oral potassium supplementation, total body exchangeable potassium may not increase significantly.

4. In cases in which diuretic treatment must be maintained, a potassium-sparing agent should be employed.

C. When diuretics are employed, chronically hypertensive patients should receive:

1. Supplementary oral magnesium in divided doses in order to prevent hypomagnesemia. In these cases 8 mg./kg./day of magnesium should be the total daily intake.

2. Supplementary oral zinc in amounts ranging from approximately 50 to 200 mg./day. Zincuria is a frequent result of diuretic therapy, and a loss of body zinc stores may complicate diet and drug therapy through diminished taste and loss of appetite.

D. Patients should be weighed on the initial visit and on subsequent visits. Obese patients should be placed on restricted calo-

Table 9-1. **Salt Substitutes and Their Sodium and Potassium Contents**

Brand Name of Salt Substitute	Sodium		Potassium	
	mg./g.	*mEq./g.*	*mg./g.*	*mEq./g.*
Morton's Salt Substitute	1	0.044	493	12.62
Co-Salt	1	0.044	476	12.18
Adolph's Salt Substitute	2	0.09	333	8.51
Neocurtasal	100	4.40	469	12.00
Morton's Lite Salt	240	10.54	195	6.15
NaCl (reference)	410	18.00	0	0.00

rie diets aimed at achieving ideal weight gradually.

E. Hyperlipidemia should be treated concurrently as outlined on pages 126 to 127 (see also Chap. 10).

F. Vitamin supplementation is desirable when chronic diuretic therapy is employed especially because so many patients take their first day's diuretic dose around the time of meals. Oral potassium supplementation with slow-release agents has been reported to cause vitamin B_{12} deficiency with associated megaloblastic anemia.

G. All neuroplegic-type antihypertensive agents cause sodium and water retention and subsequent expansion of blood volume.

1. When neuroplegics are employed, for whatever reason, sodium restriction should be therapeutic at less than 11 mEq./day.

2. Propranolol alone initially causes approximately a 500 ml. expansion in blood volume on an ad lib salt diet, and weight gain may exceed 10 lbs. over 4 to 6 weeks.

H. Monitoring of the 24-hour urinary sodium excretion can be used as a compliance check on dietary sodium restriction. Also, serial weights will assist in assessing therapeutic efficiency of both diet and drug treatments.

I. When hypertensive patients are on a sodium-restricted diet, some care should be exercised in the choice of salt substitutes because some are fairly high in potassium and have on occasion been known to induce hyperkalemia.

1. Table 9-1 lists some of the available salt substitutes and their sodium and potassium concentrations.

J. Foods preferred on sodium-restricted diets for cardiovascular disease are listed in Table 9-2. Table 9-3 lists the foods that

Table 9-2. **Foods Preferred on a Sodium-Restricted Diet for Patients With Cardiovascular Disease***

Food	Sodium (mg./lb.)	Potassium (mg./lb.)
Apples (as purchased)	4.0	463
Apricots (fresh)	2.6	1880
Bananas (as purchased)	3.0	1275
Cherries (fresh)	8.5	1110
Corn (fresh)	1.8	1362
Dates (dried)	4.1	3587
Kidney beans (as purchased)	4.5	5896
Oranges (as purchased)	1.0	555
Pecans	1.4	1907
Plums (as purchased)	2.6	732
Potatoes	3.6	1560

*For sodium-restricted patients who are not potassium-restricted or for whom potassium intake needs to be increased

should be avoided on sodium-restricted diets.

Table 9-3. **Foods to Avoid on a Sodium-Restricted Diet**

Food	Sodium (mg./100 g.)
Asparagus (canned)	410
Caviar (pressed)	2200
Carrots (canned)	280
Cheddar cheese	700
Corned beef (canned)	1700
Kale (fresh)	110
Mayonnaise	600
Olives	2400
Peas (canned)	270
Potato chips	340
Pretzels	1700
Sauerkraut	730
Soda crackers	1100
Tomato catsup	1300
Wheatflakes	1300

K. *General Principles* for practical sodium restriction for outpatients requiring a salt intake of less than 2.5 g./day (approximately 1000 mg. of sodium per day)

1. Do not use salt in cooking or in preparing foods.

2. Do not add any table salt. If necessary for taste use a salt substitute in moderate amounts. Check the sodium and potassium contents of the salt substitute to determine the allowable amount in each case.

3. Use fresh vegetables daily, when available, except for beets, celery, kale, spinach, and turnips. Avoid all canned vegetables as much as possible, unless dietetically canned for a low-salt diet.

4. Use fresh fruit or fresh or canned fruit juices daily. Avoid the use of canned fruit unless they are dietetically canned. Do not use canned tomato juice.

5. Use unsalted butter, cheeses, and margarine. Limit the use of milk and milk products. Limit eggs to one daily.

6. Use salt-free breads and baked goods when available. Avoid the use of baking powders and self-rising flour. Avoid the use of breakfast cereals other than shredded wheat, puffed wheat, or puffed rice.

7. Use coffee, sherry, cream or root beer soda, tea, or tonic water. Whiskey also may be used in small amounts. Lemon and sugar may be used in usual amounts. Avoid the use of cocoa, broths, bouillons, canned soups, and canned extracts.

8. Use herbs for seasoning. Avoid the use of commercial salad dressings, sauces, gravies, ketchups, mayonnaise, mustard, or pickles.

9. Use fresh beef, chicken, duck, lamb, liver, tongue, and veal in moderate amounts. Avoid the use of luncheon meats and all canned, pickled, salted, or smoked meats.

10. Use fresh fish in moderate amounts. Avoid the use of shellfish and all canned, pickled, salted, or smoked fish.

11. Check the sodium content of tap water supply (ppm.) and use accordingly, or use spring water with a low-sodium content.

12. Reevaluate dietary intake periodically.

L. Table 9-4 is a sample menu that can be followed by patients on sodium-restricted diets.

M. It has been shown that middle-aged male hypertensives have an impaired glucose tolerance and a higher fasting insulin level more often than normotensive controls.

1. These differences are not explainable solely on the basis of differences in degrees of obesity between subjects in the two groups.

2. It may be necessary to restrict caloric intake in the form of carbohydrates in these patients.

Table 9-4. **Menu Plans for a 1000-mg. Sodium Diet**

Breakfast

1 serving fruit or fruit juice:
Cantaloupe slice (5–10 mg.); peaches, 3 halves (5–10 mg.); pears, 3 halves (5–10 mg.); or fruit juices, 1 cup or less (1–2 mg.). Do not use canned tomato juice.
2 slices of bread (100–150 mg. each)
2 pats unsalted margarine (0–1 mg./pat)
1 cup coffee or tea (0–2 mg. each)
2 tablespoons cream (10–20 mg.)

Substitute 1 serving of a low-salt cereal (100–150 mg.) and/or 1 egg (50–75 mg.) for 1 to 2 slices of bread accordingly.

Lunch

1 serving fish, fowl, or red meat:
Beef, 4 oz.; chicken, 3 oz.; flounder, 3 oz.; turkey, 3 oz.; or veal, 3 oz. (50–70 mg. each)
2 servings fresh vegetables:
Asparagus, 1/2 cup; barley, 1/2 cup; sweet corn, 1 ear; eggplant, less skin, 1/2 cup; green beans, 1/2 cup; onions, 1 medium; peas, 1/2 cup; green peppers, 1/4 cup; potatoes, less skin, 1 medium; winter squash, 1 cup; tomatoes, 1 medium (1–5 mg. each)
1 slice bread (100–150 mg.)
1 cup coffee or tea (0–2 mg. each) or cream or root beer soda, 8 oz. (2–10 mg.) or whiskey, 1.5 oz. (2–10 mg.)

Dinner

1 serving fish, fowl, or red meat:
Beef, 6 oz.; chicken, 4 oz.; duck, 4 oz.; halibut, raw, 5 oz.; liver, calf, 4 oz.; salmon, raw, 6 oz.; shrimp, 2 oz.; turkey, 4 oz.; veal, 5 oz. (75–90 mg. each)
3 servings fresh of dietetic canned vegetables:
1 serving of cauliflower, 1/2 cup; mushrooms, 1/2 cup; or parsley 1 oz. (5–10 mg. each)
2 servings of navy beans, 1/2 cup; broccoli, 1/2 cup; cabbage, 1 cup; carrots, 1/2 cup; or lettuce, 1/2 head (10–15 mg. each)
1 slice bread (100–150 mg.)
1 pat unsalted margarine (0–1 mg.)
1 serving dessert:
Cooked puddings, 1/2 cup (100–120 mg.) or milk chocolate, 1/2 oz. (100–120 mg.)
1 cup coffee or tea (0–2 mg. each) or cream or root beer soda, 8 oz. (2–10 mg.) or 1 cup apple, pineapple, or tangerine juice (1–2 mg. each)

Values given in parentheses are for sodium in mg.

Other substitutions may be made according to standard food table values for sodium content. Variations will be necessary in order to achieve better compliance.

Adjustments for the effects of exercise and climate may be necessary to avoid hyponatremia.

CARDIAC FAILURE

I. Definition

A. The term cardiac failure, or heart failure, refers to myocardial failure as manifested by various symptoms and physical signs produced by an underlying disease process, in which cardiac output does not meet the demands of the body.

II. Basic Principles

A. The reduced cardiac output associated with heart failure leads to a parallel decrease in renal blood flow and glomerular filtration rate. The alterations in renal hemodynamics is associated with retention of sodium and water.

B. An increased blood volume is common in heart failure ranging from a 10 to

20% increase in moderately severe heart failure to 30 to 50% in severe or refractory heart failure. Additionally, extravascular fluid volume is expanded due to increased capillary pressures.

III. Criteria for Diagnosis

A. An accurate history, including dietary history, especially of salt intake, and physical examination are important in determining the etiological factors and treatment of congestive heart failure.

B. Clinical laboratory tests identical to those for hypertensive vascular disease should be employed (see p. 131).

IV. Management

A. Generally, measures are taken aimed at increasing cardiac output or decreasing cardiac work.

B. Sodium restriction is an important therapeutic measure in the treatment of heart failure (see Tables 9-2, 9-3, and 9-4).

1. It should be employed along with diuretic therapy in an effort to eliminate excess body fluid and to maintain, as nearly as is medically feasible, the patient's edema-free or dry weight.

2. Sodium restriction in itself, to the extent of 1 to 2 g. of sodium per day, can markedly improve patients with heart failure.

3. Dietary salt restriction should be reevaluated periodically in order to avoid the occurrence of hyponatremia.

4. It is especially important to monitor sodium balance closely in severe or intractable heart failure in which salt intake often needs to be reduced below 0.5 g. or 8.5 mEq. of sodium/day.

5. If there is the occurrence of mild to moderate hyponatremia, the first step in alleviating it is to restrict daily water intake.

6. When rigorous sodium restriction is prescribed, it must include a survey of the patient's medications for their sodium content and potassium content.

a. Some over-the-counter preparations have very high sodium contents and need to be discontinued; especially to be avoided are the sodium-containing antacids and stomach remedies.

C. Thiazide, furosemide, and other potent diuretics are employed in the therapy of congestive heart failure.

1. These agents can be life-saving but also have potential deleterious side effects because they lead to significant urinary losses of potassium, magnesium, and, to a lesser degree, zinc.

2. Serum sodium and chloride levels also require monitoring.

D. Digitalis and other cardiotonics generally are of significant benefit.

1. A careful monitoring of both the electrocardiogram and the serum potassium is required to guard against the occurrence of hypokalemia.

2. Hypokalemia potentiates digitalis toxicity, which occasionally may become clinically irreversible before the total body exchangeable potassium and serum potassium are adequately restored.

E. Potassium balance needs to be maintained so that total body exchangeable potassium and serum potassium are kept in their normal ranges (serum potassium 3.5 to 5.4 mEq./L.).

1. Most patients with diuretic-induced hypokalemia require daily supplementation of potassium in the amount of 40 to 60 mEq./day.

a. Foods that are rich in potassium should be ingested to prevent the development of hypokalemia. Some of these food sources are listed in the preceding section on hypertension.

b. If hypokalemia develops, potassium solutions should be prescribed. Many products are now available.

2. Care has to be exercised so as to avoid hyperkalemia, especially when the potassium-sparing diuretics (e.g. triamterene) are employed.

F. Magnesium balance needs to be maintained (normal serum levels are 1.5 to 2.5

mEq./L.). Excessive diuretic-induced losses of magnesium can provoke cardiac arrhythmias (see p. 131 for the dosages of oral magnesium to be employed).

1. If necessary, as in the case of serious ventricular arrhythmias, parenteral magnesium may be required.

2. For magnesium infusion, a 20% magnesium solution may be employed acutely as an emergency measure, followed by an intravenous drip using a 2% magnesium sulfate solution that contains glucose and other necessary electrolyes.

G. Zinc supplementation may be required at times due to diuretic-induced zincuria (see p. 131).

SUGGESTED READINGS

Carey, R.M., *et al.*: The Charlottesville blood-pressure survey. J.A.M.A., *236:*847, 1976.

Cohn, P.F., *et al.*: Serum lipid levels in angiographically defined coronary artery disease. Ann. Intern. Med., *84:*241, 1976.

Erdos, E.G.: The kinins, a status report. Biochem. Pharmacol., *25:*1563, 1976.

Gresham, G.A.: Is atheroma a reversible lesion? Atherosclerosis, *23:*379, 1976.

Gresham, G.A.: Regression of atherosclerosis? Lancet, *2:*614, 1976.

Kannel, W.B., *et al.*: Role of blood pressure in the development of congestive heart failure: the Framingham study. N. Engl. J. Med., *287:*781, 1972.

Keys, A.: Coronary heart disease—the global picture. Atherosclerosis, *22:*149, 1975.

Kuller, L.H.: Epidemiology of cardiovascular diseases: current perspectives. Am. J. Epidemiol., *104:*425, 1976.

Laragh, J.H. (ed.): Symposium on hypertension. Am. J. Med., *61:*721, 1976.

Perry, H.M., Jr., *et al.*: The biology of cadmium. *In* Burch, R.E., and Sullivan, J.F. (eds.): Symposium on trace elements. Med. Clin. North Am., *60:* 759, 1976.

Ross, R.S.: Ischemic heart disease: an overview. Am. J. Cardiol., *36:*496, 1975.

Ross, R., and Glomsett, J.A.: The pathogenesis of atherosclerosis (First of two parts). N. Engl. J. Med., *295:*369, 1976.

_____: The pathogenesis of atherosclerosis (Second of two parts). N. Engl. J. Med., *295:*420, 1976.

Schwarz, K.: Essentiality and metabolic functions of selenium. *In* Burch, R.E., and Sullivan, J.F. (eds.): Symposium on trace elements. Med. Clin. of North Am., *60:*745, 1976.

10. PREVENTION AND TREATMENT OF HYPERLIPIDEMIA

Peter T. Kuo, M.D.

Hyperlipidemia has been established as an important risk factor in atherosclerosis. A joint committee of the American Medical Association and the National Academy of Sciences, National Research Council, has considered the association between hyperlipidemia and cardiovascular health to be sufficiently strong to recommend that measurement of plasma lipid profile become "a routine part of all health maintenance physical examinations. Such measurements should be made in early adulthood. . . ."

DEFINITIONS

I. Lipids

A. Lipids are compounds that contain in their molecular structure fatty acid or its derivative. They are insoluble in water but soluble in ethyl ether, petroleum, ether, and chloroform.

B. In human nutrition and biochemistry, the common lipids include triglycerides, phospholipids, sterols, sterol esters, glycolipids, lipoproteins, and fat-soluble vitamins.

II. Plasma Lipids

Four major classes of lipids are transported in the plasma.

A. Cholesterol

1. This steroid is closely associated with other fats in the body.

2. It circulates in the blood stream as two-thirds cholesterol ester and one-third free cholesterol.

3. It is synthesized mainly by the liver and the small intestine, although it is synthesized in practically all the tissues of the body.

4. Dietary cholesterol provides a relatively small, but significant, fraction of total serum cholesterol.

5. The major pathway of its catabolism to bile acids is limited to the liver.

   a. Hypercholesterolemia has been shown to be one of the major risk factors in the development of coronary artery disease.

B. Triglycerides (TG)

1. Triglycerides are fatty acid esters of glycerol that consist of one molecule of glycerol and three molecules of fatty acids.

2. The chemical, biochemical, and physical properties of a given triglyceride depend on the carbon chain length and the degree of unsaturation of its fatty acid components.

3. Triglycerides have been strongly implicated in the etiology of atherosclerosis.

C. Phospholipids

1. Phospholipids are the building stones of biomembranes, and they participate in the transport of cholesterol from the tissue stores.

2. They contain glycerol, two fatty acids, and a phosphated nitrogenous base—choline, serine, or ethanolamine.

D. Free Fatty Acids (F.F.A.)

1. Fatty acids in food and body triglycerides usually have an even number of saturated and unsaturated carbon atoms arranged in a straight chain with a carboxyl group at one end.

2. In plasma, F.F.A. are bound to albumin.

3. The main sources of free fatty acids in the blood are

   a. Synthesis in the liver from excessive carbohydrates

   b. Hydrolysis of absorbed fats

   c. Mobilization from the adipose tissue

III. Hyperlipidemia

A. Hyperlipidemia is the presence of excess lipid(s) in the plasma.

B. The term refers to a heterogenous group of disease states which cause disturbances in synthesis, transport, metabolism, or catabolism of lipids.

C. It may be classified according to increases in cholesterol, triglyceride, or both.

D. A major problem is to set the respective normal ranges.

1. The statistical norm of the American population has been set high to exclude the upper 5% of each age group.

2. The ideal norm is a fasting cholesterol level of 220 mg./100 ml. or less and a triglyceride level below 140 mg./100 ml.

a. A part of the total cholesterol is carried as HDL. This averages approximately 45 mg./dl. in males and 55 mg./dl. in females. The remainder of serum cholesterol is LDL cholesterol.

3. A hyperlipidemic state exists whenever these levels are exceeded.

IV. Lipoproteins

A. In living organisms, nonpolar lipids are complexed with proteins for transport in the aqueous extracellular fluid.

B. Nearly all of the cholesterol, phospholipid, and triglyceride in plasma are associated with specific globulins to form lipoprotein macromolecules.

C. They can be differentiated and classified by physical or chemical systems (refrigeration, electrophoresis, ultracentrifuge, or differential ionic precipitation).

D. Forms of Lipoproteins

1. *Chylomicrons*

a. Chylomicrons are derived from dietary fat which is absorbed from the intestines.

b. They transport exogenous triglycerides from the intestines to the blood stream.

2. *VLDL (Very Low-Density Lipoproteins)*

a. VLDL are synthesized by the liver and small bowel from F.F.A., carbohydrates, glycerol, and two carbon fragments of other dietary components.

b. They carry endogenous triglycerides.

3. *ILDL (Intermediate Low-Density or Floating β-Lipoproteins)*

a. ILDL are derived from VLDL after VLDL have been divested of a portion of their TG content and some of their proteins.

b. ILDL are present in minute amounts in healthy persons and in hyperlipoproteinemic patients, other than those with Type III abnormality where they are greatly increased (see p. 140).

Table 10-1. **The Family of Plasma Lipoproteins**

Ultracentrifugation	Chylomicron	VLDL	ILDL	LDL	HDL
Density	<0.95	0.95–1.006	<1.006	1.006–1.063	1.063–1.21
Electrophoresis (Mobility)	Origin	Pre-β	β	β	α
Size (Å)	750–10,000	300–800	250–400	200–220	75–100
% Composition					
Protein	2	10	10	25	50
Cholesterol	5	12	30	50	20
Triglycerides	90	60	40	10	5
Phospholipids	3	18	20	15	25

HDL=high-density lipoproteins

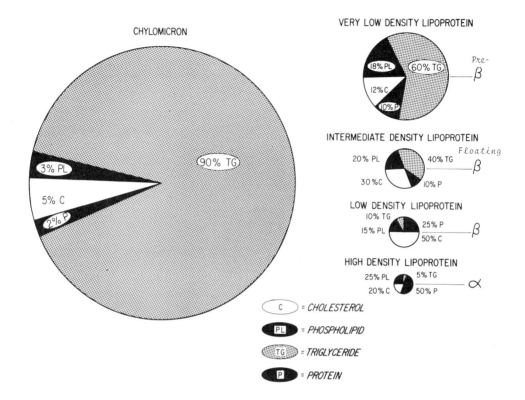

Fig. 10-1. The lipoproteins.

4. *LDL (Low-Density or β-Lipoproteins)*

a. In healthy persons, VLDL in circulation are degraded by lipoprotein lipase with removal of much of their triglycerides to form LDL by means of a transient intermediary step of ILDL transformation.

b. About 60% of the total serum cholesterol is contained in LDL.

c. LDL are removed slowly by the liver.

5. *HDL (High-Density or α-Lipoproteins)*

a. HDL probably are produced chiefly by the liver.

b. HDL transport cholesterol out of the tissues and facilitate cholesterol-ester metabolism.

E. The differentiating characteristics of the different plasma lipoprotein species are shown in Table 10-1.

GENERAL CONSIDERATIONS

I. The four major plasma lipid components of concern to clinicians are cholesterol and its esterified form, triglyceride, phospholipids, and free fatty acids.

A. Active participation of free fatty acid in physiologic and metabolic activities causes its concentration to fluctuate rapidly and widely in plasma, and, therefore, it is not a diagnostic index of hyperlipidemia.

B. Phospholipids are involved in normal cellular function and in atherogenesis, but knowledge of their contribution is quite limited. Their plasma levels do not appear to have a distinctive differential diagnostic value in the common clinical types of hyperlipidemia.

C. Most long-range epidemiologic and clinical studies have been concerned with serum cholesterol elevations in the development of atherosclerosis.

D. Recently, serum triglyceride levels have received more recognition as an independent risk factor in atherosclerosis, since hypertriglyceridemia has been associated with clinical coronary artery disease.

II. A significant increase in any one of the lipoprotein classes may result in hypercholesterolemia, hypertriglyceridemia, or in variable combinations of both.

CLASSIFICATION OF HYPERLIPOPROTEINEMIAS

I. Hyperlipoproteinemias have been classified into Types I through V, based on the differences in elevation of one or more plasma lipoprotein fractions, to assist in prognosis and to indicate appropriate nutritional therapy. These lipoprotein classes are shown diagramatically in Figure 10-1. This system recently has been modified by subdividing the original Type-II pattern into Types IIa and IIb.

A. Type I indicates a more or less "pure" increase in chylomicrons, caused by

an inborn deficiency in lipoprotein lipase (triglyceride lipase).

B. Types IIa and IIb signify an abnormal increase in LDL cholesterol. Type IIb is characterized by a combined increase in cholesterol, triglyceride, and their carriers (LDL and VLDL, with preponderance of LDL).

C. Type-III abnormality indicates an increase in floating β or a species of β-migrating VLDL (electrophoresis) which have a higher cholesterol content than the normal VLDL.

D. VLDL elevation is common in Types IV and V, but in the latter type, in addition to VLDL increase, the patient has chylomicronemia after a 12 to 14-hour fast.

II. The correlation of the five types of hyperlipoproteinemia with plasma lipid abnormalities is shown in Table 10-2.

III. Recently a combined hyperlipidemia was described. In this type, a heterogeneous array of lipoprotein patterns (Types IIa, IIb, IV, and V) was observed in family members of patients with hyperlipidemic myocardial infarction.

IV. While increases in LDL and their associated metabolic abnormalities are implicated in atherosclerosis, an increase in HDL tends to facilitate the transport of cholesterol from tissue deposits to the liver for catabolism and may have an anti-

Table 10-2. **Relationships of Plasma Lipoproteins to Hyperlipidemia**

Types		Serum Cholesterol	Serum Triglycerides
I	Hyperchylomicronemia (genetic)	⟶ or 1+	4+
IIa	↑LDL	3–4+	⟶ or 1+
IIb	↑LDL and VLDL	2–3+	2–3+
III	Floating β (ILDL)	3+	3+
IV	↑VLDL	⟶ or 1–2+	2–4+
V	↑Chylomicrons and VLDL	⟶ or 1–2+	4+

⟶=normal range
1+ to 4+ =degrees of severity
LDL=low-density lipoproteins
VLDL=very low-density lipoproteins
ILDL=intermediate low-density lipoproteins

atherogenic effect. For this reason, specific measurements of HDL are now being recommended by many authorities as a prognostic factor for coronary artery disease.

A. The greater the proportion of cholesterol carried in the low-density lipoproteins (LDL cholesterol), the greater the risk of developing coronary atherosclerosis.

B. Conversely, the higher the ratio of HDL cholesterol to LDL cholesterol, the lower the risk of developing coronary artery disease.

V. Familial Hyperlipidemia.

A. Familial hyperlipidemia has been classified into three types: hyupercholesterolemia, hypertriglyceridemia, and combined hyperlipidemia.

B. Table 10-3 shows the correlation between the six types of hyperlipoproteinemia and the three familial hyperlipidemia classification systems.

C. Since clinical experiences indicate that a large number of coronary artery disease patients manifest mild to moderate increases in plasma cholesterol, triglyceride, and their transporting lipoproteins (LDL and VLDL), this "mixed" nonfamilial hyperlipidemia is also listed in the table for comparative study.

HYPERLIPIDEMIA

I. Incidence and Transmission

A. Familial hypercholesterolemia (Type-II hyperlipoproteinemia) is the most common hyperlipidemia in children.

B. Hypertriglyceridemia (Type-IV abnormality) is the most frequently encountered in adolescents and adults.

C. Both of these genetic types are shown to be of autosomal dominant transmission.

II. Serum Cholesterol and Triglyceride Levels

A. The ideal norms for serum triglyceride and cholesterol in Americans eating a regular diet should range below 140 mg./dl. and 200 mg./dl. respectively. The ideal norm for LDL cholesterol should range

Table 10-3. **Hyperlipoproteinemia vs Hyperlipidemia Systems of Classification**

Hyperlipidemia Genetic Types*	Hyperlipoproteinemia Phenotypes†	Plasma Lipids		
		Cholesterol	Triglyceride	LDL Cholesterol
—	Type I	Normal or medium high	Very high	Low or normal
Familial hypercholesterolemia	Types IIa and IIb	High	Normal or mild increase	High
—	Type III	High	High	Normal or mild increase
Familial hypertriglyceridemia	Type IV	Normal or mild increase	High	Normal
Familial hypertriglyceridemia	Type V	Normal or mild increase	High	Normal
Combined hyperlipidemia	Types IIb or IV (family members with Types IIb, IV, and V)	High normal or high	High normal or high	High or normal
Mixed hyperlipidemia	Types IIb, III, IV (II+IV)	Normal or high	High	Normal or high

*Goldstein's classifications
†Fredrickson's classifications

below 170 mg./dl., after the commonly adopted automated procedures is standardized against the original manual method.

B. A child born and living in the U.S. or Europe should be considered to have hyperlipidemia when his serum cholesterol or TG exceed 190 mg./dl. or 120 mg./dl., respectively.

C. The truly ideal norm for serum cholesterol in adults may be as low as 150 to 170 mg./dl., as observed in underdeveloped countries, where the incidence of atherosclerosis is far lower than in the Western world.

D. Some authorities contend that the normal serum lipid values should be allowed to rise with advancing age, and they have set an age-adjusted lipid level.

1. The value of this definition of normality is difficult to measure, since atherosclerosis may not produce clinical symptoms in some persons for prolonged periods of time.

2. Normal serum lipid levels, like weight norms, should probably be considered the same for adults of any age.

III. Differential Diagnosis

A. Prior to the institution of any form of therapy, secondary causes should be diagnosed.

B. Among the more common conditions to be excluded are: hypercholesterolemia due to hypothyroidism or occult diabetes mellitus, alcohol-induced hypertriglyceridemia, hepatic and renal diseases, and side effects of certain drugs.

C. A more complete list of these conditions follows.

Secondary Causes of Hyperlipidemia

Metabolism and physiology
   Weight gain in adults
   Pregnancy
   High CHO, high calorie diet
Diet
   High saturated fat
   Alcohol-induction
   High calorie and high CHO

Medication
   Estrogens
   Contraceptive pills
   Steroids
   Thiazides
Disease
   Hypothyroidism
   Diabetes
      Insulin deficient
      Adult onset type
   Renal disease
      Nephrosis
      Chronic failure
   Obstructive jaundice
   Porphyria
   Dysproteinemia

D. Treatment of a secondary hyperlipidemia should be directed to the basic disease.

E. If the basic disease is managed successfully, the blood lipid abnormality will be automatically corrected.

DIETARY TREATMENT OF HYPERLIPIDEMIA

I. General Considerations

A. Diet is recognized as one of the chief environmental determinants of serum cholesterol and triglyceride levels and is the keystone of therapy for all types of hyperlipidemias.

B. High cholesterol, saturated fat, and sugar intakes have been linked conclusively with serum cholesterol and triglyceride elevations and increased morbidity and mortality from coronary artery disease (CAD).

C. Reducing the quantities of these dietary substances would produce a drop in serum lipids and perhaps a lowering of the incidence of coronary artery disease (CAD).

D. Dietary saturated fats and cholesterol have been shown to alter the function of the platelets and to increase their tendency to aggregate and induce thrombosis.

E. Platelet aggregation could be reduced by a diet with a high polyunsaturated fat to saturated fat ratio.

F. Although a high caloric intake has an inconsistent effect upon the adipose tissue mass of a person, it would act to aggravate hyperlipidemia, diabetes, and hypertension.

G. Other dietary factors such as greater amounts of ascorbic acid, α-tocopherol, vegetable sterols, and fiber have been considered to be desirable. The therapeutic role of these items is not yet clear, but it is safe to assume that deficiency of essential vitamins is not desirable.

H. Prevention of Hyperlipidemia

1. Atherosclerosis is not peculiar to older persons. There is ample autopsy evidence of significant atherosclerosis occurring during the first two decades of life in clinically healthy persons.

2. It has been found that the combination of elevated cholesterol and TG carries a high risk of coronary artery disease.

3. These observations suggest the desirability of screening infants and children for hyperlipidemia to initiate long-term control of hyperlipidemic children.

4. Diet should be emphasized in the treatment of hyperlipidemic children.

I. In order to achieve a significant reduction or normalization of serum lipid value in a given patient, the dietary therapy should be tailored to the type of lipoprotein abnormality demonstrated.

II. Type-I Hyperlipoproteinemia Diet

A. Deficiency in chylomicron glyceride hydrolyzing enzyme-lipoprotein lipase (triglyceride lipase) in Type-I abnormality, markedly delays the "clearance" of absorbed dietary fat from the blood stream to produce massive chylomicronemia.

B. This causes abdominal crisis, acute pancreatitis, and eruptive xanthoma.

C. Severe dietary fat restriction is required to reduce chylomicronemia.

1. In most instances, daily dietary fat (saturated or unsaturated) intake should be reduced from the average 80 to 100 g. to 20 to 30 g. to lower serum triglyceride concentration to levels below

1,000 mg./dl. and thus prevent attacks of abdominal crisis.

2. Because the fat content of meat is high, intake should be limited to 3 to 4 oz. of lean meat per day. Preferably, white meat of fowl and low-fat fish should be substituted for meat.

3. Total caloric intake can be augmented by extra carbohydrates and supplemental medium-chain triglycerides (MCT; see MCT diet, Chap. 12). MCT are absorbed by means of portal circulation and are not incorporated into chylomicrons.

III. Type-II Hyperlipoproteinemia Diet

A. In familial hypercholesterolemia (Type IIa), it is imperative to lower cholesterol intake to below 250 to 300 mg./day and to lower saturated fat content of the regular American diet by 50 to 70%.

B. Substituting moderate amounts of polyunsaturated oils for saturated fat has been recommended to accomplish additional hypocholesterolemic effect.

1. The ratio of polyunsaturated to saturated fatty acids in the regular American diet is estimated at 0.3:1.0.

2. The ratio of polyunsaturated fat to saturated fat should be raised to 1.5:1.0 to 2.0:1.0 for optimal beneficial effect.

C. When pure hypercholesterolemia is accompanied by mild to moderate serum triglyceride elevation (Type IIb), additional measures should be taken to control overweight (if present) and to curb the intake of alcoholic beverages and foods high in carbohydrate, especially simple sugars.

IV. Type-III Hyperlipoproteinemia Diet

A. Although weight reduction is desirable in the treatment of any type of hyperlipoproteinemia, it is especially important in patients with Type-III abnormality, the majority of whom are moderately overweight.

B. Weight reduction can best be accomplished by prescribing a 35 to 40% low-carbohydrate diet with emphasis on the restriction of alcohol, cereals containing sugar, desserts, snacks, and soft drinks.

C. This dietary modification is also effective in the control of other types of hyperlipidemia (hypertriglyceridemia in particular).

D. Moderate reduction of cholesterol intake by restricting egg yolk and rich dairy products is recommended for patients who continue to manifest hypercholesterolemia while on a relatively low-carbohydrate diet.

V. Type-IV and Type-V Hyperlipoproteinemia Diet

A. Chylomicrons and VLDL share a common enzyme system for their clearance from the blood stream.

1. An increase in non-fat caloric intake could induce a Type-V pattern (VLDL elevation and chylomicronemia) in a patient with severe Type-IV abnormality (VLDL elevation only).

2. For this reason, both Types IV and V can be managed with the same dietary plan.

B. Weight reduction of overweight patients to their ideal body weight, if possible, is of primary importance.

1. Reduction of carbohydrate calories to 35 to 40% of total daily calories is recommended to attain and maintain lean body weight.

2. In milder cases, the use of diet alone could result in reverting hypertriglyceridemia to the range of normal.

C. Controlled metabolic studies show that if calorie-dense simple sugars and sugar-containing foods and drinks were eliminated from the diet, most patients would be able to tolerate the regular amount of carbohydrate calories supplied by bulky starchy foods customarily consumed in three regular meals.

1. It is estimated that this simple dietary maneuver, coupled with omission of snacks of dehydrated carbohydrate preparations, should lower the total carbohy-

Table 10-4. **Principles of Dietary Plans Used in the Treatment of High Coronary-Disease-Risk Hyperlipidemias**

Types of Hyperlipidemia (Hyperlipoproteinemia)	Dietary Modifications				
	Cholesterol	Saturated Fat	Poly-unsaturated	Carbohydrates	Alcohol
Hypercholesterolemia (Type IIa)	<250 mg./day No egg yolk, rich dairy products, organ meats	↓4+ of meat More fish and fowl	↑Corn- or safflower oil or polyunsaturated margarine	Regular amounts	Cocktails not excessive
Hypertriglyceridemia (Type IV)	<350 mg./day 2–3 eggs/week Low in dairy products	↓2+ of meat More fish and fowl	Regular amounts	↓4+ No simple sugars	↓4+ Occasional cocktail
Combined or "Mixed" Hyperlipidemia	<350 mg./day 2–3 eggs/week No rich dairy products or organ meats	"	↑Corn- or safflower oil or unsaturated fat margarine	↓3+ No simple sugars	↓3+ Cocktail once/week

↓and the accompanying numbers (1–4+)=mild–moderate–severe degrees of reduction.

drate intake to about 125 to 150 g./day, which is adequate for maintenance of normal metabolism and nutrition.

2. In addition to their high caloric value, it has been postulated that fructose and sucrose (with its fructose moiety) can promote greater glyceride synthesis and can facilitate weaker glyceride clearance from the blood stream than glucose (derived from starches).

D. Alcohol is known to exert a profound influence on lipid metabolism through a number of lipogenic and lipolytic mechanisms involving the hepatic and adipose tissues.

1. An alcohol-induced hyperlipemia has been differentiated from the common carbohydrate-induced form.

2. It is advisable for the hypertriglyceridemic patients to stop having daily cocktails and to limit alcohol intake to one or two drinks on weekends.

VI. Principles of the dietary treatment of the three types of hyperlipidemia that are known to increase the risk of coronary artery disease are tabulated in Table 10-4.

VII. Table 10-5 gives the details of a low-cholesterol-, low-saturated-fat-, and low-simple-carbohydrate diet which can be given to patients with hypertriglyceridemia and combined or mixed hyperlipidemia (e.g., Types IIb, III, IV, and V). This diet also can be used for hypercholesterolemia (Type-II hyperlipoproteinemia), except that carbohydrates need not be limited unless there is a weight problem. Alcohol should still be used with discretion. In Type IIa, cholesterol should be restricted to 300 mg. per day.

DRUG TREATMENT OF HYPERLIPIDEMIA

I. Indications

The primary indication for treatment of hyperlipidemia is to prevent atherosclerosis and its complications.

A. The benefits of treatment are not conclusively proven.

B. Possible adverse side effects of antilipemic drugs are not completely understood. Such drugs should be used with caution.

C. There could be a justification for prescribing long-term drug treatment provided that:

1. Diagnosis of a primary hyperlipidemia known to predispose to premature atherosclerotic arterial disease has been made.

2. A thorough trial of dietary therapy has been made and maintained, even if the alteration from baseline level has been minimal.

D. The physician should advise continual adherence to the specific diet, while an appropriate drug is added to the program for synergistic effect.

E. Non-adherence to dietary treatment is not an indication for the use of a drug in its place, because the question of compliance will remain.

F. Satisfactory control of lipid abnormality is impossible to accomplish with the use of currently available drugs alone.

G. When a partial (about 15 to 20%) hypolipemic response is already accomplished by dietary therapy, an antilipemic drug may be used to further normalize the elevated levels.

II. Rationale

A. The rationale for drug treatment of hyperlipemia when diet alone is not successful goes beyond the prevention and treatment of coronary artery disease.

B. It includes:

1. Reduction of chylomicronemia to prevent attacks of abdominal crisis with or without acute pancreatitis

2. Lowering the VLDL, ILDL, and LDL concentrations to facilitate clearance of eruptive, palmar, tendinous, and tuberous xanthomas for cosmetic and functional reasons

C. Tables 10-6 and 10-7 give the choice of drug(s) according to the types of hyper-

(Text continues on p. 148)

Table 10-5. Low-Cholesterol-, Low-Saturated-Fat-, and Low-Simple-Carbohydrate Diet

Principle: This diet is designed to lower cholesterol and other blood fats associated with cardiovascular disease in carbohydrate-sensitive persons with high blood lipid levels.

General Rules:

1. The diet is to be ordered specifically for the individual patient. This is a very basic diet, and alterations are made by the physician according to the severity of the lipemia.

2. The diet is to reduce sucrose, fructose, lactose or, glucose intake. Total carbohydrate content is 125 to 150 g./day.

3. Fats and oils with a high degree of short- or medium-chain fatty acids are to be avoided (saturated fats and coconut oil).

4. Alcohol consumption is restricted or eliminated as directed.

5. Any commercially packaged or prepared foods containing butter, coconut oil, milk solids, cream, or sugar should be used sparingly.

6. There is no restriction on the normal use of either the amount or kind of proteins or oils (except excessive meat fats and butterfat) unless the total calorie level is to be reduced.

7. Snacks between meals and after dinner should be avoided.

Include Each Day	
Food Group	*Amount*
Vegetables Group A (leafy)	As desired
Vegetables Group B (starchy)	1 serving, as side-dish
Bread or substitute	1-2 servings
Eggs	Egg white or yolk-free egg substitute
Meat, fish, fowl	Red meat 2-3 times a week; mainly fish and fowl
Fat	Unsaturated fat and unsaturated fat margarine for cooking and bread-spread.

Suggested Daily Meal Plan	
Breakfast	
Unsweetened vegetable or tomato juice	Small glass
Cereals	Cooked cereals or 1–2 slices of bread
Egg substitute	1–2
Fat	Corn, safflower, soya oil (margarine) for bread-spread or cooking
Beverage	Coffee/tea, black
Meat or substitute	3–4 oz. fowl, sardine, salmon, smoked fish
Dinner	
Soup, broth base	1 bowl
Meat or substitute	4–5 oz. fish or fowl
Vegetables Group A	As desired
Vegetables Group B	1 serving
Bread	1–2 slices
Fat	Corn oil, oleo (unsaturated fat)
Beverage	Coffee/tea, black
Dessert	Avoid dessert or have 1 piece fresh fruit
Supper	
Soup, broth base	1 bowl
Meat, fish, fowl	4–6 oz. meat or substitute
Vegetables Group A	As desired
Vegetables Group B	1 serving
Fat	Corn oil/oleo for bread-spread and cooking
Bread	1–2 slices
Beverage	Tea/coffee, black
Salad	Oil and vinegar
Dessert	Fresh fruit, 1 piece

Table 10-5. **Low-Cholesterol-, Low-Saturated-Fat-, and Low-Simple-Carbohydrate Diet** *(Cont.)*

	Foods Allowed	*Foods Omitted*
Beverages	Coffee, tea, decaffeinated beverages, unsweetened carbonated beverages, unsweetened Kool-Aid, skim milk	All milk and milk products; sweetened drinks and fruitades; yogurt; sweetened cocoa
Bread	Corn–1/3 cup Cooked cereal–1/2 cup Matzo, plain or wheat –1 wafer Bread–1 slice Bagel–3/4 Potato, white–1/2 cup Potato, sweet–1/4 cup Rice, cooked–1/2 cup Spaghetti, cooked–1/2 cup Dried beans and peas, cooked–1/2 cup Flour–3 tbsp. Parsnips–2/3 cup Lima beans, fresh or frozen–1/2 cup	Cereals that contain sugar, milk solids, graham crackers, muffins, biscuits, cornbread, pancakes, waffles, fritters, all others that contain sugar, milk solids, butter, sweetened cocoa
Cheese	None	All
Desserts	Sugar-free gelatin desserts; occasionally one piece of fresh fruit a day	All containing sugar, cream, milk and milk solids, butter, coconut, egg yolk (e.g., pies, cakes, pastries, sherbet, ice cream, cookies)
Eggs	One daily, maximum, prepared with allowed fat.	Any in excess of one daily and prepared with milk, cream, butter
Fats	Margarine—not to contain milk solids or coconut oil, mayonnaise, vegetable oils, salad dressing—not containing sugar or coconut oil	Coconut oil, butter, margarine containing milk solids or coconut oil, sugar-cured bacon, peanut butter, sugar-coated nuts
Fruits	One piece a day	All
Soups and sauces	Broth base soups made with foods allowed	All soups and sauces made with milk or cream, sauces containing sugar
Sweets	None	All candy, jelly, honey, molasses, marshmallows, syrups
Vegetables	Refer to Group A-Group B exchange servings below.	All if prepared with butter or saturated margarine or cream sauce, glazed or containing sugar
Miscellaneous	Vinegar, herbs, spices, artificial sweeteners (not containing lactose), dill pickles, catsup (may be used sparingly), dry unsweetened cocoa	Peanut butter, coconut, sweet relish, artificial sweeteners that contain lactose, non-dairy milk, sugar-coated nuts
Meat, fish, fowl	All meats, fish, fowl that are not omitted, lean fresh pork	Any sugar-cured, pickled, or containing sugar, luncheon meats, scrapple, frankfurters

(Continued)

Table 10-5. **Low-Cholesterol-, Low-Saturated-Fat-, and Low-Simple-Carbohydrate Diet** *(Cont.)*

Vegetables		
Group A (Leafy; Amounts not restricted)		
Asparagus	Eggplant	Radishes
Broccoli	All greens	Sauerkraut
Cabbage	Lettuce	String beans
Cauliflower	Mushrooms	Summer squash
Celery	Okra	Tomato juice, unsweetened
Cucumbers	Pepper	
Group B (Starchy; Amounts restricted) (Serving of 1/2 cup)		
Beets	Green Peas	Winter Squash
Carrots	Onions	Turnips

lipoproteinemia, their therapeutic dosages, possible side effects, and drug interactions.

III. Mechanisms of Action of Commonly Used Hypolipemic Drugs

A. Drugs That Increase Lipoprotein Catabolism

    1. Cholestyramine

        a. This is a water-insoluble resin that exchanges chloride ion for bile acids at the level of the small intestine.

        b. The drug forms an insoluble complex with bile acids to increase the enterohepatic cholesterol degradation and its excretion as acidic steroids (bile acids).

        c. This increased cholesterol catabolism probably accelerates the catabolism of LDL.

        d. Recent studies suggest that, in familial hypercholesterolemia (Type-II abnormality), there is a defect in cellular (cholesterol) LDL binding, leading to decreased rate of LDL catabolism, as well as increased rate of cholesterol synthesis.

        e. Hence, cholestyramine is the drug of choice for patients with familial hypercholesterolemia (Type-IIa abnormality).

    2. Colestipol

        a. This is a new synthetic organic bile acid sequestrant copolymer.

        b. It is insoluble in water.

        c. Like cholestyramine, it acts to lower serum cholesterol by increasing fecal excretion of bile acids and to increase cholesterol turnover, which is followed by reduction in plasma LDL level.

        d. In cross-over study, colestipol at 20 g./day and cholestyramine at the same dosage have essentially the equivalent effect.

    3. Dextrothyroxine

        a. This is the dextrorotatory isomer of *l*-thyroxine.

        b. Dextrothyroxine lowers serum cholesterol chiefly by increased cholesterol catabolism and increased LDL removal but with a lower hypermetabolic effect than thyroxine.

        c. At higher dosages of 6 to 8 mg./day, usually required for hypolipemic effect, the drug can significantly elevate body metabolism, aggravate myocardial ischemia, and initiate cardiac arrhythmia.

        d. Use of the drug should be limited to hypercholesterolemic patients who have not yet developed any significant cardiovascular disease.

    4. β-Sitosterol

        a. This is an older preparation which may increase LDL catabolism by means of fecal cholesterol loss. A few persons, however, may absorb plant sterols and cause increased cholesterol levels and xanthomata.

        b. It contains a mixture of plant sterols that acts to inhibit cholesterol absorption by a competitive mechanism.

c. The recently improved formula is recommended for the treatment of Type-II hyperlipoproteinemia, but the hypocholesterolemic effect is relatively mild.

B. Drugs That Decrease Lipoprotein Production

1. *Clofibrate (Atromid-S)*

a. Clofibrate is a branched-chain fatty acid ester.

b. The most important action of the drug is thought to be an inhibition of VLDL synthesis and secretion by the liver.

c. Since several other effects upon lipid metabolism have also been demonstrated, these may contribute to the resultant hypolipemic effect.

d. The precise mechanism of action of clofibrate is not fully understood at this time.

e. It has been shown to be of clinical value in the control of Type-III hyperlipoproteinemia and to have an adjunctive role in the treatment of hypertriglyceridemia or Type-IV hyperlipoproteinemia.

f. While clofibrate lowers VLDL triglycerides and VLDL cholesterol, it tends to increase LDL cholesterol in some patients.

g. Its value in treating Type-II abnormality (pure hypercholesterolemia) is limited.

2. *Nicotinic Acid*

a. Nicotinic acid is a metabolic product of tryptophan and a member of the B-vitamin group.

b. The hypolipemic dosage of nicotinic acid is many times higher than that prescribed for its vitamin effect. This causes extreme flushing, itching, and other annoying side effects. Some tachyphylaxis to these symptoms develops after a few weeks.

c. In large doses, nicotinic acid probably works by several mechanisms to lower serum lipid concentration.

(1) One of the best known actions of the drug is in inhibiting lipolysis of triglycerides from the adipose stores to decrease the free fatty acid flux to the liver for triglyceride and VLDL synthesis.

(2) Experimental studies show that nicotinic acid inhibits cholesterol synthesis and facilitates catabolism of VLDL and chylomicrons.

d. If it can be tolerated by the patient, it is useful in a wide variety of hyperlipidemias—Types IIa, IIb, III, IV, and V.

3. *Para-aminosalicylic acid (PAS)*

a. This is a well-known antituberculous drug.

b. A purer preparation is obtained by recrystallizing it in vitamin C, PAS-C (Hellwig).

c. The preparation, well tolerated by patients with Type-IIa and -IIb hyperlipoproteinemias, reduces both serum cholesterol and triglyceride concentrations.

d. One of the pharmacological activities of the drug is to inhibit hepatic cholesterol and triglyceride synthesis.

4. *Probucol (Lorelco)*

a. This is a new drug which appears to have a moderate cholesterol-low-

Table 10-6. **Hypolipemic Drugs (Increase Lipoprotein Catabolism)**

Drug	Indications	Dosage	Drug Interactions	Side Effects
Cholestyramine	↑LDL (Type II)	12–32 g./day	Decreased absorption of digitalis, thyroid	Nausea, constipation
Colestipol		15–30 g./day	Warfarin	Steatorrhea
Sodium dextrothyroxine (Choloxin)	↑LDL or ILDL (Types II, III)	4–8 mg./day	Increased Coumadin effect	Increased metabolism
Sitosterol (Cytellin)	↑LDL (Type II)	30 ml. four times a day	—	Nausea, vomiting, diarrhea

ering action. Its effect on triglycerides is variable.

b. Its mechanism of action is not fully understood.

b. Its principal effect is in lowering LDL cholesterol (primary hypercholesterolemia). It may be effective where other drugs have not been.

d. A rise in triglycerides may occur while on probucol therapy, especially when all dietary measures have not been strictly complied with.

EFFICACY OF ANTILIPEMIC THERAPY

I. Data suggest that antilipemic therapy is clinically of value.

A. There is a slow but definite exchange of cholesterol between the plasma and the atherosclerotic lesions.

B. In early lesions, the lipid deposits can be removed within a reasonable period of time.

1. Experiments on rhesus monkeys have shown that animals fed American Heart Association prudent diets developed few or no significant arterial lesions as compared with animals fed typical high-cholesterol high-fat American diets.

2. There is radiographic evidence of regression of atherosclerotic lesions in the peripheral arteries after hypolipemic therapy.

C. The author and his co-workers performed serial coronary arteriograms on 12 well-controlled atherosclerotic and hyperlipidemic patients and on a group of matched controls, over a period of 8 years.

1. The lesions of 10 treated patients remained essentially stable.

2. The treated patients also showed significant improvements in both subjective and objective symptoms of ischemia.

3. Two patients in the untreated control group have died, and all in this group have shown clinical and laboratory evidences of deterioration.

4. It is the author's opinion that permanent alteration in dietary habits and the maintenance of lean body weight were the main ingredients for success in the treated patients.

D. There are other reports of success, such as the improvement of peripheral arterial circulation in Type-III patients by investigators from the National Heart and Lung Institute.

E. Dramatic results have been obtained in a small number of patients undergoing ileal bypass operations, continual plasma exchange, and portacaval shunt, where the procedure corrected the hyperlipidemia.

II. The data on improvement in human

Table 10-7. **Hypolipemic Drugs (Decrease Lipoprotein Synthesis)**

Drug	Indications	Dosage	Drug Interactions	Side Effects
Clofibrate (Atromid S)	↑ILDL (Type III) ↑VLDL (Types IV and V)	2 g./day (1 g. twice daily)	↑Hypoprothrombin effect of Coumadin	Nausea, diarrhea, myositis
Nicotinic acid	↑ILDL, ↑VLDL ↑LDL	1–6 g./day	Exaggerated vasodilating and hypotensive effects of ganglionic blocking agents	Flushing, nausea diarrhea, hepatotoxicity, ↓glucose tolerance
Para-amino-salicylic acid	↑LDL	6–10 g./day	Effect nullified by alcohol	Nausea, diarrhea, hypothyroidism
Probucol (Lorelco)	TLDL (Type II)	500 mg. twice daily	No effects on coumadin	Diarrhea, nausea, flatulence

atherosclerosis are still far too few to have reached statistical significance, although the data so far available are encouraging.
III. There is reason to believe that primary prevention would be more effective than secondary intervention measures.

A. Data obtained from autopsy studies on children and young adults have shown conclusively that coronary artery disease begins in early life and progresses at variable rates toward eventual occlusion of the coronary and cerebral vessels.

B. One of the more effective ways to prevent disability and death due to atherosclerosis would be early detection and control of hyperlipidemia in children with family histories of this disorder.

C. Pediatricians and nutritionists are placing increased emphasis on early diagnosis and on early use of dietary management of hyperlipidemia for the prevention or retardation of atherosclerosis and its complications.

D. Diet alone, and not hypolipemic drugs, should be used in treating children and adolescents with hyperlipidemia unless they have familial hypercholesterolemia, (Type IIa).
IV. Experience gained from treating hyperlipidemia for primary and secondary prevention of atherosclerosis suggests a need for fulfilling the following conditions.

A. Accurate identification of the specific type of hyperlipidemia in terms of lipoprotein(s) abnormality and the underlying metabolic-genetic abnormality

B. Diet therapy which is specific for the control of the apparent lipid-lipoprotein abnormality

C. Identification and treatment of secondary hyperlipidemia, by attending to the primary disorder.

D. Modification of the regimen on the basis of subsequent alterations in the serum lipoprotein pattern following the initial diet therapy program.

E. If the lipid abnormality is of the primary type, and if it does not show satisfactory response to the prescribed diet, the dietary therapy should be supplemented, but never liberalized, with a hypolipemic drug chosen for its specific action, to obtain a synergistic effect. Not infrequently, both a drug which increases lipid catabolism and one that decreases lipid synthesis may be required.

F. Therapy should be individualized to include control of all other known major risk factors which are present (e.g., smoking and hypertension).

G. The diet regimen should be maintained for life when there is a known disturbance in lipid-lipoprotein metabolism.

11. SURGICAL NUTRITION

George L. Blackburn, M.D., Ph.D.

Baltej S. Maini, M.D.

Bruce R. Bistrian, M.D., M.P.H., Ph.D.

Joanne E. Wade, R.D.

Significant advances in diagnostic methods, surgical techniques, postoperative monitoring, and care of critically ill patients have favorably altered morbidity and mortality. For optimal results, however, nutritional therapy should be an integral part of present-day life support systems. Basic knowledge in this field is essential in order to formulate a rational approach to surgical nutrition.

I. Metabolic Response to Injury

A. Significant changes in body metabolism occur secondary to trauma, surgical injury, and infection and are characterized by a biphasic hormonal response (Fig. 11-1).

B. Acute Phase

1. In the acute phase, the hormonal profile is mediated through the sympathetic nervous system and is associated with the release of substrate-mobilizing hormones.

2. Associated anorexia produces a low-calorie- and low-protein dietary intake, which, together with a glucocorticoid-induced catabolism of peripheral protein, results in a negative nitrogen balance.

3. The mobilization of skeletal muscle has purposes other than simply providing precursors for gluconeogenesis and increasing urea nitrogen excretion.

    a. This phenomenon probably represents a redistribution of body reserves to meet the amino acid requirements for the synthesis of acute phase proteins.

    b. This response is in contrast to that seen in starvation without injury, in which initial losses are largely from labile visceral protein sources. Only after approximately 4 days of starvation does considerable mobilization of skeletal protein begin to occur.

4. Glucocorticoids and other hormones antagonize the action of insulin in the peripheral tissues during the acute phase with the participation of polypeptides, kinins, and leukocytic endogenous mediators.

    a. This hormonal interaction leads to a temporary sacrifice of carcass protein

	"Ebb Phase"	"Flow Phase" → Convalescence	
		"Acute Phase"	"Adaptive Phase"
DOMINANT FACTORS:	Inadequate circulation	Catecholamines	Glucocorticoid
SYMPTOMS:	Hyperglycemia Hyperlactic	Hyperglycemia	Hyperglycemia
		Low insulin	High insulin
	Hyperacidemia		

When compared to equivalent *Food Deprivation WITHOUT Trauma:*

Fat Mobilization is:		Activated	Curtailed
Nitrogen Losses:		May be less!	Increased

Fig. 11-1. Metabolic response to injury. The sequence of hormone and substrate changes during injury are depicted. (Blackburn, G.L., and Bistrian, B.R.: Nutritional care of the injured and/or septic patient. Surg. Clin. North Am. *56[5]:* 1197, 1976)

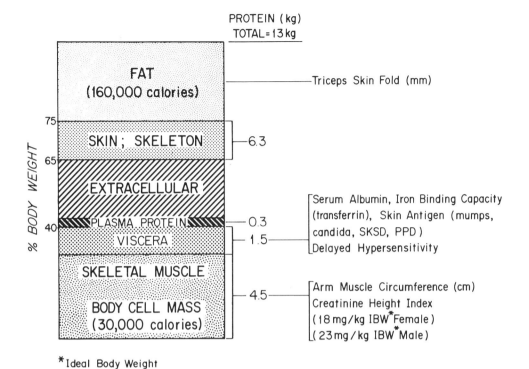

Fig. 11-2. Nutritional assessment for protein-calorie malnutrition based on distribution of body tissue compartments. (Blackburn, G.L., *et al.*: Nutritional and metabolic assessment of the hospitalized patient. J. Am. Soc. Parenteral Enteral Nutr., *1*:11, 1977)

in favor of maintaining an abundance of circulating energy substrates.

    b. Accompanying this response is the mobilization of fat reserves as free fatty acids to meet cellular energy demands.

  C. Adaptive Phase

    1. An adaptive phase follows, during which cellular mechanisms adapt to changes in the nature and sources of energy.

    2. A fall in blood glucose and urinary urea nitrogen excretion, appearance of ketone bodies, and low levels of circulating catecholamines and glucocorticoids are noted.

    3. The appearance of this phase is dependent upon

      a. Degree of hypermetabolism

      b. Presence or absence of sepsis

      c. Associated nutritional deficits

    4. Substantial nutritional repletion during the adaptive phase is possible. This leads to ultimate recovery.

  D. The goals of a well-designed nutritional therapy plan, considering the metabolic responses associated with injury are

    1. Minimizing catabolism in the acute phase

    2. Restoration of body cell mass, particularly the visceral compartment, during the adaptive and recovery phases.

II. Nutritional and Metabolic Assessment

  A. The wide prevalence of protein-calorie malnutrition in hospitalized patients has been noted.

    1. Up to 50% of surgical patients are moderately or severely malnourished.

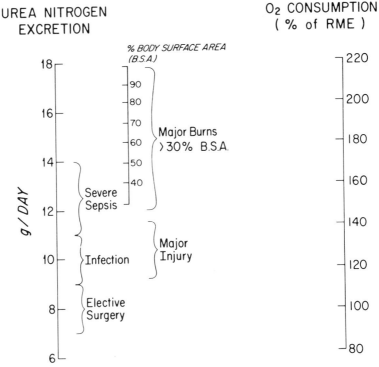

Fig. 11-3. Rates of hypermetabolism estimated from urinary urea nitrogen excretions. Energy expenditure can be estimated by urea nitrogen measurements in aliquots of 24-hour urine collections. During stress, including infection, 12 to 16% of the caloric expenditure is provided by amino acid oxidation during a low-protein or protein-free diet, thus forming the foundation for this relationship. (Schneider, H. (ed.): Nutritional Support of Medical Practice. Hagerstown, Harper & Row, 1977)

2. It is now generally well accepted that the presence of malnutrition significantly affects the hospital course of patients and directly influences mortality and morbidity.

B. A nutritional and metabolic assessment includes evaluation of skeletal muscle, visceral protein- and fat reserves, and the catabolic rate.

1. A diagrammatic representation of the distribution of body fuels is made in Figure 11-2.

C. Lean Body Mass

1. A simple, but accurate method of assessing the skeletal muscle compartment is to measure mid-arm muscle circumference.

2. Estimation of the creatinine-height index (CHI) also indicates the status of muscle stores and is a very sensitive indicator of protein depletion in cachectic or marasmic states.

3. Although height-weight index gives a reasonable estimate of a patient's nutritional status, its accuracy is limited in the presence of edema.

D. Fat Stores

1. Measurement of the triceps skin fold gives a clinically useful estimate of subcutaneous fat reserves.

E. Visceral Protein

1. In stress conditions, rapid and substantial visceral protein loss can occur.

a. The severity is indicated by depletion of the secretory proteins, albumin and transferrin.

2. The cellular immune system also reflects the functional state of the visceral protein component.

a. Immune competence is estimated by the total lymphocyte count and by delayed cutaneous hypersensitivity to common recall antigens (streptokinase-streptodornase, mumps, and Candida).

F. Nutritional repletion is assessed by estimating the nitrogen balance in addition to secretory proteins and immune competence.

1. Rather than the standard time-consuming and expensive Kjeldahl's method for measuring total nitrogen, nitrogen balance can be determined clinically by the formula:

Nitrogen balance = (nitrogen in) − (nitrogen out) =

(protein intake in grams ÷ 6.25) − (24-hour urinary urea N+4)

Where 4 represents a constant for skin, fecal, and urinary non-urea nitrogen losses.

G. Rate of Hypermetabolism

1. Measurement of the 24-hour urinary urea nitrogen excretion enables one to estimate the actual metabolic expenditure (see Fig. 11-3; Table 11-1).

Table 11-1. **Classification of Surgical Patients According to Catabolic State**

Degree of net catabolism	(N obg)* g. urea N/day	% Increase of RME over BEE†
1° Normal	< 5 g.	None
2° Mild	5–10 g.	0–20
3° Moderate	10–15 g.	20–50
4° Severe	> 15 g.	> 50

*N obg: Obligate nitrogen loss expressed in g. urea Nitrogen/24 hours in a patient with no or minimal (< 20 g.) intake and 3 days of at least 100 g. carbohydrate.

†Energy expenditure is expressed as % increase of the Resting Metabolic Expenditure (RME) over calculated Basal Energy Expenditure (BEE).

(Rutten, P., Blackburn, G.L., Flatt, J.P., Hallowell, E., and Cochran, D.: Determination of optimal hyperalimentation rate. J. Surg. Res., *18:*477, 1975)

2. The Harris-Benedict equations, which take into account age, height, weight, and sex, give an estimate of the energy expenditure under basal conditions without stress or food.

3. The ratio of actual metabolic expenditure to basal energy expenditure is a reflection of the degree of catabolic stress.

H. The comprehensive nutritional and metabolic profile (see Fig. 11-4) forms the basis for determining the type of nutritional therapy and thus permits an accurate assessment of the rate of nutrition in determining the patient's hospital course.

I. A period of 2 to 3 weeks is necessary for an objective response to nutritional therapy, due to the rates of protein turnover that limit the rate of nutritional repletion.

III. Choice of Nutritional Therapy

A. A large variety of protein and non-protein calorie sources are available to the surgeon/nutritionist.

B. An optimal nutritional support plan can be formulated after considering the following:

1. Category and extent of malnutrition

2. Degree of hypermetabolism

3. Protein and calorie requirements

4. Goal of nutritional support (i.e. maintaining the patient in a fed or semi-starved state)

5. Presence of a functioning gastrointestinal tract

6. Appetite

7. Route of delivery of nutrients

8. Presence of specific organ dysfunction necessitating restriction of one or more nutrients

C. Caloric Requirements

1. A flow chart, or logic tree, is depicted in Figure 11-5. This chart will facilitate the design of a rational nutritional therapy on an individual basis.

2. The delivery of calories in parent-

SUMMARY (CHECK)			
STANDARD PARAMETERS	90%	60-90%	60%
Weight/Height			
Triceps Skinfold			
Mid Upper Arm Circumference			
Mid Upper Arm Muscle Circumference			
Albumin			
Creatinine Height Index			
Lymphocyte Count			
Iron Binding Capacity/ Transferrin			
Cellular Immunity SK/SD			
Other Candida			
D.N.C.B.			

Nutritional or Metabolic Status (Check)

90% Standard   Not Depleted
60-90%   Moderately Depleted
60% Standard   Severly Depleted

TYPE OF PROTEIN CALORIE MALNUTRITION (CHECK)

Acute Visceral Attrition (Kwashiorkor-like)
     (Wt/Ht, TSF, AC, AMC, CHI preserved; Albumin and Transferrin acutely depressed)

Adult Marasmus (Cachexia)
     (Wt/Ht, TSF, AC, AMC, CHI depressed; Albumin and Transferrin preserved until late)

Intermediate States

Acute Visceral Attrition Superimposed on Adult Marasmus
     (Wt/Ht, TSF, AC, AMC, CHI depressed; Albumin and Transferrin rapidly and acutely depressed)

PRIMARY DIAGNOSIS

Fig. 11-4. Comprehensive nutritional and metabolic profile. This detailed assessment allows an accurate evaluation of the role of nutrition in a patient's hospital course.

eral feeding at a rate of 40 to 45 Cal./kg./ day and of adequate protein (1.5 g./kg.) will produce positive nitrogen balance in patients who are mildly to moderately catabolic.

3. Oral intakes of 35 to 40 Cal./kg./ day also will result in positive nitrogen balance.

4. The difference in caloric efficiency between oral and parenteral feeding is related to route of entry (portal vein as opposed to central vein) and to the obligatory lipogenesis that occurs secondary to hyper-insulinemia from the constant infusion of dextrose.

5. Caloric intakes greater than 40 Cal./kg./day, in the form of hyperalimentation solutions, can result in hypermetabolism.

a. However, intakes in excess of 45 Cal./kg./day may be required in patients with severe burns.

D. Protein Requirements

1. Utilization of dietary protein is less efficient during stress than during convalescent periods.

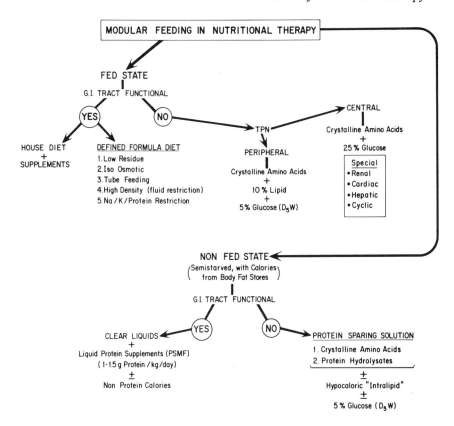

Fig. 11-5. Logic tree depicting the use of feeding modules in nutritional support (PSMF = protein-sparing modified fast). (Schneider, H. (ed.): Nutritional Support of Medical Practice. Hagerstown, Harper & Row, 1977)

2. Therefore, it is necessary to provide 16% of the calculated calorie needs (1.5 g./kg./day) from protein. The remaining calories coming from non-protein sources will make a nitrogen-calorie ratio of 1:150.

3. Although optimal in most clinical situations, this nitrogen-calorie ratio should be reduced to 1:450 or 1:700 in nitrogen accumulation disorders, such as renal or hepatic failure. The protein intake in uremia may thus have to be reduced to 4% to 6% of diet calories.

4. Routine hospital diets, which provide 8% of the calories as protein (1:300, nitrogen-calorie ratio), can maintain lean body mass and nitrogen balance in conva-

lescent patients. Conventionally defined formula diets also provide such a 1:300, nitrogen-calorie ratio.

5. In the oral high nitrogen diets used in stress and in mild to moderate hypercatabolism, this ratio is altered to 1:150, with protein contributing 16% of the total caloric intake.

6. Taste, osmolarity, digestibility, and specific disease states have to be considered when designing such therapy.

7. There is no universal formula for enteral feeding or parenteral nutrition that is applicable to all patients. With the above general rules, however, significant results can be expected in most clinical situations.

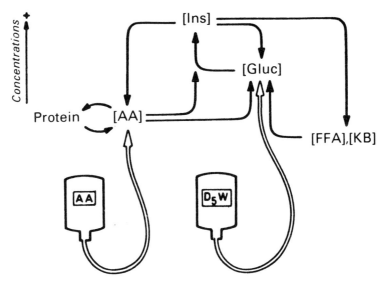

Fig. 11-6. The metabolic fuel regulatory system and protein-sparing therapies. The effects of carbohydrate and protein on the concentration of metabolic fuels and circulating insulin are depicted. (AA=3% amino acids, D₅W =5% dextrose in water, FFA=free fatty acids, KB=ketone bodies, Ins= insulin, Gluc=glucose). (Blackburn, G.L., Flatt, J.P., and Hensle, T.W.: Peripheral amino acid infusions. *In* Fischer, J. (ed.): Total Parenteral Nutrition. Boston, Little, Brown & Co., 1976)

IV. Nutritional Support in Pediatric Patients

A. Calorie Requirements

1. In newborn infants, caloric needs represent the highest concentration (cal./kg.) seen in humans..

2. The average basal metabolic requirement is approximately 50 Cal./kg./day, with an additional 25 Cal./kg./day for spontaneous activity and an additional 30 to 40 Cal./kg./day for weight gain and anabolism.

3. Once the infant's weight reaches 10 to 20 kg., the resting metabolic requirements decrease to 50 Cal./kg./day. This is similar to adult requirements.

B. Protein Requirements

1. For growing infants, protein needs are 3 to 4 g./kg./day.

2. However, nitrogen balance can be produced at levels of 2.5 g./kg./day.

3. When an infant's weight exceeds 20 kg., protein requirements decrease to 1.5 g./kg./day.

V. Protein-Sparing Therapy

A. Rationale

1. The interrelationships of protein, fat, and carbohydrates during fasting and semi-starvation were approximated in a model developed by Blackburn and Flatt (Fig. 11-6).

2. During starvation, protein stores are increasingly spared as part of a normal physiologic response, while the body progressively adapts to the use of non-protein calories (i.e. free fatty acids and ketone bodies) as major fuels.

3. During stress and semi-starvation with carbohydrate-containing diets, protein-sparing may be diminished because of increased circulating insulin levels and the

presence of peripheral insulin resistance. The body will use alternate fuels from skeletal and visceral protein during periods of hypocaloric intake.

4. In the well-nourished person, this effect may be justified, since the normal response to injury in the presence of starvation precludes effective incorporation of exogenous nutrients in the immediate post-injury phase.

5. In the malnourished patient undergoing the stress of disease, surgery, or infection, failure to minimize the catabolic phase of injury may adversely affect the final outcome.

6. In such starved states, substantial amounts of body protein can be spared by the parenteral infusion of amino acids.

   a. This method allows the maintenance of protein synthesis, particularly in the visceral compartment, and the mobilization of body fat stores.

   b. It is not essential that glucose be excluded from the amino acid solution.

   c. However, the tolerance of peripheral veins to hyperosmolar solutions (< 600 mOsm./ml.), the limits of fluid intake (< 3 L./24 hours), and the mineral (< 280 mOsm./ml.) and protein requirements (1.5 g./kg./day) for maximal nitrogen sparing, effectively limit the use of glucose in the solution.

B. Amino Acid Infusion

1. There is considerable data to show that amino acid infusion represents an excellent means to preserve body cell mass of patients in the starved state.

2. It remains the clinician's responsibility to decide the duration of this therapy.

3. Amino acids are administered as 1.0 to 1.5 g./kg. ideal body weight per day.

   a. This should be delivered at an acceptable osmolarity (< 600 mOsm.) for a peripheral vein infusion that includes electrolytes (sodium 60 to 150 mEq., potassium 60 to 80 mEq., phosphate 35 mEq., and calcium 9 mEq./day) and vitamins.

C. Monitoring the Metabolic Response

1. Estimations of urinary ketones and the blood sugar are routinely carried out and serve as excellent monitors of the metabolic response.

2. In this metabolic state, the failure to develop ketonuria in 2 to 3 days, accompanied by hyperglycemia (> 100 mg./100 ml.), indicates carbohydrate intolerance and insulin resistance common to deep sepsis and major stress.

3. Occasionally, patients may exhibit a mild metabolic acidosis, that is easily corrected by the addition of sodium acetate to the amino acid mixture.

4. A transient and minimal elevation of blood urea nitrogen may occur and poses no problems.

D. Oral Protein Therapy

1. When necessary or desirable, protein can be provided orally rather than parenterally.

2. It may be necessary to convert from amino acid infusions to forced feeding regimens if the stress-producing condition persists.

3. On the other hand, many patients may have adequate palliation and reversal of early malnutrition with appropriate protein-sparing therapy with amino acid solutions.

4. The patient's clinical status coupled with nutritional assessment criteria and estimation of the degree of hypermetabolism provide important guidelines for change of therapy (Fig. 11-7).

VI. Intravenous Hyperalimentation

A. Basic Principles

1. The development of total parenteral nutrition (TPN) has proved to be a major advance in the surgeon's constant efforts to deal with new problems that arise with increased survival from disease.

B. Indications

   1. *Preoperative Repletion*

   a. Planned major surgery in malnourished patients can have an improved outcome with proper preoperative nutritional support.

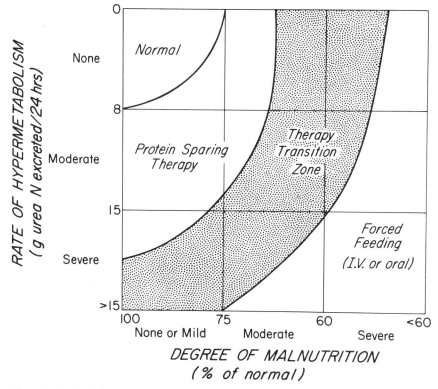

Fig. 11-7. Criteria for designing nutritional support therapy. Malnutrition and hypermetabolism is assessed by established criteria (see text). If restoration of the "fed state" is not possible, palliation may occur with protein-sparing therapy. Many patients with advanced malnutrition require forced feeding programs at the onset. (Blackburn, G.L.: Nitrogen metabolism after surgical trauma. J. Am. Soc. Parenteral Enteral Nutr., *1*:21, 1977)

b. Pharyngeal tumors, carcinoma of the esophagus, obstructing gastric tumors, and diseases of other systems which accompany malnutrition (i.e. cardiac, renal, or hepatic cachexia) are common indications.

2. *Postoperative Care*

a. Many patients who require preoperative repletion need to continue on TPN, particularly in the face of sepsis and major injury.

b. In others, postoperative complications accompanying multisystem failure may necessitate intravenous hyperalimentation.

c. Maintenance of body cell mass is

the goal of TPN when the stress response is great.

3. *Intestinal Fistulas.* With the advent of TPN, the mortality from intestinal fistulae has been reduced from the 40 to 60% range to approximately 4 to 9%.

4. *Inflammatory Bowel Disease.* Significant improvement in the outcome of granulomatous disease of the intestine has been reported, while in ulcerative colitis, the role of TPN is supportive.

5. *Cancer.* In cancer patients receiving hyperalimentation, there may be an enhanced response to surgery, radiotherapy, and chemotherapy.

6. *Burns.* The delivery of large

amounts of calories (often in excess of 45 Cal./kg./day) and protein is possible with central venous hyperalimentation. This has marked success in the treatment of patients with extensive burns.

7. *Short Gut Syndrome.* Survival of these patients is now a reality because most can be managed with TPN programs at home.

C. *Methodology*

1. *Central Venous Hyperalimentation (Usual Technique)*

a. Hypertonic (25%) dextrose and a 4.25% amino acid solution is delivered into the superior vena cava cannulated through an infraclavicular subclavian vein catheter.

b. The rate of delivery is gradually increased to 2000 to 3000 ml./24 hours over a 2 to 3 day period, in order to allow the body to adjust adequately to the high glucose load.

c. Typical hyperalimentation orders including composition of the hyperalimentation fluid and recommended metabolic monitoring are listed below.

Hyperalimentation Orders

Central Line: (Confirm position of catheter by radiograph in Superior Vena Cava)
_____ml. hyperalimentation (unless otherwise specified, the solution will be 4.25% FreAmine, 25% glucose) or _____% FreAmine, _____% glucose
Additive usually required, please specify:
_____mEq./day sodium chloride (60 to 150 mEq./day)
_____mEq./day potassium chloride (60 to 100 mEq./day)
_____mEq./day calcium gluceptate (9.0 mEq./day)
_____mEq./day magnesium sulfate (8.1 mEq./day)
_____mEq./day potassium phosphate (30 to 45 mEq./day)
_____mEq./day sodium acetate (40 mEq./day)
_____mEq./day potassium acetate
_____2 ml./day vitamins B and C (2 ml. daily Tuesday through Sunday)
_____2 ml. multivitamins (2 ml./week, Mondays)
_____μg. vitamin B_{12} (50 to 100 μg./week, Mondays)

_____mg. folic Acid (0.5 to 1.5 mg./week, Mondays)
_____units/L. regular insulin
_____units/L. heparin sodium (1000 to 2000 units/L.)
_____ml./day trace mineral mix (2 ml./day)
Rate of Infusion
_____ml. per hour
Laboratory Tests
Daily c.b.c. and Chem 6
Weekly Chem 12
Collect 24-hour urine for urea nitrogen, creatinine, sodium and potassium twice a week. Transferrin, and skin tests every 3 weeks
Weight (daily/every other day)
Accurate Intake and Output

---

d. Vitamin and mineral cofactors should be provided in adequate quantity. The known daily mineral requirements are listed below.

Daily Trace Element Requirements (Parenteral Use)

Zinc	2	mg./day
Manganese	0.4	mg./day
Copper	1	mg./day
Chromium	0.2	mg./day
Iodine	0.05	mg./day

---

2. *Hyperalimentation (Techniques Using Intralipid)*

a. Peripheral method

(1) Intralipid, a 10% soybean oil emulsion with egg yolk phospholipids and glycerol, is administered with amino acids and 5% dextrose through a peripheral vein. Extensive experience with this product in Europe preceded the availability of Intralipid for general use in the U.S. in 1975.

(2) Although the complications of long-term central venous catheterization, hypertonic glucose, and essential fatty acid (EFA) deficiency are avoided, use of Intralipid cannot be extended to patients with significant hypermetabolic states due to the inability to provide sufficient calories with limited fluid volumes.

b. Central method

(1) Intralipid can also be used to provide calories required in excess of estimated resting energy expenditure (i.e. those calories beyond 30 Cal./kg./day).

(2) Thus, if 5 to 6 Cal./kg./day are provided as protein and 20 to 25 Cal./kg./day as glucose, optimal TPN would be obtained by the administration of 1000 to 1500 ml. of 10% Intralipid (20 to 25 Cal./kg./day).

(3) Central venous catheterization would still be essential to avoid hyperosmolarity.

c. Complications due to Intralipid are limited to minor disorders of platelet adhesiveness, febrile reactions, and, occasionally, liver dysfunction.

d. Intravenous fat emulsions should be avoided in patients with disorders of fat metabolism and hyperlipidemias.

D. Complications of Central Venous Hyperalimentation

1. Numerous complications have been described with central venous hyperalimentation. They are briefly listed and the management described in Table 11-2.

2. Strict antiseptic measures must be emphasized with central venous hyperalimentation to maintain sterility of the catheters.

3. A significant number of critically ill patients on TPN are febrile because of a coexisting source of infection (lungs, urinary tract, peritoneum). Prior to removal of the subclavian catheter, septic foci elsewhere must be ruled out, the diagnosis established by blood cultures, and the catheter replaced 48 hours after removal.

4. Leukocytosis and glucose intolerance often precede the clinical appearance of catheter-related sepsis.

Table 11-2. **Complications of Central Venous Hyperalimentation and Guidelines for Management**

Complication	Management
Pneumothorax Hemothorax	Removal of catheter, needle aspiration ? closed thoracotomy
Subclavian vein thrombosis	Removal of catheter, add heparin to hyperalimentation (HA) solution
Hyperglycemia	Add insulin to HA solution, capillary blood glucose every 6 hours
Hyperosmolar nonketotic hyperglycemia	Slow or stop HA infusion, insulin, treatment of associated fluid and electrolyte disorders.
Metabolic acidosis	Decrease sodium chloride in solution and substitute sodium acetate
Hypokalemia	Potassium in adequate amounts (especially during anabolic or recovery phase)
Hypophosphatemia Hypomagnesemia Hypocalcemia	Appropriate supplements daily
EFA deficiency	500 ml. Intralipid twice weekly ? Cyclic hyperalimentation
Trace mineral deficiency	Appropriate supplements daily
Catheter sepsis	Establish diagnosis, remove catheter after other sources of sepsis have been ruled out, and reinsert catheter after 48 hours

(Blackburn, G.L., Maini, B.S., and Pierce, J.: Nutrition in the critically ill patient. Anesthesiology, *47*:181, 1977)

E. Cyclic Hyperalimentation

1. The standard practice of continuous hyperalimentation with hypertonic dextrose provides a constant stimulus for insulin secretion and subsequent lipogenesis and glycogenesis.

2. This results in fat and glycogen deposition in the liver and elevation of hepatic enzymes.

3. Cyclic hyperalimentation provides parenteral feeding with hypertonic dextrose and amino acids for approximately 12 hours each day. During the remaining period, dextrose-free solutions (saline or 3% amino acids) are provided.

4. This allows the development of a postabsorptive state, facilitating the mobilization and utilization of calories stored as fat during the hypertonic dextrose infusion.

5. There is often recovery from liver dysfunction and improvement in visceral protein synthesis.

6. Patients on long-term TPN in the hospital also benefit from this technique.

7. An additional advantage may be the possible mobilization of essential fatty acid (EFA) stores during the dextrose-free phase, which will delay the onset of EFA deficiency.

F. Special Uses for Intravenous Hyperalimentation

1. Renal Failure

a. A low-protein diet of high biologic value with excess calories may cause a lowering of blood urea nitrogen (BUN) in patients with azotemia.

b. This principle is utilized in the treatment of postsurgical acute renal failure by intravenous hyperalimentation.

c. Lower BUN levels, easier control of electrolyte problems, less frequent dialysis, and improved mortality have been noted.

d. Fluid requirements are adjusted as indicated by the conversion from the oliguric to the diuretic phase, and the protein intake is guided by BUN and creatinine levels.

e. A protein intake of 20 to 30 g./day with a nitrogen-calorie ratio of 1:450 to 1:700 seems best tolerated.

f. In patients with an intact gastrointestinal tract, defined formula diets (Aminaid) with the same N-cal. ratio (nitrogen largely provided as essential amino acids) may be used.

g. In order to produce optimal results, renal failure hyperalimentation with low-protein regimens should be initiated early in the course of acute tubular necrosis.

h. Recovery is signalled by a lowering of BUN and creatinine, the correction of hyperphosphatemia and hypermagnesemia, and the gradual increase of potassium requirements suggesting anabolism.

2. Hepatic Failure

a. In liver failure, an inability to effectively metabolize the aromatic amino acids (tryptophan, tyrosine, and phenylalanine) results in elevated blood levels of these compounds.

b. When semi-starvation regimens are employed—as is so often the case—the serum levels of branched-chain amino acids (leucine, isoleucine, and valine) are lowered due to increased peripheral utilization.

c. Parenteral nutrition should provide sufficient calories to meet energy requirements and, at the same time, should alter the amino acid composition (low in aromatic amino acids and high in branched-chain amino acids). This may speed the recovery from hepatic failure.

d. In addition, such a formula may provide an optimal synthesis of brain neurotransmitters, the metabolism of which is altered in hepatic encephalopathy.

3. Cardiac Disorders

a. The presence of protein-calorie malnutrition in patients with prolonged circulatory failure from heart disease is associated with a poor response to cardiac surgery.

b. Reversal of the malnourished state over a period of 3 to 4 weeks preoperatively can considerably improve the outcome from major cardiac surgical procedures.

G. Use of Intravenous Hyperalimentation in Children

1. Total parenteral nutrition has proved to be an invaluable adjunct in the management of infants with chronic diarrhea and anomalies of the gastrointestinal tract.

2. There is also an important role of TPN in the management of low-birth-weight infants.

3. Central venous hyperalimentation for children is used with guidelines similar to those used for adults.

a. In infants, however, the catheter is inserted through the internal jugular vein and threaded into the superior vena cava.

b. The proximal end is brought through a subcutaneous tunnel to exit through a stab wound in the parieto-occipital area of the scalp.

c. This makes care of the catheter much easier, and meticulous asepsis is maintained.

d. The septic complications are minimal in expert hands, and problems related to essential fatty acid deficiency, metabolic acidosis, and mineral deficiency should be monitored.

e. Requirements of up to 100 to 125 Cal./kg./day may be satisfied by this method, and a standard TPN solution could employ protein (2.5 g./kg.), glucose (25 to 30 g./kg.), and fat (4 g./kg.) every day.

4. Intravenous fat emulsions can be employed in children when needed.

a. The provision of 40 ml./kg./day of 10% Intralipid with 10% dextrose and 3% amino acids (85 ml./kg./day) provides 125 ml./kg./day.

b. This makes the administration of 80 Cal. and 25 g. protein/kg./day relatively easy.

c. Two infusion pumps and all other precautions observed with the intravenous lipid technique are employed.

d. Peripheral veins, with or without venesection, may be utilized.

VII. Enteral Hyperalimentation

A. Whenever possible, the gastrointestinal tract should be utilized for feeding programs.

B. It is likely that the oral route is associated with better visceral protein synthesis.

C. Currently available products for enteral nutrition enable one to formulate dietary prescriptions to accomodate most clinical situations (see Tables 12-1, 12-3, and 12-5).

1. These products differ widely in their sources of protein, calories, and fat but, by and large, provide about 1 cal./ml. in their recommended concentrations.

2. The usual nitrogen-calorie ratio provided is 1:300, which is altered to 1:150 in the high-nitrogen diets.

D. Defined formula diets frequently are used for enteral hyperalimentation (see Table 12-1).

1. They are low in residue because carbohydrates are provided in the monosaccharide and oligosaccharide forms to facilitate digestion.

2. Protein is often provided either as amino acids or protein of high biologic value.

3. Fat is usually minimized in such diets because fat digestion is often impaired in a variety of disease states. However, enough fat is added to prevent EFA deficiency.

E. A second group of diets falls into the category of meal replacements. These are of particular value in nasogastric and gastrostomy tube-feeding programs in convalescent patients (see Table 12-5).

F. A third group consists of meal supplements, which are used in patients who need the extra caloric and protein intake during periods of hospitalization, stress, and recovery from semi-starvation (see Tables 12-1 and 12-5).

G. Precautions

1. Monitoring of patients on enteral feeding requires constant nutritional assess-

ment with parameters similar to those in TPN. Hyperglycemia and hyperosmolar, non-ketotic coma have been described with enteral feeding.

2. While many enteral feeding products usually provide vitamins and minerals in adequate amounts, this is not invariably true. Formulas should be ascertained, and appropriate supplements should be administered if indicated.

3. Nitrogen and calorie requirements vary from patient to patient. No single diet is adequate for all hospitalized patients. Feeding modules of protein, fat, and carbohydrate can be provided in order to formulate an optimal feeding program.

4. In cases of pancreatic insufficiency, effective digestive enzymes may be added (e.g., Viokase, Cotazym, J and J Digestive Aid) to promote absorption. This may also obviate the need for a predigested diet in these patients.

5. Special needs should be met—sodium and protein restriction in renal failure, high-carbohydrate diet in liver failure, and high calories per unit volume in heart failure.

6. Most diets require that the feedings be started at low concentration. The desired volume is reached first, followed by a gradual increase in the concentration.

   a. This allows the intestines to slowly adapt to the high osmolar load.

   b. In cases in which diarrhea is persistent, parasympathomimetic agents may be mixed with the formula for easy administration and quick control.

ORAL FEEDINGS AFTER SURGERY

I. Head and Neck Surgery

A. The patient with head and neck cancer must not only deal with the psychological aspects of his disease but must also deal with day-to-day living. The provision of nutrients, especially protein and calories, is necessary to insure preservation of lean body mass (LBM) strength and to insure

good response to medical or surgical therapies.

B. To provide adequate nutrients, the parenteral or enteral route may be utilized.

1. It is necessary, at all times, to provide each nutrient in its required amount, including during transitional phases (parenteral to enteral formula to food).

C. The patient with head and neck cancer has many problems in feeding him- or herself orally.

1. Depending on the location of the cancer, the patient may experience difficulty in masticating, swallowing, and salivating.

2. Treatment therapies themselves may produce glossitis, mucositis, and facial muscle weakness, thereby causing difficulty in chewing or swallowing.

3. Glossectomy and mandibulectomy make the swallowing of food initially difficult.

4. In each of these instances the patient must be taught new methods of feeding.

D. Initially the patient may be fed with a pharnygostomy or gastrostomy feeding tube.

1. The possibility of aspiration, however, may necessitate the use of a feeding jejunostomy or placing a nasogastric feeding tube beyond the pylorus into the duodenum.

E. The following facts should be heeded when the patient is to start oral foods:

1. The patient will be apprehensive about taking oral foods.

2. He will require soft, moist foods perhaps starting off with nonirritating liquids and gradually advancing to ground foods and eventually to soft solids.

3. The diet should be given in very small, frequent feedings, served in an appetizing manner.

4. These patients often are able to tolerate liquids of thick consistency rather than thin fluids.

5. Foods, especially soft solids, must be moist and nonirritating (for example, gravies and sauces on finely ground meats,

potatoes, and alkaline-type pureed fruits— applesauce, pears, and peaches).

6. Tube feeding and these moist, soft solids work well when combined together.

F. It is important to provide protein and calories along with vitamins and minerals.

1. To provide the sufficient protein and calories, patients are given small, frequent feedings of protein- and calorie-containing foods with the avoidance of low- and empty-calorie foods and beverages.

2. This means that such items as coffee, tea, vegetables (unless in cream sauce or combined with soft protein sources), low-calorie tonics, and fruits (unless in heavy syrup or served with cream or milk) are to be avoided.

3. If patients desire coffee, fortified milk flavored with coffee can be served.

G. Emphasis must be placed on small, frequent meals that are served in a pleasant way.

1. It is psychologically important for the patient to realize that he can eat these small quantities.

2. Gradually, as confidence in taking small meals increases and appetite improves, additional increments in meal size can occur.

3. This is a progressive process, and the positive attitude shown by staff and the patient's family is necessary.

H. Milk products tend to coat the mucous lining of the mouth and to increase phlegm.

1. Initially patients may find it necessary to avoid milk and milk drinks because of this.

I. Careful preparation of food is necessary.

1. For example, all bones must be removed from fish to prevent choking.

2. Flavors should be intensified to increase stimulation of taste sensors, but they should not cause irritation to mouth.

3. Toast, crackers, cookies, and breads, although hard and crunchy, can be softened by having the patient dunk these items in a beverage.

4. Often foods can be combined to give a soft, mushy consistency (e.g., ground meat mixed with mashed potatoes and vegetables).

J. The approximate composition of the sample diet outlined in Table 11-4 is:

Carbohydrate	256 g.
Protein	100 g.
Fat	94 g.
Calories	2270 g.

K. The diet is limited in fiber content.

Table 11-3. **Foods Allowed After Head and Neck Surgery**

Milk*	Milk drinks: fortified milk—additions of skim milk powder to milk. Yogurt, puddings made with milk
Eggs	Soft scrambled, poached, omelets, egg salad (no celery or onions), boiled, custards
Cheese	Cottage cheese, processed cheese
Meat, Fish, and Poultry	Any type: ground, flaked, pureed; added to soups, casseroles
Starches	Potatoes (mashed, boiled, scalloped), rice, spaghetti, noodles, cooked cereals, baby cereals, cooked barley, soft breads, muffins with extra jelly and butter, zwieback, rusk, toast—which may be dunked into hot beverages to soften
Fruits (alkaline)	Apricots, applesauce, peaches, pears, and bananas. All pureed if necessary
Vegetables†	Soft cooked vegetables, pureed if necessary
Fats	Butter, margarine, cream, cream cheese, oil, mayonnaise, dressings
Desserts	Egg custards, puddings, fruit shortcake, ice cream (if patient can tolerate cold)
Miscellaneous	Honey, jelly (no jam, preserves, or conserves), syrups, sugar

*If tolerated
†To increase calories, use cream, extra butter or margarine, melted cheese or other sources.

L. Table 11-3 lists the foods to be used after head and neck surgery.

M. Table 11-4 lists a meal plan and sample menus to be used after head and neck surgery.

II. Foods Allowed After Gastric Surgery

A. After gastric surgery, patients generally have difficulty tolerating osmotic loads, of carbohydrate especially.

1. In addition, the combination of fluids with the solid portion of meals tends to increase dumping syndrome.

2. To avoid these two symptoms, a diet of limited carbohydrate, high protein, and high fat is recommended, along with the ingestion of fluids either 30 minutes prior to the meal or 30 minutes after solids; not together.

B. Milk may or may not be tolerated and should be started in puddings or custards.

1. It is important to note that these desserts should be homemade because packaged puddings and desserts contain higher amounts of carbohydrate.

C. Meals should be divided into six feedings initially.

Table 11-4. **Meal Plan and Sample Menu for Patients After Head and Neck Surgery***

	Meal Plan	Amount	Sample Menu
Breakfast	Fruit	1/2 cup	1/2 banana, mashed, with
	Milk†	4 oz.	1/2 cup fortified milk and
	Miscellaneous	Any amount	2 tsp. sugar
	Protein	2 oz.	Cheese omelet (1 egg, 1 oz. cheese, and fat)
Midmorning	Starch	1/2 cup or 1 slice	1/2 cup cooked cereal with
	Milk†	4 oz.	1/2 cup fortified milk and honey
Lunch	Protein	2 oz.	2 oz. white fish with cream sauce
	Starch	1/4 cup or 1/2 slice	1/4 cup cooked baby noodles with butter
	Vegetable	1/4–1/2 cup	1/4 cup mashed butternut squash
	Miscellaneous	Any amount	with brown sugar
	Fat	Any amount	Butter and cream sauce
	Beverage	Any amount	1/2 cup apricot nectar
Midafternoon	Protein	1/4 cup; 1 oz.	1/4 cup cottage cheese
	Fruit	1/2 cup	1/2 cup canned peaches (may be pureed)
2 hours later	Protein	1 oz.	1/2 cup custard
	Milk†	4 oz.	1/2 cup fortified milk, flavored†
Supper	Protein	2 oz.	2 oz. finely ground beef with 2 oz. of gravy
	Starch	1/4–1/2 cup	1/4 cup mashed potato made with
	Milk†	4 oz.	1/2 cup fortified milk
	Fat	Any amount	2 tsp. butter
	Dessert	Any amount	1/2 cup junket
	Beverage	Any amount	1/2 cup pear nectar
Evening snack	Milk†	4 oz.	1/2 cup fruit yogurt
	Beverage	Any amount	1/2 cup peach nectar

*Approximate Composition:

Carbohydrate	256 g.	Fat	94 g.
Protein	100 g.	Calories	2270

†If tolerated

D. All feedings should contain a protein source for satiety and a fat source to help delay gastric emptying.

E. If the patient's intake is limited because of anorexia or the inability to ingest sufficient nutrients as food, the following measures are recommended:

1. Avoid low- and empty-calorie foods and beverages (coffee, tea, tonics, and broth).

2. Try commercially available feeding modules to increase calories through protein fat.

3. Try smaller, more frequent meals.

F. Table 11-5 lists the foods allowed after gastric surgery.

G. Table 11-6 presents a feeding plan and sample menus for patients who have had gastric surgery.

III. Foods Allowed Following Cholecystectomy

A. Following cholecystectomy, patients may require a low—fat diet for approximately 3 months. A regular diet after this period is generally well tolerated.

B. Meals should be planned initially for

Table 11-5. **Foods Allowed After Gastric Surgery**

	One Serving Is:
Milk*	
Plain or in cooking	8 oz.
Eggs	
Boiled, poached, scrambled, omelet	1 egg
Cheese	
Cottage cheese	2 oz.
Pasteurized process, hard	1 oz.
Meat, Fish, and Poultry	
All types, baked, broiled, boiled, or combined with other allowed foods to make simple casseroles	1 oz.
Starches	
Potatoes, rice, noodles, spaghetti	1/2 cup
Enriched white bread, plain soft roll	1
Crackers (graham, uneedas, and arrowroot)	3
Angel or sponge cake	1 slice
Cooked cereal	1/2 cup
Dry cereal (none with sugar-coating)	3/4 cup
Fruits	
All unsweetened juices	1/2 cup
Initially, all cooked or canned fruits (unsweetened); gradually add fresh fruit	
Vegetables	
First 2 weeks—cooked asparagus tips, green beans, carrots, beets, chopped spinach, and mashed butternut squash.	1/2 cup
Avoid all vegetables which may cause flatulence (cabbage, broccoli, and brussel sprouts)	
Two weeks after surgery, new vegetables may be tried (shredded lettuce)	1/2 cup
Fats	
Butter, margarine, oil	1 tsp.
Cream cheese	2 tbsp.
Cream	2 tbsp.
Crisp bacon	1 strip
Salad dressing	1 tsp.
Desserts	
Plain cakes, junket, cookies, homemade pudding	As desired

*If tolerated.

six small feedings until the patient can gradually resume prior eating pattern.

1. If nutrient intake of food is limited because of anorexia, it may be necessary to limit intake of low- and empty-calorie foods and beverages (coffee, tea, and broth).

2. Commercially available liquid preparations may be used to supply additional calories as carbohydrate, protein, or fat.

C. Table 11-7 lists the foods allowed after cholecystectomy.

D. Table 11-8 presents a meal plan and sample menus for postcholecystectomy patients.

IV. Foods Allowed After Intestinal Surgery

A. Postoperative patients who have had bowel surgery are begun on soft, low-bulk diets.

1. This type of diet limits the amounts of foods that will increase fecal residue,

Table 11-6. **Meal Plan and Sample Menu for Patients After Gastric Surgery***

	Meal Plan	Amount	Sample Menu
Breakfast	Protein	2 servings	2 soft boiled eggs
	Starch	1 servings	1 slice white toast
	Fat	Any amount	2 tsp. margarine
30 minutes after meal	Beverage	4 oz.	1/2 cup warm milk
Midmorning	Protein	2 servings	1/2 cup cottage cheese
	Fruit	1 serving	1/2 cup unsweetened apricots
	Starch	1 serving	3 uneedas
30 minutes after meal	Beverage	Any amount	Tea, sugar substitute
Lunch	Protein	4 servings	4 oz. broiled steak
	Starch	1 serving	1/2 cup boiled rice
	Vegetable	1 serving	1/2 cup green beans
	Fruit	1 serving	1/2 fresh banana
	Fat	Any amount	Margarine
30 minutes after meal	Beverage	Any amount	Tea, sugar substitute Dietetic gelatin
Midafternoon	Protein	2 servings	2 oz. cheese
	Starch	1/2 serving	3 saltines
30 minutes after meal	Beverage	Any amount	Dietetic ginger ale
Supper	Protein	4 servings	4 oz. lamb chop
	Starch	1 serving	Potato with parsley
	Vegetable	1 serving	1/2 cup peas
	Fruit	1 serving	1/2 cup unsweetened applesauce
	Fat	Any amount	Margarine
30 minutes after meal	Beverage	Any amount	Tea, sugar substitute Dietetic gelatin
Evening snack	Protein	1 serving	1 oz. American cheese
	Starch	1/2 serving	3 saltines
30 minutes after meal	Beverage	Any amount	Dietetic ginger ale

*Approximate Composition:

Carbohydrate	150 g.	Fat	110 g.
Protein	120 g.	Calories	2070

especially fiber, which consists of cellulose, pectin, gums, lignin, and agar-agar and is found in fruits, nuts, vegetables, and cereal grains.

2. It is insolvent to chemical action in the bowel.

3. All fruits and juices except bananas and peeled apples and all vegetables except potatoes are to be avoided.

4. Gradually, as the patient begins to tolerate various foods, fruits, juices, and vegetables may be added in small quantities.

B. Patients who have had intestinal surgery may not be able to tolerate milk and milk products.

1. Milk is eliminated from the diet in the first week and gradually reintroduced in the form of cooked milk products.

C. No indigestible fiber is contained in animal protein sources.

1. Meats should be lean and should contain no gristle.

2. Milk, fats, and certain carbohy-

drates increase fecal volume but do not contribute to fiber content.

D. Meals initially should be given in small, frequent feedings—generally six equal feedings.

1. This enables the gastrointestinal tract to become accustomed to food and allows the postoperative patient an opportunity to gradually increase oral intake.

2. If intake of nutrients as food is limited because of anorexia, it may be necessary to limit the amounts of low- and empty-calorie foods and beverages (tea, coffee, and broth).

3. In addition, commercially available feeding modules may be utilized to supply additional calories as carbohydrate, protein, or fat.

E. Table 11-9 lists foods allowed after intestinal surgery.

F. Table 11-10 shows a food plan and sample menus for a low-bulk diet to be used after intestinal surgery.

Table 11-7. **Foods Allowed After Cholecystectomy (Low-Fat Diet 25 to 40 g.)**

Milk	Skim milk, 2% milk, skim milk yogurts, puddings made with skim milk, "cream" soups made with skim milk
Eggs	Boiled, poached, scrambled (with no additional fat); limit to 3 servings per week Egg white as desired
Cheese	Low-fat cottage cheese Low-fat pasteurized cheeses
Meat, Fish, and Poultry	Baked, broiled, boiled fish, poultry, veal, lean pork Baked, broiled, boiled beef, lamb; limit to 5 servings per week Baked, broiled liver; limit to 1 serving per week Avoid all luncheon meats, capon, duck, corned beef, spare ribs, and ground beef with greater than 20% fat content.
Starches	Potatoes, rice, noodles, spaghetti, lima beans, corn, barley, cooked cereals, dry cereals, plain breads, crackers, zwieback, rusk, melba toast, muffins. No biscuits, no French, Italian, or Vienna breads
Fruits	All types allowed except avocados and nuts
Vegetables	All types allowed except those made with cream sauces
Fats	Limit to 3 tsp. per day Butter, margarine, oil, mayonnaise, salad dressing, cream, cream cheese Bacon (1 strip)
Desserts	Plain angel cake, plain cookies, water ices, ice milk, meringues, gelatin
Miscellaneous	Honey, sugar, jelly

Table 11-8. **Meal Plan and Sample Menu for Patients After Cholecystectomy***

	Meal Plan	*Amount*	*Sample Menu*
Breakfast	Fruit	4 oz.	Orange juice
	Protein	1 oz.	2 scrambled egg whites
	Starch	Any amount	1 slice white toast
			1/2 cup oatmeal
	Beverage	Any amount	8 oz. skim milk
	Fat	None	None
	Miscellaneous	Any amount	Sugar, jelly
Midmorning	Milk	1 serving	8 oz. skim milk, junket
Lunch	Soup	4 oz.	4 oz. fish chowder (skim milk)
	Protein	4 oz.	4 oz. broiled chicken breast
	Starch	Any amount	1/3 cup corn
			French bread
	Vegetable	Any amount	Asparagus
	Fruit	Any amount	Baked apple
	Fat	1 serving	1 tsp. margarine
	Beverage	Any amount	Gingerale
Midafternoon	Starch	Any amount	3 graham crackers
	Milk	Any amount	4 oz. skim milk
Supper	Protein	4 oz.	4 oz. baked haddock with tomato sauce
	Starch	Any amount	Mashed potato
			Italian bread
	Vegetable	Any amount	Broccoli
	Fruit	Any amount	Fresh fruit cup
	Fats	1 tsp.	1 tsp. margarine
	Beverage	Any amount	Tea, sugar
Evening snack	Milk	1/2 cup	Skim milk, fruit, or yogurt
	Starch	Any amount	2 sugar cookies

*Approximate composition: Carbohydrate, 289 g.; Fat, 43 g.; Protein, 103 g.; Calories, 1955

Table 11-9. **Foods Allowed After Intestinal Surgery**

Milk*	1 cup per day to be used alone or in cooking
Eggs	Boiled, poached, scrambled, plain omelet
Cheese	Mild, semisoft or hard cheese
Meat, Fish, and Poultry	All types: baked, broiled, boiled. Simple casseroles with other allowed foods
Starches	Potatoes (without skin), rice, spaghetti, noodles, cooked cereals, dry corn and rice cereals, enriched white bread, soft rolls, melba toast, plain crackers, zwieback, rusk
Fruits	First 2 weeks—bananas only After 2 weeks—peeled apples (fresh), cooked or canned applesauce, peeled apricots, peaches, pears, plums, ripe honeydew melons or cantaloupes*
Vegetables	First 2 weeks—none After 2 weeks—cooked asparagus tips, beets, carrots, mushrooms, mashed butternut squash, any pureed vegetable, shredded lettuce
Fats	Butter, margarine, cream, crisp bacon, cream cheese, mayonnaise, non-dairy creams, oil, gravies, sauces
Desserts	Plain cakes, cookies, gelatins, water ices. If milk is tolerated—custard, plain puddings, and ice cream
Miscellaneous	Creamy peanut butter, honey, sugar, jelly (no jam, preserves, or conserves)

*If tolerated

Table 11-10. **Meal Plan and Sample Menu for Low-Bulk Diet for Patients After Intestinal Surgery***

	Meal Plan	Amount	Sample Menu
Breakfast	Fruit	4 oz.	1/2 cup cooked applesauce
	Protein	1 oz.	Scrambled egg
	Starch	Any amount	1 slice white toast
	Fat	Any amount	2 tsp. butter or margarine
	Milk†	4 oz.	1/2 cup whole milk
	Miscellaneous	Any amount	Jelly, sugar
Midmorning	Starch	Any amount	1/2 cup oatmeal
	Protein	Any amount	1/4 cup non-dairy cream
	Miscellaneous	Any amount	Sugar or honey
Lunch	Protein	3 oz.	3 oz. sliced turkey
	Starch	Any amount	2 slices white enriched bread (turkey sandwich)
	Fat	Any amount	Mayonnaise
	Dessert	Any amount	Tapioca pudding
	Beverage	Any amount	1/2 cup milk
Midafternoon	Protein	1 oz.	2 tbsp. creamy peanut butter
	Starch	Any amount	3 melba toast
	Miscellaneous	Any amount	Jelly
	Beverage	Any amount	Gingerale
Supper	Soup	Any amount	Chicken noodle with 1 oz. additional chicken added
	Protein	4 oz.	Broiled filet of sole
	Starch	Any amount	Noodles, soft roll
	Vegetable	1/2 cup	Cooked beets
	Fat	Any amount	Margarine or butter
	Dessert	Any amount	Angel cake with frosting
	Beverage	4 oz.	1/2 cup milk
Evening snack	Protein	4 oz.	1/2 cup cottage cheese
	Fruit	1/2 cup	1/2 cup peaches
	Starch	Any amount	3 arrowroot cookies

*Approximate Composition:
  Carbohydrate   264 g.   Fat   105 g.
  Protein   110 g.   Calories   2441
†If tolerated.

SUGGESTED READINGS

General Reading

Ballinger, W.F., (ed.): Manual of Surgical Nutrition. Philadelphia, W.B. Saunders, 1975.

Fischer, J.E., (ed.): Total Parenteral Nutrition. Boston, Little, Brown & Co., 1976.

Ghadimi, H. (ed.): Total Parenteral Nutrition: Premises and Promises. New York, John Wiley & Sons, 1975.

Winters, R.W., and Hasselmeyer, E.G., (eds.): Intravenous Feeding in the High Risk Infant. New York, John Wiley & Sons, 1975.

White, P.L., and Nagy, M.E. (eds.): Total Parenteral Nutrition. Acton, Mass. Publishing Science Group, 1974.

Nutritional Assessment and Malnutrition

Bistrian, B.R., Blackburn, G.L., Hallowel, E., and Heddle, R.: Protein status of general surgical patients. J.A.M.A., 230:858, 1974.

Bistrian, B.R., Blackburn, G.L., Vitale, J., Cochran, D., and Naylor, J.: Prevalence of malnutrition in general medical patients. J.A.M.A., 235:1567, 1976.

Blackburn, G.L., *et al.*: Nutritional and metabolic assessment of the hospitalized patient. J. Am. Soc. Parenteral Enteral Nutr., 1:11,1977.

Copeland, E.M., McFadyen, B.V., Jr., and Dudrick, S.J.: Effect of intravenous hyperalimentation on established delayed hypersensitivity in the cancer patient. Ann. Surg., 184:60, 1976.

Jelliffe, D.B.: The Assessment of the Nutritional Status of the Community. Geneva, World Health Organization, 1966.

Sokal, J.E.: Measurement of delayed skin-test responses. N. Engl. J. Med., *293:*501, 1975.

Protein-Sparing Therapy

Blackburn, G.L., Flatt, J.P., and Hensle, T.W.: Peripheral Amino acid infusions. *In* Fischer, J. (ed.): Total Parenteral Nutrition. Boston, Little, Brown & Co., 1976.

Blackburn, G.L., Maini, B.S., and Pierce, J.: Nutrition in the critically ill patient. Anesthesiology, *47:* 181, 1977.

Freeman, J.B., Steginic, L.D., Fry, L.K., Sherman, B.M., and DenBesten, L.: Metabolic effects of amino acid vs. dextrose infusion in surgical patients. Arch. Surg., *110:*916, 1975.

Greenberg, G.R., Marliss, E.B., Anderson, G.H., Langer, B., Spence, W., Tovee, E.B., and Jeejeebhoy, K.N.: Protein-sparing therapy in post operative patients: Effect of added hypocaloric glucose or lipid. N. Engl. J. Med., *294:*1411, 1976.

Hyperalimentation

Abel, R.M., Abbott, W.M., Beck, C.H., Jr., Ryan, J.A., Jr., and Fischer, J.E.: Essential L-amino acids for hyperalimentation in patients with disordered nitrogen metabolism. Am. J. Surg., *128:* 317, 1974.

Blackburn, G.L., and Bistrian, B.R.: Nutritional care of the injured and/or septic patient. Surg. Clin. North Am., *56:*1195, 1976.

Deitel, M., and Kaminsky, V.: Total nutrition by peripheral vein—the lipid system. Can. Med. Assoc. J., *111:*1, 1974.

Dudrick, S.J., MacFayden, B.U., and VanBuren, C.T.: Parenteral hyperalimentation: Metabolic problems and solutions. Ann. Surg., *176:*259, 1972.

Dudrick, S.J., Wilmore, D.W., Vars, H.M., and Rhoads, J.E.: Long-term total parenteral nutrition with growth, development, and positive nitrogen balance. Surgery, *64:*134, 1968.

Gibbons, G.W., Blackburn, G.L., Harken, D.E., Valdes, P.J., Moorehead, D., and Bistrian, B.R.: Pre- and post-operative hyperalimentation in the treatment of cardiac cachexia. J. Surg. Res., *20:* 439, 1976.

Kaminski, M.V., Jr.: Enteral hyperalimentation. Surg. Gynecol. Obstet., *143:*12, 1976.

Maini, B., Blackburn, G.L., Bistrian, B.R., Flatt, J.P., Page, J.G., Bothe, A., Benotti, P., and Rienhoff, H.Y.: Cyclic hyperalimentation: An optimal technique for preservation of visceral protein. J. Surg. Res., *20:*515, 1976.

Rutten, P., Blackburn, G.L., Flatt, J.P., Hallowell, E., and Cochran, D.: Determination of optimal hyperalimentation rate. J. Surg. Res., *18:*477, 1975.

Zohrab, W.J., McHattie, J.D., and Jeejeebhoy, K.N.: Total parenteral alimentation with lipid. Gastroenterology, *64:*583, 1973.

12. NUTRITION AND UPPER GASTROINTESTINAL DISORDERS

William J. Klish, M.D.
Corinne Mamo Montandon, M.P.H., R.D.

Significant advances have been made in the nutritional management of disorders of the gastrointestinal tract. It is not sufficient to know only what diet to prescribe in a specific disease state, it is equally important to know why and how that diet should help.

BASIC PRINCIPLES

I. Diseases of the gastrointestinal tract amenable to dietary manipulation generally can be divided into three major categories.

A. Diseases which interfere with the digestion of nutrients, such as pancreatic or biliary insufficiency

B. Diseases which interefere with the absorption of nutrients, such as celiac disease or carbohydrate intolerance

C. Diseases which interefere with the delivery of nutrients to the appropriate absorptive site, such as abnormalities in motility or the short-bowel syndrome

II. It is important to decide into which major category a particular disease fits, because the choice of nutritional therapy differs with each category.

A. In diseases of digestion, an elemental diet should be considered because these "predigested" diets will circumvent the need for hydrolysis by pancreatic enzymes and miscellarization of fat by bile acids.

B. Diseases of absorption require changes in diet.

1. The specific nutrient being malabsorbed should be reduced or removed from the diet.

2. The interval between feedings may have to be decreased to maximize the efficiency of a reduced absorptive surface.

C. Diseases which interfere with the delivery of nutrients require some alterations in the mechanics of feeding whether it be by tube feeding or by parenteral nutrition. All too frequently, elemental diets are fed to patients who fall into the latter two categories resulting in complications inherent in the use of these products.

III. There is no substitute for sound judgment and a basic knowledge of diets when selecting a nutritional program for an ill patient.

A. Patients who are put on special diets for prolonged periods should receive specific detailed instructions on their diets by a skilled dietitian or physician.

B. When patients are well informed about their diets, their compliance increases dramatically.

SPECIFIC DISORDERS AMENABLE TO DIETARY MANIPULATION

I. Esophagus

A. Esophageal Reflux and Hiatus Hernia

1. Definition

a. A group of esophageal disorders characterized by the recurrent escape of gastric contents into the esophagus without associated belching or vomiting

2. Basic Principles

a. Esophageal reflux with or without hiatus hernia represents a physiologic disorder of the lower esophageal sphincter in which the sphincter pressure may be exceeded by intragastric pressure, allowing stomach contents to enter the esophagus.

b. This may result in the regurgitation of gastric contents and in nutrient losses.

c. Esophageal reflux without hiatus hernia is frequent in infancy but usually improves with age and should not be considered pathological unless other symptoms such as aspiration, pneumonia, or failure to thrive coexist.

d. Esophageal reflux with hiatus hernia is common in older persons.

3. *Dietary Management*

a. Feeding habits should be altered in an attempt to decrease reflux.

b. A supine position should not be allowed after eating or during sleep.

c. Garments or positions that increase intra-abdominal pressure should be avoided.

d. Meals should be small, and food should be avoided for about 4 hours before retiring.

e. Although no specific diet is recommended, foods should be avoided which increase gastric acidity or which initiate symptoms.

f. Infants should be burped frequently and not allowed to eat rapidly and ingest air. The thickening of infant formulas with cereal is sometimes helpful.

g. Severe cases often do not respond to these mechanical measures and may require surgical intervention.

B. *Achalasia With or Without Diffuse Spasm*

1. *Definition*

a. Derangement of esophageal motility resulting in a failure or relaxation of the lower esophageal sphincter

2. *Basic Principles*

a. Difficulty in swallowing and regurgitation of retained esophageal contents are the primary symptoms.

b. These abnormalities may result in severe nutritional deficiencies if they are left untreated.

3. *Dietary Management*

a. There is no specific diet recommended.

b. Very hot or very cold food may trigger esophageal spasm.

C. *Reflux Esophagitis*

1. *Definition*

a. Inflammation of the esophagus secondary to the reflux of gastric contents

resulting in substernal pain and, on occasion, hematemesis

2. *Basic Principles*

a. Same as reflux and hiatus hernia

3. *Dietary Management*

a. The general management is the same as for reflux.

b. In addition, antacids are used to neutralize gastric contents.

II. Stomach

A. *Peptic Ulcer*

1. *Definition*

a. Ulceration of the stomach or duodenum which results in symptoms of pain, bleeding, and, occasionally, obstruction

2. *Basic Principles*

a. Even though the causal relationship between acid-pepsin secretion and peptic ulcer is poorly understood, therapy for this disorder is directed at the reduction of gastric secretion and the buffering of the secretory products.

b. It is to this end that both surgical and medical treatment is directed.

3. *Dietary Management*

a. Classic diets such as bland or Sippy diets for peptic ulcer disease are generally not advocated by gastroenterologists today.

b. However, foods should be restricted which cause gastric irritation or induce acid secretion without any neutralizing effect.

(1) These include alcohol, beverages containing caffeine such as coffee and certain cola drinks, tea, and specific irritants such as aspirin or other salicylates.

(2) The patient should be advised to avoid any specific food or spice which induces pain.

(3) Bedtime snacks are not encouraged because of their ability to delay the appearance of a basal secretory state thus producing higher nocturnal acidity.

B. Chronic Atrophic Gastritis
1. Definition
a. Diffuse atrophy of the gastric mucosa with loss of gastric gland cells and infiltration of the mucosa with chronic inflammatory cells
2. Basic Principles
a. Symptoms of this disease tend to be mild.
b. The mucosal atrophy frequently results in an inability to secrete intrinsic factor, which is necessary for the absorption of vitamin B_{12}. This results in pernicious anemia.
3. Dietary Management
a. No specific diet is helpful.
b. Monthly intramuscular injections of vitamin B_{12} are required for patients with malabsorption of this vitamin.
C. Hypertrophic Gastritis (Ménétrier's Disease)
1. Definition
a. A pathological condition characterized by massive enlargement of the gastric mucosal folds and hyperplastic surface mucous cells
2. Basic Principles
a. Hyperplasia of the mucosal surface of the stomach results in an increased loss of plasma proteins into the gastrointestinal tract.
b. These proteins are hydrolyzed by the proteolytic enzymes present in the lumen of the gut, and the majority are reabsorbed as amino acids.
c. Even though total nitrogen tends to stay in balance, the liver may not produce albumin rapidly enough to prevent the development of edema.
3. Dietary Management
a. A high-protein diet may be necessary to replace enteric losses (see p. 182).
D. Dumping Syndrome
1. Definition
a. Gastrointestinal symptoms, including nausea, eructation, epigastric fullness, cramping, vomiting, and diarrhea, which result from the rapid introduction of hyperosmolar solutions from the stomach into the proximal jejunum
2. Basic Principles
a. This syndrome is most frequently the result of gastric surgery such as a subtotal gastric resection (Billroth II) or vagotomy and pyloroplasty.
b. With the recent introduction of the hyperosmolar elemental diets, this syndrome can be seen in patients with normal G.I. tracts who are fed these diets by tube.
3. Dietary Management
a. In postsurgical patients, high-protein, low-carbohydrate diets will usually alleviate symptoms.
b. If at all possible, when tube feedings are required, they should be instituted with isotonic diets (see Table 12-1 and Elemental Diets, p. 192).

III. Small Intestine

A. Acute Enteritis
1. Definition
a. A clinical syndrome characterized by the acute onset of watery stools in a greater volume than normal
2. Basic Principles
a. Acute enteritis is caused by microorganisms or toxic substances which interfere with the function of either the small or large intestine.
b. Those that confine their effects essentially to the small intestine can be divided into two groups depending upon whether they interfere with the absorptive function of the intestinal mucosa or with the secretory mechanism.
(1) Absorptive diarrheas tend to be less severe, and they frequently result in a transient lactose intolerance. Fecal volume decreases when the patient is made NPO (nothing by mouth).
(2) Secretory diarrheas tend to be more severe, and fecal volume does not change with decreased oral intake.
c. A schematic of the differential diagnosis is shown in Figure 12-1.

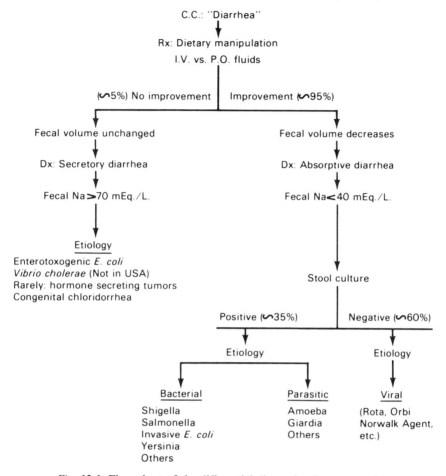

C.C.: "Diarrhea"

Rx: Dietary manipulation
I.V. vs. P.O. fluids

(∿5%) No improvement | Improvement (∿95%)

Fecal volume unchanged

Dx: Secretory diarrhea

Fecal Na > 70 mEq./L.

Etiology
Enterotoxogenic *E. coli*
Vibrio cholerae (Not in USA)
Rarely: hormone secreting tumors
Congenital chloridorrhea

Fecal volume decreases

Dx: Absorptive diarrhea

Fecal Na < 40 mEq./L.

Stool culture

Positive (∿35%) | Negative (∿60%)

Etiology | Etiology

Bacterial | Parasitic | Viral
Shigella | Amoeba | (Rota, Orbi
Salmonella | Giardia | Norwalk Agent,
Invasive *E. coli* | Others | etc.)
Yersinia
Others

Fig. 12-1. Flow chart of the differential diagnosis of acute enteritis.

3. Dietary Management

a. The dietary management of diarrhea should be aggressive.

b. Patients should not be made NPO with intravenous fluids for longer than 12 to 24 hours after which clear liquids, full liquids, and, finally, a regular diet is instituted.

c. This progression in diet should take no longer than 72 hours.

d. Maintaining a patient NPO or on clear liquids for an extended period results in significant and unnecessary weight loss. This is especially true in infants.

e. Infants frequently develop a transient lactose intolerance following an episode of acute enteritis and must be carefully observed for this problem when a lactose-containing formula is reintroduced.

B. Regional Enteritis (Crohn's Disease)

1. Definition

a. Regional enteritis is a chronic inflammatory disease of the intestinal tract characterized by inflammation with granulomas extending through all layers of the intestinal wall.

2. Basic Principles

a. This disease can present with a

wide variety of clinical symptoms including pain, diarrhea, melena, fever, and failure to thrive.

b. It is usually a discontinuous disease of the gut, and the symptoms depend on which portion of the intestinal tract in involved.

c. Specific nutrients such as vitamin B_{12} may be malabsorbed depending on the location of the disease.

d. In the pediatric age group, the disease is frequently heralded by a failure to grow.

e. Strictures and fistulous tracts are frequent complications.

3. Dietary Management

a. Strict attention should be paid to balancing the diet because of the marginal nutritional status of many of these patients.

b. Adequate replacement of protein in the diet, as well as calcium and iron, is essential. This can be done by increasing dietary protein (e.g., additional meats, eggs, and dairy products) or with a supplement of a prepared high-protein drink.

c. In patients with strictures or fistulas, a low-residue diet is helpful (see p. 183).

C. Celiac Disease (Gluten-Sensitive Enteropathy)

1. Definition

a. Celiac disease is the permanent intolerance of dietary wheat, rye, oat, or barley gluten, which results in histologic abnormalities of the jejunal mucosa and malabsorption.

2. Basic Principles

a. Gluten, a water-insoluble protein found in wheat, rye, barley, and oats, has the ability to interact in a toxic manner with the intestinal mucosa of patients with celiac disease.

b. This results in damage to the mucosa characterized by villous atrophy and infiltration of the lamina propria mucosae with chronic inflammatory cells.

c. Malabsorption of all nutrients results in chronic diarrhea, weight loss, and multiple specific nutrient deficiencies.

d. The symptoms can be totally reversed by removing gluten from the diet.

3. Dietary Management: Gluten-free diet (see also pp. 185, 190)

a. Cereal and bakery products made from wheat, barley, rye, and oats are prohibited.

b. Care must be exercised to avoid commercial products which use wheat or other gluten-containing flour as a filler.

D. Whipple's Disease

1. Definition

a. Whipple's disease is an uncommon systemic disease presenting with malabsorption, fever, skin pigmentation, anemia, arthritis, endocarditis, and central nervous system involvement.

b. It is characterized by the infiltration of glycoprotein-laden macrophages and small rod-shaped bacilli in involved tissues.

2. Basic Principles

a. Because the pathogenesis of this disease is related to a bacteria, antibiotics such as penicillin or tetracycline are the treatment of choice.

b. The severe malabsorption in this disease results in profound weight loss and multiple nutrient deficiencies which must be corrected.

3. Dietary Management

a. A high-protein and -calorie diet, supplemented with multiple vitamins, should be instituted until normal weight is achieved.

b. Vitamin D and calcium should be given until the steatorrhea resolves to prevent the occurrence of tetany due to the loss of calcium from saponification with the fat in the stool.

c. Iron should be supplemented in anemic patients.

E. Short-Bowel Syndrome

1. Definition

a. Surgical resection of a portion of the small intestine compromising the absorptive surface, which results in malabsorption

2. Basic Principles

a. Resection of small segments of the small intestine usually causes no symptoms because of the reserve capacity of the intestine for absorption.

b. Significant malabsorption results if more than 50% of the small intestine is removed.

c. When less than 30% of the intestine remains in an adult or less than 30 cm. in an infant, the resulting malabsorption may be life threatening.

d. Removal of the ileocecal valve significantly increases the risk of catastrophic malabsorption.

e. The portion of the small intestine that is resected also is important because some nutrients are absorbed at specific levels.

f. As an example, bile acids and vitamin B_{12} are absorbed in the distal portion, whereas calcium and iron tend to be absorbed proximally.

g. Because the remaining intestine tends to compensate by hypertrophy of villi and increased diameter, symptoms may decrease with time.

3. Dietary Management

a. Management is directed at utilizing the remaining intestinal surface with maximal efficiency.

b. Frequent small feedings lead to maximal utilization of the diet ingested.

c. A continuous nasogastric drip may be necessary if the symptoms are very severe.

d. Total parenteral nutrition is helpful immediately following surgery to allow total healing prior to feeding.

e. Elemental diets may be utilized to enhance absorption because they do not require a digestive phase. Care must be taken however not to stimulate an osmotic diarrhea (see Elemental Diets, p. 192).

F. Lactose Intolerance

1. Definition

a. The inability to efficiently absorb lactose (milk sugar) resulting in gastrointestinal symptoms

2. Basic Principles

a. Lactose intolerance may be acquired secondary to acute intestinal mucosal diseases such as acute enteritis, celiac disease, or inflammatory bowel disease.

b. Primary lactose intolerance may be the consequence of a specific enzyme deficiency which seems to have an insidious onset within the first decade after birth.

c. Secondary lactose intolerance generally is transient, whereas the primary lactose deficiency seems to be permanent.

d. Unabsorbed lactose may exert a direct osmotic effect in the small bowel and colon, or it may be fermented by intestinal bacteria giving rise to the formation of organic acids.

e. These fermentation products can enhance the osmotic effect as well as possibly be a direct irritant to colonic function.

f. The resulting symptoms may include nausea, vomiting, flatulence, and diarrhea.

g. Because the symptoms are dose related, lactose-intolerant patients usually have no difficulty with small amounts of milk sugar.

3. Dietary Management

a. A lactose-restricted diet is indicated. This is designed to provide a minimum amount of lactose (8 g. or less per day). Labels of food products should be checked for addition of milk, lactose, or milk solids. Foods listing these should be avoided, or small amounts may be used with discretion, if tolerated. Lactalbumin, lactate, and calcium compounds are salts of lactic acid and do not contain lactose.

b. Many adults with this problem subconsciously restrict lactose in their diet, even though they are unaware of the causal relationship.

c. A lactose-restricted diet is low in calcium. It is adequate, however, in all other nutrients (see pp. 182, 186).

G. Intolerance to Carbohydrates (Other Than Lactose)

1. Definition

a. The inability to absorb other carbohydrates such as sucrose, isomaltose, maltose, trehalose, glucose, or fructose, which results in symptoms similar to lactose intolerance.

2. Basic Principles

a. Malabsorption of carbohydrates other than lactose is seen far less frequently than lactose intolerance.

b. Sucrase-isomaltase and trehalase deficiencies exist as specific congenital disorders.

c. Congenital glucose-galactose intolerance has also been reported.

d. Infants may acquire a combined carbohydrate intolerance following severe intestinal disorders such as acute enteritis or necrotizing enterocolitis.

e. This syndrome, which has been called intractable diarrhea of infancy or acquired monosaccharide intolerance, is reversible with proper dietary management.

f. Infants with intractable diarrhea present with failure to thrive due to the severe malabsorption associated with this syndrome.

3. Dietary Management

a. In diseases with specific disaccharidase deficiencies, foods containing those disaccharides in large quantities are to be avoided.

b. For example, sucrase-isomaltase deficiency requires a decrease in foods high in sucrose content.

c. Trehalose is a disaccharide commonly found in fungi. Persons with trehalase deficiency, therefore, cannot tolerate eating mushrooms.

d. Congenital glucose-galactose malabsorption is treated with a low-carbohydrate diet. Sucrose and all foods high in carbohydrate are to be avoided (see Chap. 16 for food exchange lists).

e. Infants with acquired monosaccharide intolerance are best treated with a modular diet (see Modular Formulas pp. 195, 197).

H. Intestinal Lymphangiectasia

1. Definition

a. Intestinal lymphangiectasia is a generalized disorder of the intestinal lymphatics resulting in a protein-losing enteropathy.

b. It is characterized by edema, hypoproteinemia, lymphocytopenia, and mild gastrointestinal symptoms.

2. Basic Principles

a. The pathogenesis of the transudation of plasma proteins in this disease is thought to be related to increased intestinal lymphatic pressure with dilatation of the vessels and discharge of lymphatic fluid into the bowel lumen.

b. The lost protein is subsequently digested by intestinal enzymes and reabsorbed with only a marginal loss of protein.

c. Ingested fat stimulates lymphatic flow in the gut, since it is transported to the bloodstream by way of the thoracic duct after absorption.

d. Therefore, dietary fat is poorly absorbed and may increase the symptomatology in this disease.

3. Dietary Management

a. Since medium-chain triglycerides can be transported directly into the portal venous system without utilizing the lymphatics, an MCT (medium-chain triglyceride) diet is therapeutic (see MCT diet, pp. 192, 194).

I. Abetalipoproteinemia

1. Definition

a. A rare congenital disease characterized by hypolipemia, acanthocytosis, fat malabsorption, cerebellar ataxia, and accumulation of lipid droplets in the intestinal mucosal cells

2. Basic Principles

a. The basic defect in this disease is related to the inability to transport preformed triglycerides from within the intestinal mucosal cells and the liver.

3. Dietary Management

a. Even though no treatment can arrest the central nervous system complications of this disease, an MCT diet may be helpful in managing the other symptoms (see MCT diet, pp. 192, 194).

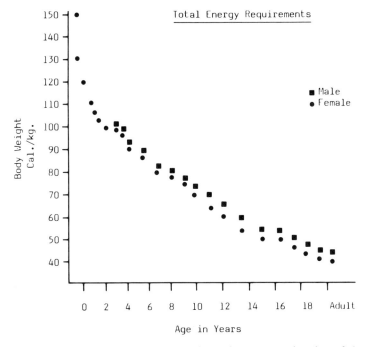

Fig. 12-2. This graph is designed to give only an approximation of the caloric requirements. Disease or a change in activity may change the patient's demand for energy.

IV. Allergic Gastroenteropathy

A. Definition

1. A rather indistinct clinical syndrome characterized by various gastrointestinal symptoms, including pain, diarrhea, melena, nausea, and vomiting, which are precipitated by specific foods

B. Basic Principles

1. Diagnosis of this disorder is difficult because of the variability of symptoms and the lack of good antigens for specific allergy testing.

2. Poor correlation between the available skin testing materials and oral challenges exists.

3. Until present testing methods are improved, this should remain a diagnosis of exclusion.

   a. Sensitivity to food often may be diagnosed by eliminating known or suspected food allergies.

4. The most common food allergies are:

   a. Fruits, especially apples, bananas, berries, grapes, pineapples, oranges, and rhubarb

   b. Vegetables, especially corn and tomatoes

   c. Fats, especially nuts and cream cheese

   d. Protein foods, especially eggs, fish, pork, shellfish, peanut butter, corned beef, and cheese

   e. Chocolate, cocoa, strong spices, garlic, and highly seasoned foods

C. Dietary Management

1. If a specific food antigen can be identified, it should be excluded from the diet.

2. Infants with casein hypersensitivity should be fed formulas made of soy protein or hydrolyzed protein (see Table 12-3).

3. Hypoallergenic diets, which elimi-

nate all food allergens, should be monitored carefully to insure that they are adequate to fulfill the nutritional requirements of the patient.

SPECIAL FEEDING TECHNIQUES

I. Basic Principles

A. The large majority of patients require no special feeding technique.

B. If the patient can feed orally, it is best to allow him to do so.

C. Only in those patients who will not eat, or cannot eat, are other feeding methods appropriate.

II. Tube Diets

A. Whenever tube diets are prescribed, the volume should be based upon the caloric requirement of the patient.

B. Normal values for the total energy requirements for all ages are detailed in Figure 12–2 and Table 2-1.

III. Methodology of Nasogastric and Nasojejunal Tube Feeding

A. This is the technique of choice in a patient whose gastrointestinal tract is intact, but who, for other reasons, cannot ingest adequate calories.

B. The only contraindications to tube feeding are those diseases which result in ileus.

C. Feedings can be given intermittently or continuously depending upon the underlying disease.

D. Intermittent feedings should be delivered slowly, and volumes should be kept relatively small to prevent regurgitation.

E. Care should be taken not to allow the tube to enter the duodenum, where delivery of the feeding would cause a dumping syndrome.

F. If vomiting becomes a problem with nasogastric feeding, the tube should be passed down into the proximal jejunum, and the nutrients should be delivered directly into the small intestine.

1. Continuous infusion is necessary to prevent an osmotic diarrhea when using the nasojejunal feeding technique.

G. Complications from these techniques include nasal erosions and sinusitis and are directly related to the length of time the tube is in place.

1. Changing tubes and alternating sides of the nose every few days will help minimize these complications.

2. The use of silastic tubes also helps alleviate these problems.

IV. Gastrostomy and Jejunostomy

A. The surgical placement of the feeding tube through the abdominal wall directly into the stomach or jejunum should be considered if tube feeding will be required for more than several months.

B. This technique is much less irritating to the patient, and the tube can be hidden from sight when not in use.

C. The same principles apply to these techniques as to the nasal tubes.

V. Total Parenteral Nutrition (TPN)

A. This technique should only be used when gastrointestinal function is not sufficient to provide an adequate caloric intake.

B. The details of this procedure are discussed in the chapter on hyperalimentation (see Chap. 20).

DIETS USED IN CLINICAL PRACTICE

I. High-Protein Diet

A. A high-protein diet is sometimes recommended for use in patients with protein-calorie malnutrition and patients with diseases with increased protein losses, such as protein-losing enteropathy or the nephrotic syndrome.

B. A high-protein diet constitutes a diet in which approximately 20% of the calories are protein.

C. Increasing the protein to greater than 20% is not recommended because the renal solute load of a diet higher than this could be hazardous.

D. By increasing the amount of milk, milk products, eggs, meat, meat substitutes, fish, poultry, cereal, and breads in the diet, the requirements for a high-protein diet generally will be fulfilled.

E. When prescribing a high-protein diet, several considerations should be made.

    1. Adequate caloric intakes should be prescribed.

    2. Protein should supply approximately 20% of the total calories; the remaining calories should come from both fat and carbohydrate.

    3. The major source of protein in the diet should be from animal sources, which have a higher biological value than plant sources.

Rough Estimates for Use in Estimating Proteins in Foods

Animal protein	Plant protein
7 to 9 g.:	7 to 9 g.:
1 oz. meat, fish or poultry	2 tablespoons peanut butter
8 oz. milk	$\frac{1}{2}$ cup cooked dried beans (legumes)
1 egg	1 cup green peas
1 oz. cheese	$\frac{1}{4}$ cup shelled peanuts or sunflower seeds
$\frac{1}{4}$ cup cottage cheese	
$\frac{1}{2}$ cup baked custard	
1 frankfurter (8–10 to the pound)	2 g.:
	1 slice bread
3 g.:	4 graham crackers
$\frac{1}{2}$ cup ice cream	8 saltine crackers
2 thin slices cooked bacon	$\frac{1}{2}$ cup rice, noodles, spaghetti, cereal
	$\frac{1}{2}$ cup potatoes
	$\frac{1}{2}$ cup cooked cereal
	$\frac{1}{2}$ cooked greens, broccoli
	$\frac{1}{4}$ cup pecans
	1 g.:
	$\frac{1}{2}$ cup other vegetables and fruits

F. Protein calculations for a 70 kg. male whose caloric needs have been determined to be 2100 are:

    20% of 2100 Cal. = 420 Cal.

    4 Cal./g. of protein = 420/4 or 105 g. of protein

II. Low-Residue Diet

A. This diet is planned to avoid chemical and mechanical irritation of the gastrointestinal tract by the use of foods low in indigestible carbohydrates, connective tissue, and organic acid content.

B. A minimal-residue diet is helpful in reducing symptoms in diseases of the small intestine which produce strictures such as in regional enteritis and in the treatment of enterocutaneous fistulas.

C. Minimal residue is achieved by restricting all fruits, vegetables, milk products, and whole grains from the diet.

    1. This diet may be deficient in vitamin A, vitamin C, calcium, riboflavin, and iron, so if it is used for any period of time, supplements are required.

D. An alternate way to obtain a minimal-residue diet is by use of elemental diets.

    1. These diets are completely absorbed in the proximal small intestine.

    2. Table 12-1 lists the composition of commercially available elemental diets.

III. Lactose-Restricted Diets

A. A lactose-restricted diet is easily achieved by avoiding milk and milk products (see Table 12–2).

    1. The only exception to this rule is hard aged cheese because the lactose in cheese is converted to lactic acid through aging.

B. A lactose-free diet would include avoidance of all foods and medications which contain lactose as an additive.

    1. Total exclusion of lactose from the diet is usually not necessary because symptoms from lactose intolerance are a dose-related phenomenon.

    2. The average patient can ingest small amounts of lactose without experiencing any problems (see also Lactose Intolerance, p. 179).

Table 12-1. Composition of Commercially Available Elemental Diets
Composition/1000 ml.

Product (Company)	Source of Cho	Source of Pro	Fat	% of Calories Cho	Pro	Fat	Osmolarity mOsm/L	Calcium (mg.)	Phosphorus (mg.)	Iodine (µg.)	Magnesium (mg.)	Zinc (mg.)	Sodium (mg.)	Potassium (mg.)	Chlorine (mg.)	Copper (mg.)	Iron (mg.)	Iron (mg.)
Flexical (Mead Johnson)	Sucrose, oligosaccharides citrate	Hydrolyzed casein + methionine tryptophan and tyrosine	Soy Oil, MCT Oil (20%), soy lecithin	61.00	9.00	30.00	723	600	500	75	200	10	350	1250	1000	1.0	9.0	10.1
Vivonex (Eaton)	Glucose, oligosaccharides	Pure crystalline amino acids	Safflower oil	90.20	8.50	1.30	Flavored 610–678 Unflavored 500	445	445	80	194	6.9	860	1170	1803	1.1	5.6	1.0
Vivonex HN (Eaton)	Glucose oligosaccharides	Pure crystalline amino acids	Safflower oil	80.96	18.26	0.78	850–920	267	267	48	117	4.2	771	702	1858	0.7	3.3	0.6
Precision LR (Doyle)	Maltodextrin, sucrose, citrate	Egg albumin (pasteurized egg white solids)	Soy oil, mono- and diglycerides (as stabilizer)	89.80	9.50	0.70	525	526	526	79	211	7.9	632	789	1000	1.1	9.5	0.08
Precision MN (Doyle)	Maltodextrin, sucrose, citrate	Egg albumin (pasteurized egg white solids)	Soy oil, mono- and diglycerides (as stabilizer)	59.00	13.00	28.00	395	500	500	75	200	7.5	850	750	900	1.0	9.0	3.1
Precision HN (Doyle)	Maltodextrin, sucrose, citrate	Egg albumin (pasteurized egg white solids)	Soy oil, mono- and diglycerides (as stabilizer)	83.00	17.00	0.40	557	333	333	50	134	5.0	933	867	1133	0.7	6.0	0.04
Resolve (Hospital Dietary Products)	Dextrose	Synthetic amino acids	Corn oil, mono- and diglycerides	66.10	8.90	25.00	1516	375	417	0	133	3.9	417	472	0	0.8	10.0	20.8

C. This diet is deficient in calcium, and children and pregnant or lactating women should be given calcium supplements.

1. This can be easily accomplished in children by offering them a lactose-free milk substitute, such as a soy-based formula, or by use of a calcium supplement, such as Neo-calglucon.

2. Pregnant or lactating women should also be supplemented while on this diet with a dose of 400 to 500 mg. calcium per day. There are many commercial preparations of calcium available (see the PDR).

IV. Other Carbohydrate-Restricted Diets

A. Infants with intractable diarrhea may develop intolerance to carbohydrates other than lactose.

1. This may include intolerance to sucrose, maltose, and, occasionally, glucose.

2. A formula must be selected which avoids the particular sugars which produce symptoms.

3. Table 12-3 lists the available infant formulas with their composition.

B. Because intractable diarrhea with carbohydrate intolerance is a reversible disease, an attempt should be made to reinstitute a more normal formula after symptoms have been controlled for several months.

V. Gluten-Free Diet

A. Gluten is a water-insoluble protein moiety found in the cereal grains, wheat, barley, rye, and oats.

B. This substance is toxic to the intestinal mucosa of patients with celiac disease or adult non-tropical sprue.

C. Treatment of this disease is based upon the avoidance of gluten because even small amounts of this substance can cause symptoms.

1. Cereals and bakery products made from wheat, barley, rye, and oats must be eliminated from the diet (see Table 12-4).

D. A gluten-free diet may be difficult to achieve because commercial products such as frankfurters, sausage, cold cuts, soups, and baked beans frequently use wheat flour as a filler.

E. Professional counselling by a trained dietitian may be necessary in some instances to achieve an adequate gluten-free diet.

F. Because this diet does not meet the recommended dietary allowances for iron and thiamine for certain age groups, supplementation is sometimes required.

G. Because of the restrictive nature of this diet, the diagnosis of celiac disease and non-tropical sprue should not be made casually.

VI. Nutritional Supplements

A. Various products have been designed for the purpose of supplementing a patient's caloric intake or providing him with complete nutrition by means of a nasogastric tube when gastrointestinal function is normal, but mechanical problems interfere with the ingestion of sufficient food.

B. Patients who benefit from these products include those who cannot eat because of coma, ventilators, or oropharyngeal disease, or those who require more calories than they can ingest because of anorexia or hypermetabolic disease states such as chronic infection.

C. Examples of these products include Ensure, Sustacal, Isocal, Nutri-1000 Liquid, and Formula 2 (see Table 12-5).

D. Most of these products are based on milk or milk protein with various kinds of carbohydrates and fats added to increase the caloric content to 30 cal./oz. Cutter's Formula 2 is a defined blenderized diet.

(Text continues on p. 191.)

Table 12-2. Lactose-Restricted Diet

Individuals vary in their ability to utilize lactose. Those who are lactase deficient or who have a transitory lactose intolerance are often able to consume small amounts of milk and its products. Some can only tolerate milk in cereal or in their coffee, and others cannot tolerate lactose in any form. This latter situation, however, is rare.

Milk is the most important food item in the diet of the infant and young child. It is the major source of protein, calcium, phosphorous, riboflavin, vitamin A, vitamin D, and water. For infants, it is also the major source of calories. When milk is removed from the diet, great care must be taken to replace the nutrients. A lactose-free formula, such as fortified soy, should be substituted for milk. Most often an older child who has acquired a "taste" for milk refuses proprietary formulas. In this event, he should be given supplemental calcium, riboflavin, and, in some instances, vitamin A and vitamin D. Protein food items, such as meat, poultry, fish, and peanut butter, should be used to replace milk protein. Water or juices can be used as a beverage. Whole grain and enriched breads and cereals, leafy dark green vegetables, liver, and other lean meats contain riboflavin. However, until a child consumes a variety of foods in substantial amounts, riboflavin should be supplemented to the diet.

For those who can tolerate limited amounts of lactose, the following food items are generally accepted without symptoms:

Cultured products such as buttermilk and yogurt
Cheese
Milk and milk solids contained in such products as bread, hot bread, cake, sherbet
Margarine and butter
Milk treated with commercial enzymatic products that hydrolyze the lactose

Food items generally omitted include all those in which milk or milk products are the main constituent.

Milk, whole, skim, and low-fat
Milk drinks (malted milk, milk shakes, chocolate milk)
Creamed soups and sauces, hot chocolate, ice cream, and pudding

Lactose-Free Diet

For those persons who cannot tolerate any lactose, a diet in which lactose is eliminated should be prescribed. The patient must become label conscious because many processed foods contain some lactose in many forms, such as milk, milk solids, curds, and whey. (Those foods containing lactalbumin, lactic acid, and calcium lactate are allowed because these substances are chemically different from lactose.)

	Foods Allowed	*Foods Not Allowed*
Beverages	Fruit juices, soft drinks made without lactose, coffee, tea, fortified soy formulas can be substituted for milk if accepted.	Milk and milk drinks, instant chocolate drinks, cultured milks (unless tolerated), powdered soft drinks, instant coffee or tea with added lactose.
Meat, poultry, fish, meat substitutes	Beef, veal, lamb, pork, chicken, turkey, fish, shellfish, glandular meats. Salmon and sardines with bones, and oysters are good calcium sources. Bake, broil, boil, or fry without adding milk, butter, or bread crumbs containing milk. Legumes, nuts, and nut butters.	Weiners, bologna, lunch meat, commercially breaded meats and fish (i.e., fish sticks), all types of cheese including American, blue, cheddar, cottage, roquefort, cheese spreads, casseroles made with milk or commercial soups containing milk, creamed foods. Check label of canned legumes and peanut butter for added lactose.
Eggs	Hard- or soft-cooked, fried or scrambled without adding butter, milk, or cream.	Eggs in cream sauce or cooked with milk.
Vegetables	Any fresh, frozen, or canned. Prepare without butter, cream, soups. (Broccoli and the dark leafy greens such as turnips, mustard, and collard greens are good sources of calcium.)	No cream sauces, butter, commercially prepared sauces containing milk, butter, or lactose-containing foods. Some instant potato products and french fries have added lactose. Check labels.

186

Table 12-2. **Lactose-Restricted Diet** *(Continued)*

	Foods Allowed	Foods Not Allowed
Potatoes and substitutes	White or sweet potatoes, rice, noodles, macaroni, spaghetti	Foods cooked with cheese, white sauce, or canned or frozen soups containing milk, lactose, whey, or curds. Packaged dry mixes with milk, lactose, whey, or curds added, convenience and cheese dinners.
Fruit	Fresh, canned, frozen, dried.	Check labels for lactose.
Breads	Some commercial french breads are made without milk—check label. Hot water cornbread made without milk. Homemade bread made without milk, butter, whey, curds.	Commercial breads containing milk solids, butter, or margarine with whey, lactose, curds. Rolls, biscuits, commercial bread mixes, corn mixes, waffles, pancakes, coffee cake, doughnuts.
Cereals	Cooked cereals made without milk: oatmeal, farina, grits, cream of wheat, cream of rice pettijohns. Ready-to-eat cereals (check labels). Those generally lactose-free: cornflakes, puffed rice, puffed wheat, shredded wheat, Rice Krispies. Many patients, especially children, like ready-to-eat cereals plain or with fruit juice.	Many ready-to-eat cereals are presweetened and contain, along with sugar, lactose. Check labels of ready-to-eat and instant cereals for added lactose. Cereals should be eaten without milk, cream, or milk products added.
Fats	Margarine without added milk solids, shortening, oil, some non-dairy cream substitutes.	Butter, margarine with milk solids added, cream. Non-dairy cream substitutes with added lactose.
Soups	Broth, homemade soup made with tomato or broth as base. Check labels of commercially prepared soups.	Cream and milk soups such as cheese or potato soup, oyster or clam chowder; commercially prepared soups with added lactose.
Desserts	Fruits, plain or fruited gelatin dessert without milk, angel food cake, fruit ices, fruit tapioca, and fruit pie (do not season with butter). Cookies made without butter, margarine without milk solids or milk, sherbet made without milk solids or lactose.	Custard, puddings, cream tapioca, butter cakes and cakes containing milk, lactose, milk solids, whey; crusts made with milk, French pastries made with butter and milk; cookies made with butter, milk, or margarine containing milk solids, ice cream.
Miscellaneous	Salt, pepper, sugar (cane or beet, white or brown), honey, jam, jelly, spices, herbs, cocoa, candy made from foods allowed, marshmallows, meat sauces and gravies with cornstarch or potato.	Check contents on labels of all commercially prepared products. Commercially prepared sauces unless prepared from foods allowed on list.

Table 12-3. **Composition of Infant Formulas**
Composition/100 ml.

Product (Company)	Source of Cho	Source of Pro	Fat	Normal Dilution	Cal./oz. Normal Dilution	Pro (g.)	Fat (g.)	Cho (mEq.)	Na (mEq.)	K (mEq.)	Ca (mg.)	P (mg.)	Fe (mg.)	Chloride (mEq.)	Magnesium (mg.)	Zinc (mg.)	Solute Loads Renal mOsm./100 ml.	Solute Loads Intestinal mOsm./kg. H₂O	Indications
Human Milk					20	1.2	3.8	7.0	0.7	1.4	33	15	0.15	1.1			10.1		
Cow's Milk					20	3.3	3.7	4.8	2.7	3.7	138	96	0.1	2.9	13		27.7	275	
Milk-based Formulas																			
Enfamil (Mead Johnson)	Lactose	Skim milk	Soy oil, coconut oil	1:1 or 1 measure:2 oz. H₂O	20	1.5	3.7	7.0	1.2	1.8	54	46	0.14*	1.3	5	0.4	12.8	299	Routine infant feeding
Similac (Ross)	Lactose	Skim milk	Soy oil, coconut oil, corn oil	1:1 or 1 measure:2 oz. H₂O	20	1.6	3.6	7.2	0.96	1.7	57	43	tr.†	1.58	4	0.5	10.5	290	Routine infart feeding
Similac PM 60/40 Liquid (Ross)	Lactose	Electro-dialyzed whey, sodium caseinate	Coconut oil, corn oil	1:1	20	1.6	3.8	6.9	0.7	1.5	40	20	0.26	0.71	4	0.4	9.2	281	60% Lactalbumin: lactoglobulin, 40% Casein: Indicated for infants needing lower renal solute load
S-M-A (Wyeth)	Lactose	Skim milk, whey	Coconut oil, oleo oil, soy oil, safflower oil	1:1	20	1.5	3.6	7.2	0.7	1.4	44	33	1.27				11.6	300	Routine infant feeding
Soy-based Formulas																			
ProSobee (Mead Johnson)	Sucrose, corn syrup solids	Soy protein isolate, L-Methionine	Soy oil	1:1	20	2.5	3.4	6.8	1.8	1.9	78	52	1.2	1.17	7	0.5	26.3	258	Milk sensitivity or lactose intolerance, galactosemia
Mull-Soy (Syntex)	Sucrose	Soy flour	Soy oil	1:1	20	3.2	3.7	5.3	1.6	3.6	125	83	1.04	1.6	8	0.8	24.4	236	" "

	Carbohydrate	Protein	Oil	Dilution														Indications
Neo-Mull-Soy (Syntex)	Sucrose	Soy protein isolate, L–Methionine	Soy oil	1:1	20	1.8	3.5	6.4	1.6	2.3	83	63	1.04		8	0.3	15.8	253	″
Nursoy (Wyeth)	Sucrose, corn syrup	Soy protein isolate	Oleo oil, soy oil, safflower oil	1:1	20	2.3	3.6	6.8	0.83	1.5	65	46	1.2						″
Isomil (Ross)	Sucrose, corn syrup solids, corn starch	Soy protein isolate, L–Methionine	Corn oil, coconut oil, soy oil	1:1	20	2.0	3.6	6.8	1.3	1.8	70	50	1.2	1.5	5	0.5	12.6	253	″
Cho-Free (Syntex)	None	Soy protein isolate, L–Methionine	Soy oil	1:1 (12.8% CHO Sol.)	20	1.8	3.5		1.6	2.3	88	68	0.83	0.9	8	0.5	15.6	509	Disaccharide or monosaccharide intolerance
Meat-based Formulas																		
MBF (Gerbers)	Sucrose, modified tapioca starch	Beef hearts	Sesame oil	1:1.5	17	2.9	3.3	4.2	0.8	1.0	101	67	1.5	0.73	4		19.0	147	Milk sensitivity or lactose intolerance, galactosemia
Special Formulas																		
Lofenalac (Mead Johnson)	Corn syrup solids, tapioca starch	Specially processed hydrolyzed casein	Corn oil	1 Measure:2 oz. H₂O	20	2.2	2.7	8.7	2.0	2.6	94	65	1.2	2.3	8	0.4	19.6	457	Phenylketonuria
Nutramigen (Mead Johnson)	Sucrose, tapioca starch	Enzymatically hydrolyzed casein	Corn oil	″	20	2.2	2.6	8.6	1.7	2.6	94	65	1.2	2.3	8	0.4	19.6	484	Sensitivity to intact proteins of milk
Portagen (Mead Johnson)	Corn syrup solids, sucrose	Sodium caseinate	MCT oil, corn oil	″	20	2.4	3.3	7.8	1.7	2.6	67	53	1.2		14	0.4	18.5	236	Fat malabsorption, disaccharide intolerance
Pregestimil (Mead Johnson)	Dextrose, tapioca starch	Enzymatically hydrolyzed casein	MCT oil, corn oil	″	20	2.2	2.8	8.8	1.7	2.3	90	73	1.2	2.3	8	0.4	19.4	627	Disaccharide intolerance

*Enfamil c̄ Iron = 0.85 mg. Iron
†Similac c̄ Iron = 1.2 mg. Iron

Table 12-4. **Gluten-Restricted Diet**

General Information

Foods made from the cereal grains—wheat, oats, rye, and barley—are omitted in this diet. These grains are ubiquitous in the American diet, and efforts to avoid them must be thorough. Flour or meal from rice, potato, soy, and corn are used for making breads, cakes, cereals, pastries, and thickening agents. Some patients on this diet can tolerate the minute amounts of wheat protein present in wheat starch flour. This can be used in baking breads, cakes, and cookies.

Nutritional counselling should be provided by a dietitian. Along with the individualized instructional list, recipes for using the flour or meal of rice, potato, soy, and corn should be provided. Initially the patient should keep an accurate and detailed food diary. The diary should include types of foods eaten, methods of preparation, and where food was eaten. This can assist in determining the patient's understanding of the diet and should assist in directing him to long-term diet compliance.

If careful dietary assessment and clinical examination of the patient indicate inadequacies of the B vitamins and iron, they should be supplemented in the diet. In the event that the patient continues with malabsorption symptoms, other nutrients including the fat-soluble vitamins might be considered for supplementation.

Gluten-Restricted Diet

	Foods Allowed	Foods Not Allowed
Beverages	Milk, milk substitutes, fruit juices, soft drinks, tea, coffee. Initially, milk might not be tolerated. Once resumed in diet, it should be added gradually. If to be omitted, milk substitute or nutrient supplementation should be considered.	Coffee substitutes made with cereal, milk drinks mixed with malt, instant mixes with malt or cereal added, beer, ale.
Meat, poultry, fish, meat substitutes	Beef, veal, lamb, pork, chicken, turkey, fish, shellfish, glandular meats, cheese, cottage cheese, cream cheese, natural cheese, dried beans and peas, nuts, and nut butters. Bake, broil, boil, or fry without adding flour, bread coatings, or cereal grains listed in the "not allowed" list.	Any commercially prepared product containing cereals not allowed. Luncheon meat, weiners, meat loaf, sausage, meat or fish patties, and gravies usually contain one of the grain products not allowed and should be avoided unless made from pure meat. Casserole-type foods made with cereals not allowed, canned and frozen foods containing sauces thickened with flour/meal of grains not allowed. Cheese spreads containing cereal products as fillers not allowed.
Eggs	Hard or soft cooked, fried, poached, scrambled	Eggs in sauces containing cereal flours not allowed.
Vegetables	Any fresh, frozen, or canned vegetable or vegetable juice	Vegetables cooked with sauces thickened with grain products (wheat flour, etc.) not allowed.
Potatoes and substitutes	White or sweet potatoes, rice, corn, hominy, gluten-free (low protein) pastas, grits.	Noodles, macaroni, spaghetti
Fruit	Fresh, canned, frozen, dried	Check labels of fruit sauces to make sure thickening agent does not contain flours of grains not allowed.

(Continued)

Table 12-4. **Gluten-Restricted Diet** *(Continued)*

	Foods Allowed	Foods Not Allowed
Breads	Breads made from: rice flour, cornmeal, soybean flour, gluten-free wheat starch and potato starch. Waffles, pancakes and muffins can be made using grain flour/meal allowed. Corn tortillas, corn and potato chips may be used. Rice crackers made without gluten, gluten-free (low protein) breads.	Wheat flour bread, oatmeal, rye or barley breads, flour tortillas, commercially prepared biscuits, pancakes, waffles, toaster pastries, crackers made from wheat flour, wheat gluten, and cereal flours not allowed. Check labels for grain flours not allowed.
Cereals	Cereals made from rice or corn, such as cream of rice, boiled rice, corn grits, cornmeal mush. Ready to eat cereals such as corn flakes, Rice Krispies, puffed rice, rice flakes. Manufacturers publish updated ingredient lists of cereals.	All those containing wheat, wheat gluten, oats, rye, or barley, such as oatmeal, pettijohns, cream of wheat, wheat flakes, Cheerios, shredded wheat. Check labels for cereal grains not allowed.
Fats	Butter, margarine, shortening, oil salad dressing made with those cereal flours allowed.	Commercial salad dressings made with wheat flour or thickened with other restricted grain flour/meals not allowed.
Soups	Broth, home-made vegetable soups made from foods allowed; creamed soup with cornstarch or potato	Commercially prepared canned or frozen soups thickened with wheat flour, oats, barley or rye, or those containing barley.
Desserts	Fruits, plain or fruited gelatin desserts, cornstarch and tapioca puddings, home-made ice cream without flour, sherbet and fruit ices, meringue shells. Cakes, cookies, and pies can be made from allowed flours (see bread list). Grain products allowed can be made into pie crusts and cookies.	Commercial cakes, cookies, pastries, pies, puddings, ice cream
Miscellaneous	Salt, pepper, sugar (cane or beet, white or brown), honey, jam, jelly, spices, herbs, cocoa, candy made from foods allowed, marshmallows, meat sauces and gravies with cornstarch or potato.	Check contents on labels of all commercially prepared products. Commercially prepared sauces unless prepared from foods allowed on list.

E. The advantages of these products are

  1. Acceptable flavor

  2. Relatively high caloric concentration in a liquid form

  3. Low osmolality

  4. They represent a complete diet.

F. The single disadvantage is that patients frequently get bored with them because they do not offer enough variety in taste and texture.

G. Table 12-5 lists some of the available products with their compositions.

VII. Elemental Diets

A. Elemental diets are chemically defined diets made up of predigested (hydrolyzed) protein or synthetic amino acids, glucose, or sucrose as the calorie source, a small amount of fat in the form of essential fatty acids, minerals including electrolytes and the trace elements, and vitamins.

B. They are totally absorbed in the proximal gut, which is an advantage in fistulas and the short-gut syndrome.

C. They have low to no residue, which is an advantage in fistulas and lower bowel diseases such as regional enteritis or ulcerative colitis.

D. Because of the decrease in fecal production, they are helpful in diseases in which feces are a disadvantage (i.e., burns or rectal surgery).

E. They do not require pancreatic enzymes for digestion, which is helpful in pancreatitis and cystic fibrosis.

F. These diets have several disadvantages.

　1. They tend to taste bad because of the presence of the sulfated amino acids, which impart to them a sulphur-like flavor.

　2. The osmotic density of these products varies from 700 to 1500 mOsm./L., which causes an uncomfortable feeling of fullness when in the stomach and may result in an osmotic diarrhea when used improperly.

　3. The glucose they contain may be absorbed rapidly and produce hyperglycemia.

G. They are best tolerated initially at half-strength concentration and then at increasing strength over several days.

H. Because of their flavor, a nasogastric tube generally is required to deliver significant quantities of elemental diets.

I. Table 12-1 lists some of the commercially available elemental diet products and their composition.

VIII. Medium-Chain Triglyceride (MCT) Diet

A. Medium-chain triglycerides are more efficiently absorbed than long-chain fats in patients with pancreatic or biliary insufficiency and certain diseases of absorption such as intestinal lymphangiectasia and abetalipoproteinemia.

B. MCT is made up of fatty acids which vary from 6 to 12 carbons in length as compared to long-chain triglycerides (LCT) which are greater than 16 carbons in length. MCT's are partially soluble in water thereby giving them their unique properties.

C. Because they are not dependent upon bile acids for solubilization, they are utilized by patients with liver disease.

D. They are able to appose the mucosal surface because of their solubility and to be hydrolyzed by mucosal lipases, therefore, they do not require pancreatic lipase.

E. A large percentage of absorbed MCT is transported directly into the portal circulation bypassing the lymphatic channels, which are necessary for the transport of long-chain triglycerides. This decreases lymphatic flow and is useful in the management of patients with diseases such as intestinal lymphangiectasia.

F. An MCT diet restricts the amount of long-chain fat in the diet and replaces it with MCT (see Table 12-6).

　1. The natural source of MCT is coconut oil which is fractionated through steam distillation to prepare the commercial product, which is essentially 100% MCT.

　2. This product can be used to fry food or can be added to skim milk and taken as a beverage.

　3. Portagen (Mead Johnson) is a commercial MCT product which can be used as an infant formula or as an adult beverage (see Table 12-7).

G. Disadvantages of MCT diet

　1. It is not very palatable.

　2. When given in large amounts, it has a cathartic effect which occasionally limits its usefulness.

Table 12-5. Composition of Commercially Available Tube Diets
Composition/1000 ml.

Product (Company)	Type	Normal Dilution Cal./ml.	Source of Cho	Source of Pro	Fat	% of Calories Cho	% of Calories Pro	% of Calories Fat	Osmolality mOsm./kg.	Calcium (mg.)	Phosphorus (mg.)	Iodine (µg.)	Magnesium (mg.)	Zinc (mg.)	Sodium (mg.)	Potassium (mg.)	Chlorine (mg.)	Copper (mg.)	Iron (mg.)	Manganese (mg.)	Lactase (mg.)
Ensure (Ross)	Tube fdg/oral	1 Cal./ml.	Sucrose, glucose oligosaccharides	Casein	Corn oil	54.5	14.0	31.5	450 c̄ Flavor Pack 465–480	420	420	35	210	15.9	740	1270	1060	1.1	9.5	.26	0
Formula 2 (Cutter)	Tube fdg	1 Cal./ml.	Blended foods			49	15	36	300–600	1300	1100		150	5.5	450	2100		1.0	15	.2	50
Meritene Liquid (Doyle)	Tube fdg/oral	1 Cal./ml.	Milk-based formula			46	24	30	640	1500	1300	126.8	300	8.5	950	1700		1.7	16.9	3.4	56
Compleat-B (Doyle)	Tube fdg	1 Cal./ml.	Blended foods			48	16	36	500–600	500	1400	87	220	8.7	1400	1400		1.2	11.2	2.5	19
Sustacal (Mead Johnson)	Oral	1 Cal./ml.	Sucrose, glucose oligosaccharides, lactose	Skim milk, sodium caseinate, soy protein isolate	Soy oil	55	24	21	625	1000	920	139	380	14	930	2060		1.9	17	2.8	17
Isocal (Mead Johnson)	Tube fdg.	1 Cal./ml.	Glucose and glucose oligosaccharides	Sodium caseinate, soy protein isolate	Soy oil, MCT oil	50.0	13.0	37.0	350	600	500	75	200	10	500	1250	1000	1.0	9	2.5	0
Sustagen (Mead Johnson)	Tube fdg/oral	1.8 Cal./ml.	Lactose, glucose oligosaccharides, dextrose	Calcium caseinate, skim and whole milk	Milk fat	68.0	24.0	8.0		3331	2498	156	416	20.8	1249	3331		2.1	18.7	5.2	0
Nutri-1000 (Syntex)	Tube fdg/oral	1 Cal./ml.	Lactose, sucrose, dextrin, tri- and di-tetrasaccharides, dextrose, maltose	Skim milk	Corn oil	40.0	13.0	47.0	500	1200	950	79.3	200	7.9	530	1500	1200	1.1	9.5	1.3	53

Table 12-6. **Information for Medium-Chain Triglyceride Diet**

Medium-chain triglycerides (MCT), a fractionated coconut oil product, must be added to food items to replace the calories removed when long-chain triglycerides (LCT) are omitted from the diet. Commercial formulas, such as Portagen and Pregestimil, which contain MCT are available. Small amounts of LCT, as vegetable oils, are added to these formulas to provide the essential fatty acid, linoleic acid, to the diet. Both commercial formulas presently available are lactose-free, and protein is provided in the form of casein in Portagen and in the form of hydrolyzed casein in Pregestimil.

A medium-chain triglyceride formula, using skim milk as a base, can be prepared at home. A blender is essential for preparation of the formula to allow the MCT to become homogenized. The formula can be individualized to fill the infant's needs. When 3.5 g. of MCT is added to each 100 ml. of skim milk, a 20 cal./oz. infant formula containing the following components is provided:

1.8 to 2.2 g./dl. protein from the skim milk
3.5 g./dl. fat from medium-chain triglycerides (fractionated coconut oil)
6.7 to 7.5 g./dl. carbohydrate as lactose

Note: 2.5 to 5% of the total calories should come from the essential fatty acid, linoleic acid. This is best provided by adding 2 to 3 ml. of safflower oil/L. of formula.

Foods that are eaten along with the prescribed formula should be low in fat. Baby foods vary in fat content. Plain cereals, fruits, and vegetables contain minimal amounts. Meats, egg, mixed dinners, and desserts contain higher amounts of fat.

While on these formulas, infants derive over 40% of their calories from fat, 95% of which is MCT. This relationship changes as the child begins to eat table foods. Meat contains approximately 3 to 5 g. of fat per oz. Though fat in the diet may remain at 40% of the total calories, the proportion of calories from MCT drops from 95% to as low as 65% of the total fat calories. Safflower oil remains a necessary supplementation to the diet to assure an adequate intake of linoleic acid.

Many patients with fat malabsorption require supplementation with the fat-soluble vitamins, A, D, and K. Supplementation should be individualized and prescribed after careful nutritional assessment. Other nutrients to supplement are dependent on the etiology of malabsorption and could include iron, folic acid, or B_{12}.

Note: Fractionated coconut oil is a highly saturated fat and should not be used by family members who are not on an MCT diet.

The following exchange list details those foods which are allowed and not allowed for the adult on a low-fat, MCT diet.

Medium-Chain Triglyceride Diet

	Food Allowed	*Foods Not Allowed*
Beverages	Skim milk, MCT formula, evaporated skim milk, fruit juices, soft drinks, coffee, tea	Whole milk, condensed milk, evaporated whole milk, milkshakes, commercially prepared eggnog, formulas made with long-chain fats such as soy oil, corn oil.
Meat, poultry, fish, meat substitutes	Lean beef, veal, lamb, pork, chicken, turkey, fish, shellfish, glandular meat. Bake, broil, or boil. Meats can be fryed in MCT. Fat-free cottage cheese, especially prepared processed cheese food made with skim milk but without added fats or oils. Legumes such as pinto beans, kidney beans, vegetarian-style canned legumes.	Fatty meats, such as weiners, bologna, commercially prepared fried foods and frozen dinners, casserole foods made with fatty meat sauces with fat or other foods not allowed. All types cheeses except those specified Nuts, nut butters. Fats in cooking except MCT
Eggs	Three (3) eggs a week; egg whites as desired	Fried or scrambled eggs unless prepared in MCT

(Continued)

Table 12-6. **Information for Medium-Chain Triglyceride Diet** *(Continued)*

	Food Allowed	Foods Not Allowed
Vegetables	Any fresh, frozen or canned. Prepare with MCT added or sauce made with MCT and skim milk	Processed vegetables cooked with margarine, butter or sauces; avocado
Potatoes or substitutes	White or sweet potatoes, rice, noodles, spaghetti. Potatoes can be fried in MCT.	Fried, unless with MCT, creamed or whipped unless with skim milk and MCT, au gratin, unless specially prepared with special cheese, potato chips.
Fruits	Fresh, canned, frozen, dried, fruit juices	Processed or in desserts with added fats
Breads	White, wheat, french, or rye bread, enriched crackers (saltine, soda, and others low in fat)	Commercially prepared mixes, biscuits, muffins, hot breads, doughnuts, cornbread, unless made with skim milk and MCT. Tortillas unless made with MCT. Rolls with butter or margarine added, crackers made with added fats or cheeses, sesame, or other seeds.
Cereals	Cooked or ready to eat (Check labels for added fats).	Granola-type cereals with added seeds or oils, cereals with added fats or oils (Check labels).
Fats	The amount of fractionated coconut oil (MCT) used is dependent on the percentage of MCT in the diet. Safflower oil as specified.	Butter, margarine, cooking oil, shortening, cream, whipped topping, gravy, white sauce, salt pork, bacon or other meat drippings, non-dairy cream substitutes, regular coconut oil
Soups	Fat-free broth, bouillon, consomme, milk soups made with skim milk and MCT	Commercially prepared soups, either canned or frozen except bouillon cubes or fat-free broth
Desserts	Fruits, plain or fruited gelatin desserts, angel food cakes, fruit ices, sherbet made with skim milk solids, popsicles, custard or pudding made with skim milk and egg allowance. Cakes and cookies can be prepared using MCT and egg allowance.	Cake mixes, butter, oil, or shortening-based cakes, pies, commercial cookies, whipped topping, desserts, cream tapioca, commercial ice cream, iced milk
Miscellaneous	Salt, pepper, sugar (cane or beet), honey, jam, jelly, spices, herbs, catsup, mustard, vinegar, hard candy, cocoa powder, salad dressings made with MCT, popcorn made with MCT	Commercially prepared mayonnaise and salad dressings, chocolate chips and chocolate, sauces made with fats or seeds (i.e. barbecue), fried pork rinds

3. It is devoid of essential fatty acid (linoleic acid), and, when used as the exclusive fat in the diet, linoleic acid must be supplemented. This can easily be accomplished by adding a small amount (approximately 5% of the calories) of safflower oil to the diet.

IX. Modular Formula

A. Modular formula is a dietary preparation for use in treating infants with complex malabsorptive disorders.

B. With this formula, the physician can alter the quality of the various nutri-

Table 12-7. Composition of Commercially Available Specialty Products
Composition/1000 ml.

Product (Company)	Type	Normal Dilution Cal./ml.	Source of Cho	Source of Pro	Source of Fat	% Cal Cho	% Cal Pro	% Cal Fat	Osmolality mOsm./kg.	Calcium (mg.)	Phosphorus (mg.)	Iodine (mg.)	Magnesium (µg.)	Zinc (mg.)	Sodium (mg.)	Potassium (mg.)	Chlorine (mg.)	Copper (mg.)	Iron (mg.)	Manganese (mg.)
Polycose Liquid (Ross)	Calorie supplement	2 Cal./ml.	Glucose polymers derived from controlled acid/enzyme hydrolysis of corn starch	—	—	100			850	16	3			3.0	62	4	110			
Polycose Powder (Ross)	Calorie supplement	32 Cal./tbs.	Glucose polymers derived from controlled acid/enzyme hydrolysis of corn starch	—	—	100			850	14	9			6.6	122	8	234			
MCT Oil (Mead Johnson)	Medium-chain triglyceride supplement	8.3 Cal./g.			Fractionated coconut oil (94% C8-C10 fatty acids)			100												
Lonalac (Mead Johnson)	Low sodium	.67 Cal.	Lactose	Casein	Coconut Oil	28.6	20.3	47.0	259	1163	1057				20	1050				
Portagen (Mead Johnson)	MCT diet	.67 Cal./ml. / 1 Cal./ml.	Malto-dextrins and sucrose	Sodium caseinate	MCT Oil (95%) and corn oil	46.0 / 46.0	14.0 / 14.0	40.0 / 40.0	346 / 236	625 / 937	468 / 708	47 / 73	135 / 208	6.2 / 9.4	312 / 468	833 / 1249	573 / 859	1.0 / 1.6	12.4 / 19.8	2.1 / 3.1
Hycal (Beecham Labs)	Calorie supplement	2.5 Cal./ml.	Demineralized glucose	None	None	100				1					16	7				
Cal-Power (General Mills)	Calorie supplement	2.3 Cal./ml.	Deionized liquid glucose	None	None	100				3			1		30	15	7			
Amin-Aid (McGaw)	Low-protein	2 Cal./ml. calories	Malto-dextrin, sucrose	L-Essential amino acids + histidine	Modified soy bean oil	68.0	4.0	28.0	1050	<2 mEq			<2 mEq	<2 mEq	<2 mEq	<2 mEq	<2 mEq		2.1	

ents normally fed to infants, as well as the concentrations of those nutrients.

C. Infants who cannot tolerate existing proprietary formulas will often thrive on judicious use of this flexible formula.

D. The core module is comprised of only protein in the form of calcium, sodium caseinate, and electrolytes.

E. Its composition is shown in Table 12-8.

F. Infants are first challenged with the protein core and, if tolerated, are weaned onto fat and carbohydrate in a stepwise manner as shown in Table 12-9.

G. Any fat or carbohydrate may be used depending upon the infant's tolerance.

Table 12-8. **Composition of Modular Formula, Human Milk, and Milk Base Formulas**

	Modular Formula (usual concentration)	Human Milk	Milk Base Formulas* (range)
Protein (g./dl.)	2.2	1.4	1.51–3.6
Calcium (mg./dl.)	42.0	34.0	44.0–100.0
Phosphorus (mg./dl.)	32.0	14.0	33.0–80.0
Sodium (mEq./L.)	8.0	7.0	7.0–17.0
Potassium (mEq./L.)	20.0	13.0	14.0–32.0
Chloride (mEq./L.)	22.0	11.0	10.0–29.0
Magnesium (mg./dl.)	4.0	4.0	4.0–8.5
Iron (mg./dl.)	0.62	0.05	Trace–1.8
Copper (mg./dl.)	0.08	0.04	0.04–0.10
Zinc (mg./dl.)	0.32	0.30	0.20–0.42
Iodine (mg./dl.)	0.03	0.03	0.04–0.10

*Include Similac (Ross), Enfamil (Mead Johnson), SMA (Wyeth), and Similac Advance (Ross)
((Klish, W.J., Potts, E., Ferry, D., and Nichols, B.L.: Modular formula: an approach to management of infants with specific or complex food intolerances. J. Pediatr., *88*:948, 1976)

Table 12-9. **Standard Composition of Modular Formula**

Quantity/L.			g./dl.			Cal./dl.
Modular Core* (g.)	Fat† (ml.)	Cho‡	Protein	Fat	Cho	
10	–	–	0.7	–	–	2.8
20	–	–	1.5	–	–	6.0
30	–	–	2.2	–	–	8.8
30	15	–	2.2	1.4	–	21.4
30	30	–	2.2	2.8	–	34.0
30	45	–	2.2	4.2	–	46.6
30	45	10 g.	2.2	4.2	1.0	50.6
30	45	20 g.	2.2	4.2	2.0	54.6
30	45	30 g.	2.2	4.2	3.0	58.6
30	45	40 g.	2.2	4.2	4.0	62.6
30	45	50 g.	2.2	4.2	5.0	66.6
30	45	70 g.	2.2	4.2	7.0	74.6

*One tbsp. of Modular Formula weighs 5 g. which is 73.5% protein and 26.5% salts and water of hydration.
†Most oils weigh 14 g./tbsp.
‡Most sugars weigh 12 g./tbsp. in dry form.
(Klish, W. J., Potts, E., Ferry, D. and Nichols, B. L.: Modular formula: an approach to management of infants with specific or complex food intolerances. J. Pediatr., *88*:948, 1976)

X. Supplemental Vitamins and Mineral Preparations

A. Normal individuals ingesting a normal well-balanced diet do not require vitamin and mineral supplementation.

B. High-risk groups such as pregnant or lactating women, geriatric patients, and infants may require these supplements.

C. Individuals on restricted diets frequently need vitamin supplements as noted in the discussion of diets for specific disease states.

D. As a general rule, any patient recovering from a disease associated with loss of weight would benefit from supplementation until normal weight is achieved.

E. Mineral supplements, when required, are usually specific (e.g., iron and calcium). When vitamin supplementation is required, multivitamin preparations should be used.

XI. Commercially Available Specialty Products

A. A series of products has been developed to help the physician treating patients with special medical problems.

B. These products are listed below with their indications.

Product	Indication
Lonalac	Sodium-restricted diet
Portagen	Pancreatic insufficiency
Amin-Aid	Low-protein diet
Polycose	High-calorie supplement
MCT Oil	Medium-chain triglyceride supplement

C. The complete composition of these specialty products is given in Table 12-7.

D. Some of these products are not complete diets, and care must be taken with their use so as not to produce nutrient deficiencies.

13. NUTRITION AND DISORDERS OF THE COLON

George D. Ferry, M.D.

I. The Irritable Colon Syndrome

A. Definition

1. The irritable colon syndrome is characterized by recurrent abdominal pain, constipation, and/or diarrhea.

2. An alteration or exaggeration in the motor activity of the lower colon has been demonstrated in patients with this disorder, and this response is directly related to stress and emotional tension.

3. Synonyms include spastic colon, mucous colitis, and nervous diarrhea.

B. Basic Principles

1. The irritable colon is the most common chronic gastrointestinal disorder seen by gastroenterologists. There is increased frequency of colonic contractions and higher pressures, which can be directly related to symptoms.

2. Pain in the left lower abdomen may result from this increased tone in the lower colon, or from secondary distention in the more proximal bowel.

  a. Another effect of increased pressure is the excessive loss of water from the stool, and significant constipation.

  b. These patients have frequent abdominal pain and great variation in their bowel habits.

3. A second group of patients with irritable colon have only painless diarrhea, and colonic studies show a marked hypomotility in response to various stimuli.

4. Stress originating from day-to-day living is sufficient to produce chronic and recurrent symptoms in both groups of patients.

5. Although it is common to see mucus associated with the passage of stools, bleeding is unusual.

C. Criteria for Diagnosis

1. The symptoms as outlined above are suggestive of the diagnosis, but careful exclusion of more serious disorders is essential.

2. Appropriate studies include a complete blood count, sedimentation rate, proctoscopy, barium enema, stool cultures, and a careful examination for ova and parasites.

3. When diarrhea is the main presenting symptom, an upper gastrointestinal, small-bowel series, and a barium enema are indicated.

4. If all of these tests are negative, then the diagnosis of irritable colon can be made.

D. Management

1. One of the most important aspects of managing this disorder is an understanding physician and a thorough explanation to the patient regarding the many emotional factors that precipitate symptoms. A change in life-style may be essential.

2. Specific dietary changes

  a. These should be limited to avoiding foods that increase the amount of intestinal gas, such as onions, beans, melons, and cabbage. Other foods should be avoided, according to any specific intolerances suggested by the patient.

  b. Patients intolerant to the milk sugar, lactose, may get some relief by eliminating milk and ice cream from the diet, thus avoiding the increased gaseous distention and osmotic diarrhea from undigested lactose. A trial of milk elimination is worthwhile in all patients with this syndrome, but it is not necessary to eliminate cheese and other dairy products or foods cooked with milk. To provide adequate calcium (400 to 800 mg./day) a daily calcium supplement such as calcium gluconate tablets (90 mg. calcium per chewable tablet) or Neo-Calglucon (115 mg. calcium/5 ml.) can be

given, or foods high in calcium can be substituted (e.g., cheddar cheese which averages 200 mg. of calcium/oz. or broccoli,
which has 136 mg./cup).

3. Anticholinergic medications may
be of benefit during times of stress, and Pro-
Banthine in a dose of 15 to 30 mg. three or
four times daily may give some relief.
Lomotil (5 to 10 mg. three or four times
daily) is one of the most effective agents
in helping to eliminate diarrhea and
cramping.

4. Although low-residue diets were
frequently prescribed in the past, they are
generally ineffective and, in fact, might be
contraindicated in view of the increased intraluminal pressures they produce in many
patients.

   a. Because of frequent constipation,
it is often desirable to use bulk agents, such
as Metamucil or LA formula, and, in fact,
these may also help prevent the marked
variation in stools from diarrhea to constipation.

5. Tranquilizers are occasionally necessary during periods of stress but should
probably be used on an intermittent basis.

6. There is some evidence that the irritable colon syndrome may cause diverticulum formation, and long-term use of increased fiber in the diet may be beneficial in
preventing this disorder (see Constipation,
p. 205).

II. Diverticular Disease

   A. Definition
   1. Diverticulosis of the colon is a her-
niation of the mucosa through the muscular
layers of the colon.
   2. Diverticulitis is an inflammation of
the diverticuli producing fever and abdominal pain.
   B. Basic Principles
   1. Diverticuli occur most often in the
sigmoid colon and increase in frequency
with advancing age.
   2. Inflammation or diverticulitis occurs in approximately 12% of cases.

3. It has been recognized for many
years that diverticular disease is more common in the Western world, where the fiber
content of the diet is relatively low, averaging only 4 g./day. In underdeveloped countries, where dietary fiber may be 5 to 6 times
that found in the diet of industrialized societies, diverticuli are rare.

4. Large amounts of fiber in the
diet, 30 to 60 g./day, result in a large volume of intestinal contents reaching the
colon.

   a. Colonic manometric studies have
demonstrated lower pressures in the colon
when intraluminal contents are large in diameter.

   b. Small amounts of fiber present
less volume to the colon, and the colon
regularly produces higher intraluminal
pressure.

   c. High pressure over many years is
thought to be responsible for colonic
mucosa herniating through the muscle
layer, usually at the site of penetration of
nutrient arteries.

5. There are a significant number of
patients with a typical history of an irritable
colon syndrome that develop diverticular
disease, and these patients have long-
standing high pressure produced by colonic
muscle.

6. Symptoms resulting from simple
diverticuli are usually minimal, with only
occasional abdominal discomfort.

   a. Inflammation may occur at any
time in the diverticulum and may be
chronic, or acute with complications such
as perforation of the diverticulum into the
serosa or peritoneum. The perforation may
localize and heal, or develop into an abscess, fistulous tract between loops of bowel
or other organs, or peritonitis.

   b. The patients generally have left
lower-quadrant pain, fever, and tenderness
over the left side of the abdomen.

   c. They frequently develop signs of
obstruction and occasionally may have
bloody stools.

7. The presentation of diverticulitis is

often acute and at times requires surgical intervention.

C. Criteria for Diagnosis

1. Diverticulosis. This diagnosis is usually made at the time of a barium enema or at the time of proctoscopy, when the diverticulum or ostium to the diverticulum is detected.

2. Diverticulitis. The symptoms include fever, leukocytosis, left lower-quadrant pain, a history of diverticulosis, and symptoms of obstruction or peritonitis.

3. Proctoscopy may be helpful in ruling out other diseases, and colonoscopy is at times useful to rule out cancer as a cause of an obstructing lesion.

4. There are few, if any, specific barium radiographic changes in diverticulitis unless fistulous tracts are seen or unless barium is seen outside of the colon, suggesting a perforation, along with a thickening and a saw-tooth appearance of the colon. It is generally considered contraindicated to perform a barium enema in a patient who is acutely ill.

5. Differential diagnosis includes inflammatory bowel disease, such as ulcerative colitis, or granulomatous colitis, ischemic bowel disease, and cancer of the colon.

D. Management

1. Acute diverticulitis is generally managed by bowel rest, I.V. fluids, and antibiotics. Surgery may be required for acute perforation and peritonitis, or it may be required for more chronic symptoms at a time when a patient is less acutely ill.

2. The management of diverticulosis is one of prevention because the majority of patients have minimal symptoms.

3. Prevention of diverticuli rests on the assumption that the greater the amount of bulk or fiber in the diet, the less pressure can be generated in the lower colon, and the fewer diverticuli will be formed. Bulk, which holds extra water, can be added in the form of Metamucil, 1 tsp. morning and night. Alternatively, 30 to 50 g. of fiber daily may be more beneficial. (For a discussion on dietary fiber, see Constipation, p. 205.) Hemicellulose or psyllium seed preparations are useful to insure adequate bulk.

4. In those patients who do have abdominal pain, anticholinergics may be useful. However, it is desirable to avoid purgatives and colonic irritants.

5. It has been traditional for many years to avoid eating foods that contain small undigestible particles such as seeds, thinking that these may lodge in the diverticulum and lead to an acute obstruction and inflammation. Whether this is truly the case is debatable. However, this recommendation remains a reasonable dietary restriction.

III. Chronic Ulcerative Colitis

A. Definition

1. Chronic ulcerative colitis is an inflammatory disease of the colon which produces diarrhea, rectal bleeding, cramping abdominal pain, fever, and weight loss.

2. Remissions and relapses occur over many years, requiring frequent medical attention and often surgical intervention to correct or prevent complications.

B. Basic Principles

1. The inflammation of ulcerative colitis is primarily superficial, involving the colonic mucosa. The disease begins in the rectum and may involve only the rectal tissue, or it may spread to involve either part of the colon or the entire colon.

2. Colitis is a disease of young adults in their 20s and 30s. Ten to fifteen per cent of cases, however, start in childhood, and a rare case begins in the newborn period.

3. Clinical manifestations include both intestinal and extra-intestinal problems.

   a. The hyperemic, friable, and ulcerated colonic mucosa leads to significant loss of blood and loss of protein with hypoalbuminemia.

   b. If diarrhea is severe, there may be significant loss of water and electrolytes.

c. Fever and anemia are common.

4. Twenty-five per cent of children have significant growth retardation, occasionally starting before intestinal complaints are noticed.

   a. The mechanism of growth failure is partly explained by poor intake and loss of blood and protein from the ulcerated bowel, along with an increased metabolic need caused by fever.

5. Endocrine disorders, including thyroid and pituitary insufficiency, have occasionally been found in these patients but are infrequent.

6. Other systemic manifestations include arthritis, skin rashes, eye changes, and mild liver abnormalities with fatty infiltration and portal fibrosis.

7. The long-term complications include a significant incidence of carcinoma of the colon, usually after the disease has been present for 10 or more years, especially when the disease has started in childhood.

8. Abdominal pain may be absent to severe, and tenderness is often present over the left abdomen or area of the descending colon.

9. The disease occasionally progresses to a severe toxic dilatation of the colon that requires immediate surgery and has a very high mortality rate.

C. Criteria for Diagnosis

1. Proctoscopy should be performed in all patients. Edema and friability are usually seen beginning in the rectum.

2. A rectal biopsy is necessary to confirm the presence of inflammation.

3. Careful stool examinations to rule out bacterial pathogens, amebae, and other parasites are extremely important.

4. Blood studies should include a complete blood count, sedimentation rate, evaluation of liver function, and serum protein.

5. A barium enema is used to evaluate the extent of the disease and to help differentiate chronic ulcerative colitis from other disorders.

   a. In cases of many years duration, barium enema is useful to help rule out the presence of malignant lesions.

   b. Barium studies of the colon should not be undertaken in a seriously ill patient because of the high risk of perforation or development of sudden colonic dilatation or toxic megacolon.

   c. In very mild cases, barium studies may be normal.

6. An upper-G.I.- and small-bowel series should be performed in all patients to rule out Crohn's disease.

D. Management

1. There is no specific cure for ulcerative colitis other than a total colectomy. Medical management is thus aimed at controlling the symptoms, correcting nutritional problems, and reducing the frequency of exacerbations.

2. Diet has played a major role in the treatment of colitis, but emphasis has changed from a low-residue diet to a more liberal diet.

   a. Eliminating roughage seems to have little effect on preventing relapses of the disease, but it may be useful during more acute attacks of severe cramps, diarrhea, and bleeding.

   b. Milk has been implicated as a direct cause of colitis in infants and is frequently associated with increased diarrhea in adults.

   c. For this reason milk is generally eliminated from the diet early in the course of management. Reintroduction of milk in small amounts at a later time, when the patient is relatively asymptomatic, is usually well-tolerated. If lactase deficiency is present, milk should be eliminated permanently from the diet.

3. Careful attention to adequate replacement of protein in the diet, as well as calcium and iron, is essential.

   a. The adult requirement for protein is approximately 1g./kg./day. To make up for increased protein losses or poor intake, it may be necessary to increase this to 1.5 g./kg./day. In addition to increasing dietary protein with meats, eggs, and dairy products, a supplement of 8 to 16 oz. of Ensure per day adds both calories (1 cal./ml.) and protein (8.75 g. protein/8 oz.). Ensure is a liquid supplement with sucrose, polyunsaturated corn oil, and soy protein.

   b. If milk is eliminated from the diet, the daily calcium requirement of 400 to 800 mg. can be met by providing calcium gluconate tablets (90 mg. calcium) or Neo-Calglucon (115 mg./5 ml.).

   c. Iron supplementation can be given in the form of ferrous sulfate (many preparations), 50 to 65 mg. elemental iron, one to three times daily.

   4. Opiates or anticholinergics are contraindicated in severely ill patients but are useful at other times for the control of cramps and diarrhea.

   5. Occasionally, the use of bulk agents, such as Metamucil, will help decrease the number of stools per day in patients who are having just diarrhea without other significant symptoms.

   6. Salicylazosulfapyridine (Azulfidine) is the medication most frequently used to control the inflammation of colitis. Its mechanism of actions is not completely understood, but it appears to be effective in decreasing the inflammatory mucosal lesion and in preventing exacerbations of the disease when taken on a regular basis. It is not as useful in controlling disease in the acutely ill patient.

   7. Adrenocortical hormones (oral prednisone or other I.V. steroid preparations) are effective in decreasing inflammation, but they are reserved for patients who fail to respond to the above measures or who present with severe symptoms of bleeding, fever, and diarrhea.

   a. When patients require use of prednisone to control their symptoms, there is the added problem of protein catabolism from increased gluconeogenesis, which increases the difficulty in nutritional management.

   b. When steroids are used on a short-term basis to control colitis, they often produce prompt improvement, and the increased appetite that is a side effect of these drugs helps reestablish weight gain and a positive nitrogen balance.

   8. Surgical intervention is often necessary for control of severe disease that is unresponsive to the above measures and for correcting complications such as perforation, toxic megacolon, or the development of a malignancy. Surgery generally involves total removal of the colon and rectum with the creation of a permanent ileostomy. Once this is done the patient is then free of his disease and can expect no further problems from the colitis.

   9. A newer approach to treating resistant cases of colitis is a 4- to 6-week course of total parenteral nutrition (TPN) with complete bowel rest. Some patients with colitis enter a prolonged remission following TPN. This technique requires hospitalization during the procedure, and the expense and the need for an expert team approach to the use of TPN have limited its availability (see Chap. 20).

IV. Crohn's Disease of the Colon

A. Definition
   1. Crohn's disease of the colon is an inflammatory disorder of the colon that causes abdominal pain and diarrhea and may be associated with similar pathology in the small intestine.

B. Basic Principles
   1. In contrast to ulcerative colitis, Crohn's disease of the colon (transmural colitis, granulomatous colitis) may involve the entire bowel wall, including the mucosa, submucosa, and muscular layers and serosa. Because of this involvement the bowel may become narrowed from fibrosis.

   a. Regional lymph nodes also are involved in the inflammatory process.

   2. Perforation of the inflammatory lesion may lead to fistulous tracts that drain to the skin or to other loops of the bowel.

   3. The involvement in the colon is

often patchy, so that normal areas of colon occur between areas of significant inflammation. The mucosa is friable, and frequently ulcerations may be seen at the time of proctoscopy. Rectal fissures and rectal abscesses are frequently associated with the colonic disease.

4. This disease occurs in young adults and is characterized by remissions and exacerbations over many years.

5. Symptoms include severe cramping abdominal pain frequently following a meal and diarrhea. Bleeding is not as great a problem with Crohn's disease as it is with chronic ulcerative colitis.

6. Systemic signs and symptoms are frequent in this disorder and include arthritis, rashes, eye changes, and, occasionally, mild liver disease.

7. In children, there is a 25% incidence of significant growth retardation that may preceed the onset of intestinal symptoms by several years. Part of this problem may be related to decreased intake resulting from anorexia and chronic diarrhea and from protein loss from the G.I. tract.

8. The long-term complications of Crohn's disease of the colon include obstruction, fistulous tract, abscess formation, and chronic malnutrition. There is an increased incidence of colonic cancer, although this has not been as well studied and documented as chronic ulcerative colitis.

9. Malabsorption may occur when significant small bowel pathology is present. In these cases, the management becomes considerably more complicated, and malnutrition is a much greater problem.

C. Criteria for Diagnosis

1. Proctoscopic or colonoscopic findings of ulcerations, friability, or strictures in a patchy, discontinuous manner. The rectum may be completely normal.

2. Rectal biopsy confirming inflammation is helpful, and if the typical pathological lesion of a granuloma is found, this helps to confirm specifically the diagnosis of Crohn's disease of the colon.

3. Careful stool examinations to rule out bacterial pathogens, amebae, and other parasites are essential in these patients.

4. Blood work should include a complete blood count, sedimentation rate, liver function, and serum proteins.

5. If there is any suggestion of small bowel disease, appropriate absorptive studies are also indicated.

6. A barium enema will frequently show skip lesions of involved bowel and can help differentiate Crohn's disease of the colon from ulcerative colitis. If strictures are seen, this is highly suggestive of Crohn's disease.

7. An upper-G.I.- and a small-bowel series should be performed to rule out associated small-bowel pathology.

D. Management

1. As in ulcerative colitis, there is no specific cure for Crohn's disease of the colon, other than total colectomy. However, when small-bowel disease is associated with colon disease, the colectomy is not a useful procedure because the patient still has disease that will continue to cause difficulty.

2. Medical management is aimed at controlling the disease symptoms and correcting nutritional problems.

3. The use of diet and medications is essentially the same as in ulcerative colitis, and a review of the management of that condition will be instructive.

　　a. The same dietary factors are used.

　　b. The only difference in management would occur in those patients with associated small bowel disease who have evidence of malabsorption and who need specific therapeutic measures to treat that aspect of the disease.

V. Infectious Diseases of the Colon

A. Definition

1. A variety of parasites and bacterial agents cause acute and chronic colitis with diarrhea, abdominal pain, and often significant blood loss.

B. Basic Principles

1. Shigella and amebae are the organisms that more commonly cause infectious colitis by invading the colon mucosa. The infection may be acute or may become chronic lasting weeks or months with frequent relapses.

2. Diarrhea may be severe in the acute forms. Patients may present with high fever and chills, acute dehydration, electrolye imbalance, and shock.

3. In the more chronic form, it is common to see anorexia, weight loss, and increased metabolic needs from fever. Protein loss from the gastrointestinal tract may be present along with chronic bleeding.

C. Criteria for Diagnosis

1. Appropriate stool specimens both for culture and direct examination by someone trained in the recognition of parasitic diseases will lead to the appropriate diagnosis.

2. The degree of colitis can be confirmed at sigmoidoscopy or by barium radiograph, but this is often contraindicated because of the severity of the illness. They are frequently unnecessary when proper bacteriologic and parasitologic studies are available.

D. Management

1. The management of the acute infection requires intravenous therapy for fluid- and electrolyte replacement often accompanied by 1 to 3 days of no oral intake, to put the colon completely at rest.

2. Appropriate antibiotic therapy is essential and should be started as soon as the diagnosis is made.

3. Resumption of feeding by mouth should start in 1 to 3 days depending on the severity of the diarrhea and on the chronicity of the disease.

   a. In infancy, a non-lactose formula, such as soy milk, can be substituted.

   b. In older children and adults, lean meats and starches are well tolerated during recovery.

   c. Because anorexia is common, frequent feedings (four to six per day) will be helpful.

4. If the problem is chronic, a daily vitamin to provide minimum requirements and adequate protein (1 to 1.5 g./kg.; 2 to 3 g./kg. in infants) may be advisable.

5. In the young child, feeding after I.V. therapy starts with clear liquids (Pedialyte, 5% glucose, Jello, and water) and progresses in 12 to 24 hours to rice cereal, applesauce, ripe banana, crackers, or toast. Broiled lean meats and starches are then added over the next 1 to 2 days.

6. In older children and adults, liquids such as tea, beef broth, or apple juice can be started, followed by starches and lean meats. Adequate carbohydrates and protein in small frequent feedings may be tolerated well, but large amounts of fats may increase diarrhea.

7. During the recovery period four to six smaller meals per day may be tolerated better than three large ones.

8. In chronic cases, some bulk in the diet (Metamucil, 1 tsp. morning and night) may actually give more form to stools.

9. Iron replacement therapy (e.g., ferrous sulfate) may be necessary to correct the anemia from blood loss.

VI. Constipation

A. Definition

1. Constipation may be defined as the passage of very dry, hard stools, by infrequent passage of stools, or by passage of stools that are too small.

B. Basic Principles

1. Constipation can result from several disturbances in colon function.

2. Stasis and excessive drying of stools occurs when nonpropulsive segmental contractions increase pressure and drying of stool without moving colon contents into the rectum where normal defecation can occur.

   a. This pattern is seen in the irritable colon syndrome. It is aggravated by small amounts of intraluminal contents reaching the colon and producing very little stimulus to normal progressive contracting waves.

b. Ineffective motility or weak contractions in some cases may lead to stasis. Obstructive lesions, such as strictures or tumors, produce similar problems, although these are considerably less common.

c. Neurological conditions, such as Hirschsprung's disease, also lead to chronic stasis. In this disorder, there is an absence of the normal nerve endings in the colon leading to failure of relaxation of the lower colon and absence of propulsive waves through this area.

3. The second mechanism may be a more common cause of constipation and is related to the reflex stimulus indicating the need for expulsion of stool.

a. Because this neurological pathway is heavily influenced by learning experiences and is frequently ignored, prolonged periods between bowel movements occur, and chronic constipation results.

4. Other disorders may lead to infrequent passage of stools, such as anal or rectal disease associated with painful defecation.

5. Hemorrhoids and rectal fissures may result from constipation and, in turn, may make constipation worse because the discomfort causes the patient to hold on to stools.

6. The extreme in constipation is a rectal impaction, in which case the patient is unable to pass the large bolus of stool in the rectum and may experience overflow of loose intestinal contents around the impacted material.

7. In all cases of constipation except obstruction, the amount of dietary fiber may play a significant role in the prevention of the disorder.

8. Fiber adds volume and bulk to stools, and this is responsible for the stimulus to normal propulsive contractions of the colon. Without this added bulk, there is little stimulus to colonic activity, and thus, constipation results.

C. Criteria for Diagnosis

1. A good history is essential in determining the length of time that constipation has been present, what associated symptoms occur with the constipation, and whether there is dependency on laxatives.

2. Physical examination is most important in terms of a rectal exam and the detection of perianal disease.

3. Sigmoidoscopy and a barium enema are indicated in those cases with severe or prolonged constipation and when there is evidence to suggest an obstructive lesion, such as cancer or a stricture.

D. Management

1. Constipation can best be managed by careful attention to preventive measures.

2. The acute treatment of severe constipation or an impaction would include an oil-retention enema or a Fleet enema, followed by the use of mineral oil or Colace to facilitate easy passage of stool.

3. Prevention rests on good dietary and bowel habits.

a. There should be an adequate intake of dietary fiber, including bran, whole wheat, fresh fruits, and vegetables.

b. The older methods of evaluating dietary fiber are gradually being replaced by more accurate techniques.

c. Table 13-1 compares crude fiber, a relatively inaccurate measurement, and neutral detergent fiber, which includes all plant fiber except pectin.

d. Pectins are important in absorbing water and are present in significant amounts in fruits and vegetables (0.6 to 2.9% of fresh weight).

e. Although 7 to 10 g. of fiber daily may adequately relieve constipation, larger amounts, up to 30 to 50 g., have been suggested by some authors.

4. The addition of four to six glasses of water per day will help add extra fluid to the fiber and thus increase stool weight and softness of stools. The extra

bulk helps stimulate normal colon contractions.

5. Bulk agents, such as Metamucil, may be used in a dose of 1 tsp. once or twice daily to provide the same bulk and softening of stools.

6. If complicating problems such as hemorrhoids or anal fissures are present, it becomes more important to use a material that provides some lubricating effect, such as mineral oil or Colace.

7. It is extremely important to provide good counselling to the patient, not only about diet but about the need to develop a normal response to the rectal signals for elimination. This is a learned experience, and it may take weeks to months to reestablish normal bowel habits.

VII. Cancer of the Colon

A. Definition

1. Cancer of the colon is one of the most frequent malignant diseases in the U.S. and increases in frequency in older age-groups.

2. It usually involves the lower colon and frequently spreads to other organs before it is detected.

B. Basic Principles

1. Most patients with colon malignancies are in the fifth or sixth decade with an equal incidence in men and women.

2. A higher content of fat in the diet has been implicated in countries where colon cancer is common. It is speculated that bacterial alteration of fat or bile acids in the colon may produce carcino-

Table 13-1. **Foods With High Fiber Content**

Food	Average Serving*	Weight* (g.)	Neutral Detergent Fiber† (g.)	Crude Fiber* (g.)
Bread, white enriched	1 slice	23	0.49	tr
Bread, whole wheat	1 slice	23	2.21	0.4
Kellogg's All Bran	1/2 cup	28	9.26	2.3
Corn flakes	1 cup	25	1.9	0.2
Shredded wheat	1 biscuit	22	4.6	0.5
Wheat Chex (Ralston)	1/2 cup	28	4.75	0.6
Wheaties (General Mills)	1 cup	28	3.68	0.5
Grape Nuts	1/4 cup	28	3.16	–
Quaker Puffed Wheat	1 cup	12	1.01	0.2
Beans, green	1 cup	100	2.24	1.0
Beans, lima	5/8 cup	100	–	1.8
Broccoli	1 stalk	100	1.24	1.5
Cabbage	1 cup, shredded	100	1.11	0.8
Carrots	1 large	100	0.96	1.0
Lettuce, romaine	3 1/2 oz.	100	0.85	0.7
Potatoes, peeled	1	100	1.04	0.5
Potato, skin	–	100	4.3	–
Spinach, cooked	1/2 cup	90	–	0.5
Apple	1 medium	150	1.33	1.5
Apricots, raw	3 medium	100	–	0.6
Bananas	1 medium	150	–	0.8
Blackberries	1 cup	144	–	5.9
Blueberries	1 cup	140	–	2.1
Oranges	1 medium	150	0.75	0.8
Prunes, dried	5 medium	100	–	0.6
Raspberries, red, frozen	1/2 cup	123	–	2.7

*From Church, C. F., and Church, H. N.: Bowes and Church's Food Values of Portions Commonly Used. ed. 12. Philadelphia, J. B. Lippincott, 1975.
†Spiller, G. A.: Personal communication.

gens responsible for the development of cancer.

3. Absence of dietary fiber has also been suggested as a contributing factor.

a. Low fiber in the diet tends to slow the passage of stool through the colon, perhaps giving carcinogens more time to come in contact with the colonic mucosa.

b. The above are all theoretical considerations at this time, and further study is needed.

C. Criteria for Diagnosis

1. Symptoms of rectal bleeding, abdominal pain, weight loss, alteration in bowel habits, or obstruction are all suggestive of carcinoma of the colon.

2. The diagnosis can be confirmed by a barium enema and sigmoidoscopy or colonscopy.

D. Management

1. Surgical excision is the treatment of choice for most colon cancer. If the disease is widespread, a colostomy or ileostomy may have to be performed.

2. Chemotherapy and radiation therapy seem to be of little value in either primary treatment or in preoperative or postoperative care.

3. Patients may develop significant nutritional problems before or after surgery, from prolonged poor intake.

4. It may be necessary to provide calories intravenously through TPN or to provide a very low-residue diet during the preoperative phase, to prevent obstruction from large amounts of bulky stool reaching a narrowed segment of colon.

a. The lowest-residue diet can be achieved by giving one of several elemental diets (see Tables 12-1, 12-3, and 12-5) that are highly concentrated simple carbohydrate, amino acids, vitamins, and essential fatty acids. Absorption of elemental preparations occurs high in the small intestine.

b. A major disadvantage to these products is their bad taste, and feeding by nasogastric tube may be necessary.

c. The elemental diets have an extremely high osmolar load which requires

some adaptation time by the upper bowel for normal absorption to occur, and initially these diets must be diluted with gradually increasing concentration over several days.

d. Adequate nutrition has been achieved with this approach, and the elemental diet can be used until the patient has had the obstructive lesion removed.

5. Total parenteral nutrition should be considered for patients who are malnourished or who will be unable to eat for long periods of time because of the effect of surgery.

6. Prevention of colon cancer can now be discussed in terms of increasing dietary fiber and lowering the fat content of diets. This remains theoretical, however, because definitive proof for these measures is lacking.

VIII. Radiation Colitis

A. Definition

1. Radiation therapy for malignant disease may produce serious injury to the intestinal epithelium and arterioles of the colon, resulting in cell death and, eventually fibrosis and obstruction.

B. Basic Principles

1. Rapidly proliferating cells are most susceptible to damage by radiation, and the mucosal epithelial cells and endothelial cells of small arterioles undergo significant alteration following exposure to radiation.

2. There may be loss of the mucosal integrity and insufficient vascular supply, which may lead, eventually, to cellular necrosis, with resulting scarring and narrowing of the colon or chronic ulceration and blood loss.

3. In the acute phase of radiation therapy there may be nausea, vomiting, mucoid diarrhea, abdominal pain, and bleeding.

4. Later manifestations also include persistent bleeding, colic, abdominal pain, a decrease in stool caliber, and progressive obstipation suggesting a stricture or fibrosis.

C. Criteria for Diagnosis

1. A history of radiation exposure is necessary to consider this as a cause for symptoms.

2. The proof of colon disease is generally seen on barium radiographs of the colon showing ulceration or spasm, and at sigmoidoscopy, where edema and friability may be seen. The barium enema will also show evidence of stricture formation.

D. Management

1. During the acute phase treatment with sedatives and antispasmodics may be needed.

2. In the more long-term complications of radiation, the problems of anorexia and chronic blood loss may lead to malnutrition.

3. The small intestine also is frequently involved, and a variety of malabsorptive difficulties may be present that will require specific dietary therapy.

4. If only the colon is involved, a normal diet may be eaten.

5. When a stricture is present producing partial obstruction or constipation, a low-residue or elemental diet will be necessary.

6. Even in cases of significant malabsorption, an elemental diet may be sufficient to overcome the deficient absorptive state.

7. Surgery is usually required to relieve obstruction, and it is extremely important to have the patient in excellent nutritional health for proper healing of tissues following surgery. This can be accomplished by using an elemental diet, or in the case of severe malabsorption, total parenteral nutrition may be necessary (see Chap. 20).

SUGGESTED READINGS

Goldstein, F.: Diet and colonic disease. J. Am. Diet. Assoc., *60:*499, 1972.

Larsen, D. M., Masters, S. S., and Spiro, H. M.: Medical and surgical therapy in diverticular disease, a comparative study. Gastroenterology, *71:*734, 1976.

Law, D. H.: Progress in gastroenterology. Gastroenterology, *58:*1086, 1969.

Layden, T., Rosenberg, J., Nemchausky, B., Elson, C., and Rosenberg, I.: Reversal of growth arrest in adolescents with Crohn's disease after parenteral alimentation. Gastroenterology, *70:*1017, 1976.

Painter, N. S., and Burkitt, D. P.: Diverticular disease of the colon: a deficiency disease of Western civilization. Br. Med. J., *2:*450, 1971.

Painter, N. S., Truelove, S. C., Ardran, G. M., and Tuckey, M.: Segmentation and the localization of intraluminal pressures in the human colon, with special reference to the pathogenesis of colonic diverticula. Gastroenterology, *49:*169, 1965.

Reilly, J., Ryan, J. A., Strole, W., and Fischer, J. E.: Hyperalimentation in inflammatory bowel disease. Am. J. Surg., *131:*192, 1976.

Sleisenger, M. H., and Fordtran, J. S.: Gastrointestinal Disease. Philadelphia, W.B. Saunders, 1973.

Smith, J. S., and Milford, H. E.: Management of colitis caused by irradiation. Surg. Gynecol. Obstet., *142:*569, 1976.

Young, E. A., Heuler, N., Russell, P., and Weser, E.: Comparative nutritional analysis of chemically defined diets. Gastroenterology, *69:*1338, 1975.

14. NUTRITION AND THE ANEMIAS

Edward H. Reisner, Jr., M.D.

Among the nutritional factors involved in the formation of blood are iron, vitamin B_{12}, folic acid, pyridoxine, ascorbic acid, vitamin E, and minor elements, as well as protein. Thus, in both general and specific nutritional deficiency, anemia is frequently encountered.

I. Definition

Anemia is a decrease in the total red cell mass due to fewer red blood cells or to smaller red blood cells which contain less hemoglobin.

II. Basic Principles

A. Adult laboratory values of R.B.C., Hgb, HCT, and total red cell mass (RCM) fall within certain normal ranges (see Table 14-1).

B. In newborns, the values are 10 to 20% higher. They fall to normal in the first month of life and then fall below normal in the first 6 months, the period of most rapid growth. This is the so-called physiologic anemia of infancy. After 6 months, the values gradually return to levels comparable to those of adult women.

C. The average life span of the erythrocyte is 120 days, which means that each day 1/120 of the total R.B.C. mass must be replaced.

1. This amounts to about 40,000 R.B.C./mm.³ of blood, or 0.8% of the 5 million red blood cells.

2. The cells, newly released from the marrow, contain fragments of mitochondria, polyribosomes, and other organelles which can be stained by supravital dyes and which appear in a wavy reticular form; hence the name reticulocytes.

3. The reticulocyte count (RC) is usually reported as a percentage of 1000 R.B.C. counted consecutively and is usually 0.8 to 1.0%.

4. The reticulocyte count (RC) is the index of bone marrow activity and is an essential part of the blood examination of every anemic patient.

5. The driving force for the production of R.B.C. is a humoral factor produced by the kidney in response to a fall in the oxygen-carrying capacity of the blood which results from anemia or anemic hypoxia.

6. The normal response to a fall in the blood level is a rise in the reticulocyte count inversely proportional to the red blood cell count.

7. Therefore, one can determine the state of the marrow from the R.B.C. and the RC if optimal bone marrow activity for different blood levels is known.

8. A rough guide to this is shown in Table 14-2.

D. Anemia is the result of either an increased loss or destruction of R.B.C. or a decrease in their formation.

1. From the RC and R.B.C., one can

Table 14-1. **Normal Average Values for Red Blood Cells (R.B.C.), Hemoglobin (Hgb), Hematocrit (HCT), and Total Red Cell Mass (RCM) in Adults**

	Male	Female
R.B.C.	$5.1 \times 10^6 \pm 0.4$	$4.51 \times 10^6 \pm 0.4$
Hgb	15.5 g. $\pm$ 1.1	13.7 g. $\pm$ 1.0
HCT	46% $\pm$ 3.1	40.9% $\pm$ 3
RCM	26–32 ml./kg. of body weight	23–29 ml./kg. of body weight

immediately place most anemias in one of these two categories.

2. If a patient, with an R.B.C. of 3 million, has an RC of less than 2%, it is obvious that the marrow is performing less than optimally.

Table 14-2. **Optimal Bone Marrow Activity (Reticulocyte Activity) for Different Blood Levels**

Red Blood Cell Count (millions)	Reticulocyte Count (%)
3.5 to 3.0	2 to 5
3.0 to 2.5	5 to 10
2.5 to 2.0	10 to 15
2.0 to 1.5	15 to 25
< 1.5	20 or more

E. The type of blood cell that is produced by the depressed marrow is influenced by the cause of the depression.

1. Insufficient hemoglobin formation due to lack of iron or faulty heme synthesis results in the formation of thinner, smaller cells.

2. If synthesis of deoxyribonucleic acid (DNA) for mitosis is impaired without defective Hgb formation, fewer and larger cells are produced.

3. The average cell size is a cue to the cause of anemia. The mean corpuscular volume (MCV = HCT/R.B.C.) is 85 to 95 μm.^{3} normally.

4. Anemias with MCV below 80 μm.^{3} are microcytic, and those above 100 μm.^{3} are macrocytic.

a. Microcytic anemias are usually due to iron deficiency.

b. Macrocytic anemias are due to folic acid or vitamin B_{12} deficiency.

5. Normocytic anemias are due to inhibition of the marrow by chronic disease, infection, uremia, malignancy, replacement of marrow by non-blood-forming tissue, or marrow aplasia.

F. Classification of the anemia is facilitated by examination of the stained blood smear. Erythrocyte morphology is highly characteristic in microcytic and macrocytic anemias (see pp. 212, 216).

G. The examination of the bone marrow by aspiration or biopsy is an integral part of the anemia workup.

1. Marrow smears should be stained with iron stains to determine the state of iron stores and with Romanowsky stains such as Wright's-Giemsa for general morphology.

2. Specific marrow changes will be discussed in reference to the commonest nutritional deficiencies.

IRON DEFICIENCY ANEMIA

It has been estimated that 18 million people in the U.S. have some degree of iron deficiency anemia.

I. Definition

A. Iron deficiency anemia is an anemia due to inadequate intake of iron.

B. It is characterized by the production of smaller, thinner red blood cells which are deficient in hemoglobin.

II. Basic Principles

A. Iron is the basic nutritional component of heme, and, except for that present in the body at birth, iron is derived from the diet.

1. The total iron content of the body is approximately 3 to 4 g., 67% of which is in cellular Hgb.

2. Approximately 27% of total iron content is in body iron stores, most of which can be mobilized for blood formation.

3. Approximately 2.3% is in the labile iron pool and plasma en route to the marrow or storage depots.

B. Loss of iron from a person's body is almost entirely from the desquamation of iron-containing intestinal mucosal cells and amounts to about 1 mg./day.

1. During women's reproductive years, menstrual blood loss makes their monthly iron deficit about 2 mg./day.

2. Pregnant women have to provide

for the growing fetus, and their net daily loss amounts to 3 mg.

3. These iron losses must be restored each day through the diet.

C. The average American diet contains 10 to 20 mg. of iron per day, of which roughly 10% is absorbed.

1. Food iron is usually in the trivalent form and has to be reduced to the more absorbable ferrous state in the stomach.

2. It passes into the mucosal cells of the third part of the duodenum and the proximal jejunum.

3. The amount of iron entering the mucosal cell is a function of the amount outside and inside the cell membrane.

4. Absorption is enhanced by reducing agents such as ascorbic acid, gastric secretions, and alcohol.

5. It is decreased by food containing phytates, oxalates, and phosphates, which form insoluble complexes with iron.

6. Idiosyncratic ingestion of clay and starch will also interfere with iron absorption for the same reason.

7. Local or systemic infections interfere with iron absorption and transport.

8. Increased intestinal motility such as in diarrhea and surgical procedures that bypass the site of iron absorption may also lead to iron depletion.

9. Iron absorption is increased by hypoxia, anemia, and depleted iron stores, as well as by increased rates of erythropoiesis.

D. Men on a normal diet are generally safer from nutritional iron deficiency than women.

1. Women are in a state of marginal balance and require supplementation of their diet with iron during pregnancy.

E. Infants are particularly prone to iron deficiency because during the first 6 months of life, when the blood volume is expanding most rapidly, the normal infant diet consists mainly of milk, cereal, fruits, and vegetables with relatively small amounts of meat and eggs.

1. The autotransfusion of blood that the newborn receives from the placenta must last him until his diet includes adequate amounts of iron-containing foods.

2. The premature infant is at an even greater disadvantage because of his smaller RCM at birth.

3. In the first year of life, iron deficiency is so common that it has been termed the physiologic anemia of infancy.

4. In the last 15 years, supplementation of infant cereals and milk with iron has become a standard practice.

5. Infants raised on such foods have blood values much closer to those of older children.

6. Still, 25% or more of infants will be anemic.

III. Clinical Manifestations of Iron Deficiency

A. Clinical Features

1. Symptoms of iron deficiency anemia are variable, but they almost always include some measure of asthenia, ranging from mild enervation and fatigue to extreme listlessness and easy exhaustion.

2. In more severely depleted patients, sore tongue, gaseous indigestion, diarrhea, brittle spoon-shaped nails, and bizarre appetite (pica) are not uncommon.

3. Pallor is present in more severe cases.

B. Laboratory Diagnosis

1. Blood smears may be deceptive initially, but the more severe the anemia the more likely is one to find the characteristic hypochromic cells with thin rims of hemoglobin, schistocytes (fragmented cells), and elongated forms of red cells.

2. In severe cases, leukopenia is not uncommon, and platelet counts are often elevated.

3. The R.B.C. is seldom markedly depressed. (I have seen children who had been kept on a milk diet for the first 2 years of life with over 4 million R.B.C. but less than 2 g. of Hgb).

4. The MCV, MCH, and MCHC are markedly reduced.

5. Reticulocytes are subnormal.

6. Serum iron levels are generally reduced to levels below 30 μg. (normal 70 to 130 μg.) but may be normal in mild cases.

7. The amount of iron-binding protein in the blood is frequently increased (normal 150 to 300 μg./100 ml.)

C. Bone Marrow

1. The bone marrow in iron deficiency is usually hyperplastic.

2. The total number of normoblasts is not reduced, but there is a conspicuous decrease in orthochromatic forms.

3. The predominating hypochromic normoblasts appear stunted, frequently polyhedral rather than round, and with scanty amounts of cytoplasm.

4. The earliest red cell precursors are not usually increased because the maturation arrest occurs at the level of hemoglobinization, not at the state of cell division.

5. The iron stain with Prussian Blue will show decreased or absent iron stores, even in the presence of normal levels of serum iron.

D. Diagnosis

1. The diagnosis of iron deficiency anemia is not difficult, but determination of the cause may be.

2. In adult males on a normal diet, the presumptive cause is blood loss, and a thorough search for a source of bleeding should be made.

3. In all patients without an apparent site of blood loss, a careful investigation of diet peculiarities, iron absorption rates, associated infections, ingestion of starch or clay, or sale of blood to commercial blood banks must be made.

IV. Treatment of Iron Deficiency Anemia

A. The treatment is replacement with inorganic iron salts.

B. Nutritional iron deficiency can be forestalled by an adequate diet, but once anemia has developed, it is impossible to absorb enough iron from foodstuffs to correct it in a reasonable length of time.

C. There are many iron preparations on the market, but the cheapest and most effective ones are ferrous sulfate, ferrous gluconate, and ferrous fumarate.

D. In doses of 0.3 g. t.i.d., they will bring about a rise in reticulocyte levels and hemoglobin discernible after a week or 10 days of treatment.

E. Enteric-coated- and sustained-release iron remedies are more expensive, and they often carry the iron past the site of maximum absorption in the upper intestine.

F. For infants, iron drops or liquid salts are generally employed.

G. Parenteral iron is indicated only in those rare situations in which the patient can find no oral preparation that can be tolerated or in which the absorption of oral iron is impaired because of diarrhea or gastrointestinal shunts.

1. The preparations available are iron dextran (Imferon), dextriferron (Astrafer), and iron sorbitex (Jectofer).

2. Of these, the first is probably in widest use in this country.

3. It can be given intramuscularly or intravenously.

4. The intramuscular route is somewhat painful and may be attended by side effects such as hives, fever, arthralgias, and headaches.

5. With repeated injections, there is usually hyperpigmentation of the skin at the injection site.

H. Intravenous iron may cause local phlebitis.

1. The chief danger is sudden hypotension or anaphylactic shock.

2. Until patient tolerance for the drug has been established, intravenous iron should be administered very slowly with careful observation of the patient.

I. The dose of all parenteral iron preparations depends on the amount necessary to raise the hemoglobin to the desired level. Consult the package inserts that come with each preparation for the formula used to determine the appropriate dose.

MEGALOBLASTIC ANEMIA

I. Definition

A. Megaloblastic anemias are characterized by a specific type of erythropoiesis called megaloblastic.

B. This results in the formation of an abnormally large oval red blood cell, the macrocyte.

C. They are thus also known as the macrocytic anemias.

II. Basic Principles

A. The initial and essential stage in cell division is the synthesis of DNA for the replication of each chromatid. This assures each daughter cell a full complement of genetic material.

B. The coenzymes of folic acid and, less directly, vitamin B_{12} are essential for the methylation of deoxyuridine to form thymidine, the nucleotide peculiar to DNA.

C. In the absence of either of these vitamins, there is a block in DNA synthesis, which results in megaloblastic hematopoiesis.

D. This is characterized by a greater particularity of the nuclear chromatin pattern at all stages of erythroblast maturation and persistence of cytoplasmic RNA much longer than normal.

E. The result is increased formation of hemoglobin and a larger than normal cell.

F. There are parallel changes in the granulocytes—giant nuclei in the metamyelocyte stage and increased numbers of mature granulocytes with more than four segments.

G. The macrocytic red cells are more susceptible to hemolysis.

1. They have a shortened life span in normal subjects.

2. In addition, there is a poorly understood plasma hemolytic factor which disappears about 4 days after specific therapy.

H. Macrocytic anemias are due to both defective reduced rates of blood formation and to increased rates of destruction of the cells that are formed.

III. Folic Acid (Pteroylglutamic Acid)

A. Folic acid is an essential food constituent.

B. It is present in greatest abundance in green leafy vegetables, asparagus, broccoli, lima beans, certain fruits (lemons, bananas, melons), liver, kidneys, yeast, and mushrooms.

C. It consists of a pteroyl group (pteridine joined to *p*-aminobenzoic acid) conjugated with glutamic acid residues up to the number of seven.

D. Folic acid is heat-labile.

1. Among populations in which the tendency is to overcook vegetables, folate deficiency may arise despite a reasonable amount of folate in the basic diet.

E. In the natural form, folic acid is a heptoglutamate which has to be deconjugated to the monoglutamate.

1. This process commences in the upper part of the small bowel, and natural folates enter the mucosal cell in the 4 or 5 glutamate form.

2. In the cell, deconjugation to the monoglutamate continues, and the pteroyl residue begins the process of reduction by the enzyme dihydrofolate reductase to the tetrahydrofolate (THF).

F. THF is the basic active form of folic acid from which all the other folic acid coenzymes are derived.

1. Ascorbic acid apparently plays some role in this reduction.

2. The folic acid coenzymes are a group of interchangeable carriers of single carbon moieties involved in the synthesis of thymidine, purines, methionine, glycine, and serine and in the degradation of histidine.

3. 5, 10 methylene THF transfers its methylene group to deoxyuridine for the formation of thymidine and is reduced back to THF.

4. Breakdown of this reaction causes a

block in DNA synthesis and results in megaloblastosis.

G. Requirements

1. The daily requirement of folate is from 25 to 50 μg.

2. The body store of folate compounds is about 5 mg.

3. When the daily intake of folate is less than 5 μg., megaloblastic anemia develops in 3 to 4 months.

4. During pregnancy, folate requirements increase to about 400 μg./day.

5. Conditions that increase the cell turnover rate, such as hemolytic anemias and thyrotoxicosis, also increase the daily folate requirement.

H. Causes of Impaired Absorption of Folate

1. Enteropathies such as tropical sprue

2. Surgical procedures that bypass the upper small bowel

3. Some drugs such as diphenyl-hydantoin and oral contraceptives which are believed to interfere with the deconjugation of polyglutmates

I. Once absorbed, there may be interference with folate reduction caused by

1. Lack of ascorbic acid

2. Folic acid antagonists, such as methotrexate. These compete advantageously for dihydrofolate reductase because they have a greater affinity for it.

3. Alcohol also interferes with folate metabolism and absorption.

a. It is one of the commonest causes of clinical folate deficiency.

b. The mechanism by which alcohol does this is imperfectly understood.

IV. Vitamin B_{12} (Cobalamin)

A. Vitamin B_{12} is a complex planar molecule consisting of a corrin ring attached to the nucleotide 5,6 dihydrobenzimidazole.

1. The cyanocobalamin, which is the usual commercial preparation, is a highly stable form that does not occur in nature

but is easily hydrolyzed to hydroxycobalamin in the body.

2. Hydroxycobalamin is then converted to an active coenzyme form in which the hydroxyl group is replaced by a methyl group (5 methyl cobalamin) or deoxyadenosyl.

3. The B_{12} coenzymes are involved in the intermediate metabolism of folic acid and propionic acid.

4. The coenzyme methylcobalamine is involved in the methylation of homocysteine to form methionine by transport of a methyl group from 5-methyl THF.

a. Most of the folate that enters the body appears in the blood as 5-methyl THF and is converted to THF by this demethylation reaction.

b. In B_{12}-deficient patients, the levels of methyl THF rise increasingly with a resulting decrease in the amount of THF available for conversion to 5,10 methylene THF for thymidane synthesis.

c. This "methyl folate trap" theory is a good working hypothesis for the pathogenesis of megaloblastosis in vitamin B_{12} deficiency.

5. The deoxyadenosyl cobalamine coenzyme plays an essential role in the intermediary metabolism of proprionic acid, at the step converting methylamalonic acid to succinic acid.

a. In the absence of B_{12}, abnormal amounts of methylmalonic acid appear in the urine.

b. In pernicious anemia patients fed labeled proprionic acid, the label has been recovered from the myelin sheaths of peripheral nerves and the methylmalonate in the urine.

c. The crippling dorsolateral sclerosis of the spinal cord frequently seen in patients with pernicious anemia is caused by the toxicity of methylmalonate.

B. The daily average loss of cobalamin from the body is about 1.3 μg.

1. To offset this, the daily requirement is considered to be about 2 to 3 μg.

C. Vitamin B_{12} is present in animal protein, and the average American diet contains from 5 to 30 μg./day.

D. The total body stores of the vitamin are from 2000 to 5000 μg., the largest fraction of which is in the liver.

E. Even if all external sources of vitamin B_{12} were cut off, evidence of deficiency would take several years to develop.

F. Vitamin B_{12} is unique in having a highly specialized absorption mechanism.

1. Although cobalamin is freely transferable across the endothelium of the terminal ileum, which is the site of absorption in man, the small amounts of the vitamin present in foods have to be combined with an enzyme secreted by the parietal cells of the fundic region of the stomach, which is still called by the name that was given it by W. B. Castle, the intrinsic factor, or IF.

2. IF is an alkali-stable glycoprotein dimer that binds two molecules of B_{12} per dimer.

3. In a neutral pH and in the presence of Ca^{++} ions, it releases the B_{12} for passage across the intestinal cell wall.

4. In the cell, the vitamin combines with an intracellular receptor protein for 8 to 10 hours before it is once more released to cross the interior cell wall into the blood stream.

5. Here it is taken up by another protein, Transcobalamin II, and is quickly transported to the liver.

6. It remains in the liver for some time until it is released and transported by Transcobalamin I to the tissues in which it is needed.

G. Vitamin B_{12} in excess of the binding power of the transcobalamins is excreted in the urine.

H. One may wonder why Nature has made the absorption of an essential nutrient so complicated.

1. The best explanation is still the teleologic one, that the colon bacilli in the terminal ileum would consume the B_{12} present in food if the IF did not act as a shield, denying them access to it until it can be absorbed.

I. Absorption of cobalamin from food is inadequate in the absence of IF.

1. This is most commonly due to the familiar disorder of older people known as pernicious anemia in which the gastric mucosa is severely atrophic.

2. A large number of patients with pernicious anemia (P.A.) have serum antibodies to IF, and the presumption is strong that, for them at least, P.A. is an autoimmune disorder.

J. Primary dietary deficiency of B_{12} is rare in this country except among strict vegans.— *vegetarians*

1. It occurs in parts of the world where poverty or religious restrictions result in a lack of animal protein in the diet.

K. Total gastrectomy will lead to megaloblastic anemia after several years.

L. Replacement of the gastric mucosa by tumors of the fundic region may result in the picture of P.A.

M. Megaloblastic anemia may result from competitive consumption of B_{12} in the gut by colon bacteria that thrive in blind loops or surgically bypassed segments of intestine, or by B_{12}-consuming parasites, such as the fish tapeworm.

N. In patients with sprue, steatorrhea, ileal resections, or ileitis, the site of absorption may be bypassed or inadequate.

O. In chronic pancreatitis, B_{12} absorption is defective, but the mechanism of this is not clarified.

V. Diagnostic Features of Megaloblastic Anemia

A. The anemia is macrocytic with an MCV greater than 100 μm.[3].

B. In the peripheral blood smear, the oval macrocytes and hypersegmented granulocytes are characteristic.

C. In severe cases, nucleated erythrocytes, cells with nuclear fragments (Howell-Jolly bodies), and remnants of nuclear membrane (Cabot's rings) may be seen.

D. Leukopenia is common, and thrombocytopenia may occur in severe cases.

E. The bone marrow shows erythroid hyperplasia with megaloblastic red cell precursors and giant metamyelocytes in numbers inversely proportional to the blood levels.

1. In mild cases, the marrow findings may not be diagnostic.

F. Coexistent iron deficiency may mask the megaloblastic features of the marrow and the degree of macrocytosis. These may become apparent only after the patient has been treated with iron.

G. Severely anemic patients have a lemon yellow hue to their skin, which is due to the elevated indirect bilirubin in the serum.

H. The LDH levels are increased, often quite markedly.

I. Serum cholesterol is reduced.

J. Iron levels and marrow iron stores are usually normal or increased.

K. The reticulocyte count is usually very low but, occasionally, may be elevated without being followed by a rise in the blood levels.

VI. Classification of Megaloblastic Anemias

A. Megaloblastic anemias can be divided primarily into those caused by folate deficiency and those owing to vitamin B_{12} deficiency.

B. Within each category can be listed the various etiological mechanisms for the deficiency.

C. Table 14-3 presents a classification of megaloblastic anemias according to etiology.

VII. Differential Diagnosis of Megaloblastic Anemias

A. The differentiation between folate deficiency and B_{12} deficiency as the cause of a megaloblastic anemia is best made on clinical evidence and confirmed by appropriate laboratory tests.

1. If the patient is older than 60 years of age and presents with lingual atrophy and histamine refractory achlorhydria, the presumptive diagnosis is P.A.

2. The presence of ataxia and paresthesias with decreased vibratory and position sense and pyramidal tract signs makes this diagnosis practically certain.

Table 14-3. **Classification of Megaloblastic Anemias**

Folate Deficiency	*B_{12} Deficiency*
Inadequate Intake	Inadequate Intake
Malnutrition—"tea and toaster"	Vegans
Pregnancy—failure to supplement diet	
Improper Absorption	Improper Absorption
Alcoholism	Lack of intrinsic factor
Steatorrheas	Pernicious anemia—achlorhydria
Tropical sprue—enteric infection and poor diet	Gastric resection
Medications	Gastric tumors
Diphenylhydantoin	Rapid passage through gut
Contraceptive Pills	Steatorrhea
Trimethoprim	Ileitis
	Small bowel resection
	Severe sprue
Faulty Metabolism	Defective passage through gut wall
Vitamin B_{12} deficiency—methyl folate trap	Pancreatitis
Metabolic antagonists—methotrexate	Lack of succus entericus factor (Innerslund's
Alcohol	cases)
Infancy	Competitive utilization of vitamin B_{12}
Vitamin C deficiency	Blind loops of gut
Inborn errors of metabolism	Fish tapeworm infestation

3. If the anemia is due to folate deficiency, serum folate levels should be below 4 ng./100 ml. (normal 5 to 15).

4. If the anemia is due to lack of vitamin B_{12}, serum levels of B_{12} below 100 pg./100 ml. (normal 150 to 400) should be found, and many cases will show elevated folate levels.

B. Confirmation of the inability of the patient to absorb B_{12} is obtained with the Schilling radioactive B_{12} absorption and excretion test.

1. In this test, the patient is fed an oral dose of cobalamin of 0.5 μg., labeled with ^{60}Co, ^{57}Co, or ^{58}Co, which is accompanied by a parenteral injection of 1000 μg. of "cold" B_{12}.

2. The urine is collected for the next 24 hours, and, if desired, a second 1000-μg. B_{12} injection can be given, and the urine collection can be extended for another 24-hour period.

3. The principle of the test is that the large injection of B_{12} will saturate all the Transcobalamin in the blood at the time the labeled oral dose is absorbed so that it will enter the blood stream unbound and will be excreted in the urine.

4. A normal patient will excrete amounts in excess of 8 to 10% of the ingested radioactivity.

5. Less than this implies faulty absorption.

6. P.A. patients excrete less than 1% as a rule.

7. To prove that the absorption failure is due to lack of IF, the test is repeated with the labeled B_{12} accompanied by normal gastric juice or a concentrate of IF, which should restore the absorption to normal.

8. Failure of IF to correct the defect indicates some other cause for the malabsorption.

9. It is now possible to do the two stages of the Schilling test simultaneously by using two isotopes of cobalt to label the oral dose, one of which is combined with IF.

C. It is preferable to postpone the Schilling test until after the patient has been treated and is well on the way to recovery.

1. The reason for this is that the massive dose of B_{12} used in the test will produce a hematologic response even if the patient is primarily deficient in folic acid, and will obscure the diagnosis.

2. Also, many patients in relapse may have steatorrhea or sufficient intestinal pathology due to the lack of B_{12} or folate to interfere with the test.

3. This confusion can be avoided by postponing the test until the patient is well in remission.

D. Patients who are badly undernourished, chronic alcoholics, old persons who live largely on tea and toast, and patients with tropical sprue or steatorrhea may properly be suspected of being folate-deficient.

1. The serum folate level is the best confirmation of this.

a. It must be taken as soon as possible after the diagnosis is made.

b. Only a few days of normal diet or supplementation will elevate the levels of folate.

2. Contrariwise, serum B_{12} levels are not a reliable index of vitamin B_{12} deficiency because they do not reflect body stores of this vitamin. It is common to find levels of 100 pg. in non-anemic, clinically healthy, elderly people.

E. Radiographs of the gastrointestinal tract should always be done in patients with megaloblastic anemia because they may reveal the characteristic pattern of sprue, blind loops of gut, or occult gastric tumors.

F. Megaloblastic anemia of pregnancy is now an uncommon disorder in the U.S. owing to the standard practice of supplementation of the maternal diet with folate. When it occurs, it is almost always due to lack of folic acid.

G. Megaloblastic anemia of infancy is an interesting condition that was noted about 25 years ago in infants raised on an artificial formula that simulated breast milk and contained no vitamin C.

1. Some mothers who failed to add a source of ascorbate had babies who developed megaloblastic anemia which responded to folic acid.

2. When the artificial formula was fortified with vitamin C, this type of megaloblastic anemia disappeared.

3. When occasional megaloblastic anemias are encountered in infancy now, they are usually due to inborn defects in the metabolism of folic acid or the pathways of nucleoprotein synthesis.

VIII. Treatment of Megaloblastic Anemias

A. Treatment of Vitamin B_{12} Deficiency Megaloblastic Anemia

1. If the cause of the anemia is established as B_{12} deficiency because serum folate levels are normal and achlorhydria is present, adequate treatment is 100 μg. of cobalamin, intramuscularly, twice a week.

2. If combined system disease is present, daily treatment with the same dose for a week and three times a week after that is advisable.

3. These schedules should be followed until the anemia is corrected.

4. Maintenance therapy with injections of 100 μg. every 2 weeks will maintain the blood count and restore serum cobalamin levels to normal.

5. It is common practice to give such treatments at monthly intervals.

    a. Although this will keep the blood count at normal levels, the serum B_{12} levels in about one-third of these patients will be below normal limits.

    b. Patients with combined system disease should have weekly maintenance therapy for several months and twice monthly after that.

6. The use of larger doses of B_{12} is of little value because 90% of larger doses is quantitatively excreted in the urine.

7. Long-acting depot B_{12} preparations

work, but they are more expensive and have little to recommend them aside from the advantage of less frequent injections.

8. If large enough doses of vitamin B_{12} are given by mouth, even patients with P.A. can absorb enough to maintain normal blood values and serum levels.

    a. 1000 μg. P.O. weekly is an adequate dose and can be given to patients who cannot come for injections.

    b. These oral doses also can be used for patients who are traveling and don't want to be bothered with injecting themselves or finding a doctor to inject them.

B. Treatment of Folic Acid Deficiency Megaloblastic Anemia

1. Folic acid is available in 1 mg. tablets.

2. This is about 20 times the optimal daily requirement and much more than is required to restore blood values and serum levels to normal.

3. A dose of 1 mg. three times a week is more than adequate.

4. It goes without saying that poor diet, alcoholism, and other factors leading to the deficiency state should be corrected.

5. Anticonvulsant drugs and contraceptive pills may be safely resumed after the anemia is corrected if the patient is covered with enough folic acid to offset their effect on absorption.

6. Patients with sprue may require antibiotics to eliminate intestinal infections.

C. A patient with megaloblastic anemia, the cause of which is not clear, should have a therapeutic trial with a dose of B_{12} or folic acid large enough to correct a specific defect but too small to force a response by "mass action" if the anemia is due to the lack of the other one.

1. A single 25-μg. dose of B_{12} given parenterally will cause optimal reticulocyte response and blood formation in a patient with P.A.

2. Daily oral doses of 25 μg. of folic acid will cure most primary folate deficiencies but will have no effect on patients with B_{12} deficiency.

a. In order to prepare such small doses of folate, its coenzyme, folinic acid (N-5 Formyl THF), can be used. This is readily available in solution as leucovorin calcium, which is clinically used as an antidote for the folate antagonist methotrexate and which can be readily diluted.

3. The first trial should be given with the substance deemed most likely to be lacking.

4. If after a week of the therapeutic trial there has been no rise in reticulocytes, the other may be tried.

5. Occasionally patients are encountered in whom both substances are lacking (e.g., persons with P.A. who are also alcoholics, or patients who have severe tropical sprue with excessively low B_{12} levels).

D. Because both substances are involved in interrelated reactions, large doses of either one will accelerate the consumption of the other.

1. In the early days of folic acid therapy for pernicious anemia, it was observed that, although the abnormal blood picture was corrected, in some cases this was followed by a sudden appearance of severe combined system disease.

2. This is due to the fact that reactions pushed by folic acid lowered the already depleted stores of B_{12} still further until the threshhold for the appearance of spinal cord disease was reached.

3. Folic acid is not indicated in the treatment of patients with P.A. unless there is a specific reason for it and should never be given to these patients without covering doses of B_{12}.

ANEMIAS OWING TO OTHER NUTRITIONAL FACTORS

I. Starvation

A. A moderate degree of normocytic anemia was observed in liberated war prisoners and concentration camp inmates.

1. The pathogenesis of this anemia has been studied in volunteers on severely restricted diets.

2. The anemia is due to a depression of blood formation augmented by expanded plasma volume.

3. After restoration of a normal diet, it may take several months for blood levels to return to normal.

B. Children with acute protein deficiency (kwashiorkor) are usually anemic.

1. This anemia also is normocytic and responds to appropriate diets with reticulocytosis, but attainment of normal blood levels is slow.

2. Hemodilution due to hypoproteinemia aggravates the anemia and masks an increase in red cell mass.

C. A problem in assessing all nutritionally deficient patients is that under starvation conditions, multiple deficiencies of iron, folate, and other factors involved in blood formation are likely to occur.

1. Knowledge of a specific nutrient's role in blood formation is derived from animal experiments or from human volunteers on specially restricted diets.

2. Several nutrients act as cofactors in the action of other factors.

II. Pyridoxine

A. Pyridoxine, like its coenzyme pyridoxal, is essential to the synthesis of Δ-amino-levulinic acid, a precursor of heme, from glycine and succinyl CoA. When pyridoxal is lacking, there is a block in heme synthesis and an inability to utilize iron.

1. This results in increased amounts of iron in the blood and bone marrow and the presence of ring sideroblasts in the marrow.

a. These cells contain dots of blue staining mitochrondrial iron in marrow smears stained with Prussian Blue. These dots fill the periphery of the normoblasts to form a ring around the nucleus of the cell nucleus—thus the name ring sideroblasts.

2. These sideroblasts also are found in a variety of anemias in which there is a

delay in iron incorporation into heme. Thus while they are characteristically found in B_6 deficiency, their presence is not pathognomonic of that condition.

B. The failure to form hemoglobin leads to a hypochromic microcytic anemia, and this is the commonest type of anemia found in pyridoxine deficiency.

C. In about one-sixth of pyridoxine responsive anemias, however, the anemia is macrocytic, and the bone marrow is megaloblastic.

1. The explanation of this finding is that pyridoxine is indirectly involved in the thymidine synthetase pathway.

2. The coenzyme for thymidine synthesis, 5,10 methylene THF, is formed by the derivation of a methyl group from the demethylation of serine to form glycine.

3. If the heme synthesis pathway is blocked by lack of vitamin B_6, glycine formation is also blocked. If at the same time supplies of folate (THF) are low, the formation of thymidine can be sufficiently impaired to produce a megaloblastic picture.

4. These anemias are refractory to treatment with folate or cobalamin until pyridoxine is added.

D. Pyridoxine deficiency anemia and pyridoxine responsive anemia are not the same thing.

1. Vitamin B_6 deficiency anemia is usually mild and is accompanied by other manifestations of lack of pyridoxine such as glossitis, dermatitis, neuropathy, and convulsions.

   a. It responds to oral supplementation of the diet with 1 to 5 mg. of the vitamin daily.

2. Pyridoxine responsive anemia is generally more severe and is unaccompanied by other signs of pyridoxine deficiency.

   a. It requires large parenteral doses of 50 to 200 mg./day to respond.

   b. Although this treatment may lead to reticulocytosis and improved blood levels, complete hematologic remission is seldom attained.

c. This entity involves some as yet unknown breakdown in pyridoxine utilization, or the vitamin defect is superimposed on some other hematologic abnormality.

III. Ascorbic Acid

A. Vitamin C enhances the reduction of iron to the absorbable ferrous state. At the same time, patients with scurvy bleed easily. Thus hypochromic anemia from blood loss is not uncommon in adults or infants with this disease.

B. Ascorbic acid also plays a role in stabilizing the folate reductase reaction.

1. The incidence of megaloblastic anemia in infants on vitamin C deficient formulas has been referred to previously.

2. In patients with a marginal folate intake, lack of ascorbic acid may precipitate a megaloblastic anemia which will respond to folate but not to vitamin C.

3. If they have coexistent scurvy, this will respond to vitamin C, but the anemia will not improve until folate is given.

C. Some patients with scurvy have been reported to have a mild normocytic anemia which responds to vitamin C. Many, however, do not show such an anemia, so that primary anemia due to lack of ascorbic acid is a disputed entity.

IV. Vitamin E (α-tocopherol)

A. In monkeys on a vitamin E deficient diet, a type of hemolytic anemia develops which responds to α-tocopherol.

B. A similar anemia has been described in infants.

C. The red cells of humans and animals on a vitamin E deficient diet are more susceptible to hemolysis by peroxide in vitro.

D. In Jordan, a group of infants and children living under starvation conditions were found to have a macrocytic megaloblastic anemia refractory to folate, vitamin B_{12}, and vitamin C but which responded to vitamin E.

E. Patients with acanthocytosis due to

abetalipoproteinemia exhibit autohemolysis of their cells in vitro, which can be corrected by intramuscular administration of α-tocopherol (which, however, does not change the appearance of the cells).

F. The evidence suggests that vitamin E plays a role in maintaining the resistance of the red cell membrane to hemolysis, but the evidence for a role in blood formation is inconclusive.

V. Other Vitamins

A. Riboflavin deficiency in animals and human volunteers is accompanied by a normocytic anemia with hypoplastic bone marrow, which is corrected by restoration of the missing vitamin.

1. Riboflavin plays a role in the formation of red cell glutathione reductase, and some hemolytic anemias with reduced glutathione reductase levels may be due to lack of riboflavin.

B. Lack of niacin, thiamine, pantothenic acid, and biotin has been shown to cause anemia in animals, but few if any cases of these deficiencies in humans have been reported.

VI. Minerals

A. Copper deficient diets in animals have been reported to decrease iron absorption. Copper is so widely distributed in food, however, that its lack is not a significant cause of anemia in humans.

B. Cobalt deficiency in the soil leads to B_{12} deficiency in ruminants but is not known to have any pathologic effect leading to anemia in man.

C. Although zinc is present in blood cells, it is not related to blood formation, and its lack does not lead to anemia.

15. DIET THERAPY OF RENAL FAILURE

Shaul G. Massry, M.D.

Joel D. Kopple, M.D.

BASIC PRINCIPLES

I. Patients with chronic renal failure display various abnormalities that dictate adjustments in their dietary regimen.

A. These abnormalities include

1. Retention of nitrogenous waste products

2. A decrease in the ability to excrete sodium load or conserve sodium with dietary sodium restriction

3. An increase in the renal obligatory loss of water

4. A limitation in the ability to handle loads of water, potassium, or magnesium

5. Retention of phosphate

6. Hypocalcemia

7. Wasting syndrome

II. Many observations indicate that uremic serums may be toxic to a variety of biological systems.

A. There is also evidence that many of the toxic substances that accumulate in uremia are metabolic products of protein and amino acids.

B. Thus, dietary restriction of protein may improve many of the uremic manifestations.

III. Impaired anabolic responses and wasting are common in patients with chronic uremia.

A. These patients may have

1. Loss of body fat and fat-free solids

2. An increase in extracellular fluid

3. A decrease in the concentration of serum albumin and total albumin pools and in rates of synthesis and degradation of albumin

4. A decrease in the concentration of serum transferrin and certain proteins of the complement system

5. Amino acid levels in plasma similar to those noted in protein-calorie malnutrition

B. Although several factors may be responsible for the wasting syn1drome, a major cause of it is poor dietary intake.

1. Chronic illness, uremic toxicity, and intercurrent illnesses often cause anorexia and lead to poor dietary intake.

2. The ingestion of diets that are low in protein and other nutrients and the removal of protein and nutrients during dialysis contribute further to the wasting syndrome.

3. Therefore, an appropriate dietary regimen that will maintain good nutritional status is an essential component of the overall therapy of the uremic patient.

IV. Many nutrients may be lost during hemodialysis or peritoneal dialysis.

A. The nutrients lost in dialysis include

1. Free amino acids

2. Peptides and other bound amino acids

3. Proteins

4. Glucose (with the use of glucose-free dialysate)

5. Vitamins

6. Probably other bioactive compounds

B. As an example, 8 to 10 g. of essential and nonessential amino acids and 3 to 4 g. of peptides are lost in a single hemodialysis in a nonfasting patient. Protein loss during peritoneal dialysis is significant and may reach 1 to 2 g. during each 2-L. exchange.

C. The water-soluble vitamins are more dialyzable than the fat-soluble vitamins. Dialysis patients thus may have a decrease in blood levels of water-soluble vitamins if they are not given vitamin supplements.

D. It is important that these nutrient losses be considered in planning the dietary

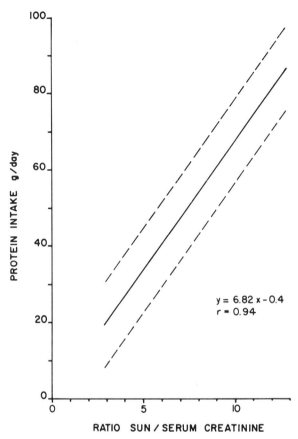

Fig. 15-1. Relation between dietary protein intake and SUN-to-creatinine ratio in chronically uremic men not treated with dialysis. The interrupted lines represent the 95% confidence limits. (Kopple, J.D., and Coburn, J.W.: Evaluation of chronic uremia: importance of serum urea nitrogen, serum creatinine, and their ratio. J.A.M.A., *227*:41, 1974)

therapy of patients maintained with chronic hemodialysis.

V. An optimal diet must prevent and correct abnormalities in fluid and electrolyte homeostasis, minimize uremic toxicity, and optimize nutritional status.

A. Adherence to a dietary regimen is the single most important factor in achieving its therapeutic effectiveness.

B. The acceptability of the diet by the patient should be a primary consideration in planning the dietary therapy. An energetic and imaginative dietician who can design nutritious meal plans that accomodate the various restrictions and, at the same time, satisfy the taste of the patient is invaluable.

C. Not infrequently, a team approach to the dietary therapy of the patient is required. Such a team may include the physician, social worker, dietician, and psychiatrist.

D. The patient should understand the importance of the dietary therapy to his welfare and should be made to view dietary restriction as an important aspect of his medical care.

DIETARY PROTEIN AND CALORIE REQUIREMENTS

I. Adult Patients Who Are Not Treated With Dialysis

A. Although dietary protein restriction may ameliorate many of the uremic manifestations, such dietary regimen may aggravate the wasting syndrome of uremia and may induce malnutrition in these patients.

B. It is, therefore, of utmost importance to choose:

1. The appropriate time in the course of renal failure when dietary protein restriction may be initiated

2. The optimal degree of dietary protein limitation

3. The biological value of the prescribed proteins

C. The biological value of a protein is defined as the ratio of the amount fed to the amount utilized in the synthesis of tissue proteins.

1. For protein to be of high biological value, it must satisfy the following criteria:

a. A large proportion of its amino acid content is essential.

b. It contains all of the essential amino acids.

c. The content of each essential amino acid must be in proportion to the minimal daily requirement for that amino acid.

2. With the use of protein of high biological value, a minimum amount of nitrogen can be ingested to provide the minimum daily requirement of various essential amino acids.

3. Protein-restricted diets containing low biological value protein do not promote anabolism to the extent that similar quantities of high biological value protein do.

4. Egg protein has the highest biological value of 0.94 on a scale of 0 to 1.0.

5. Milk products, fish, and meat provide proteins of high quality.

D. Many uremic manifestations become evident when serum urea nitrogen (SUN) approaches 90 mg./100 ml.

E. There is a direct relationship between the ratio of SUN to serum creatinine and protein intake in patients with chronic renal failure (see Fig. 15-1).

1. This relationship may help to select the optimal amount of protein intake to be prescribed to a patient.

2. For example, if one would want to keep SUN at 60 mg./100 ml. in a patient with serum creatinine of 10 mg./100 ml., the ratio of SUN to serum creatinine would be 6.

3. Using Figure 15-1, one can predict that 40 g./day would be the optimal amount of protein to be ingested by the patient.

4. The SUN-serum creatinine ratio may also be used to judge the adherence of the patient to the prescribed protein intake.

5. It should be emphasized that the relationship between protein intake and SUN-serum creatinine ratio is affected by catabolic stress, low urine volume, and probably muscle mass. Men who are wasted, woman, and children therefore may have different relationships.

6. After a change in protein intake, a period of 2 to 3 weeks is required for the serum urea nitrogen to stablize and for the SUN-serum creatinine ratio to reflect the new protein intake.

F. Several studies have shown that a daily intake of 18 to 25 g. of high biological value protein is beneficial to the patient with advanced uremia.

1. There is evidence, however, that these patients are in negative nitrogen balance and are catabolic.

2. Such severe protein restriction, therefore, is not recommended.

G. The ingestion of 40 g./day of high biological value protein by uremic patients is associated with

1. Improvement in uremic manifestations

2. A greater sense of well-being

3. Weight gain

4. Neutral or positive nitrogen balance

H. A 40 g. protein diet is clearly more satisfying and acceptable to the patient than a 20 g. protein diet. It is the most common diet used in the treatment of patients with chronic renal disease. Tables 15-1 and 15-2 provide the details of this kind of diet.

I. Male uremic patients with glomerular filtration rates greater than 5 ml./minute should not receive less than 40 g./day of high quality protein.

1. With such diets, patients with serum creatinine of 10 mg./100 ml. would have serum urea nitrogens ranging between 40 to 75 mg./100 ml.

2. Patients with serum creatinine of 15 mg./100 ml. would have serum urea nitrogens ranging between 65 to 110 mg./100 ml. on a 40 g./day protein diet (see Fig. 15-1).

3. In small male patients and in female patients the protein intake may be reduced to 35 g./day.

J. Dietary therapy alone may not be adequate in patients with glomerular filtration rates below 5 ml./minute, and dialysis therapy or transplantation should be considered.

K. It has recently been shown that diets that are very low in nitrogen but that provide essential amino acids or ketoacid or hydroxyacid analogues of the essential amino acids as the major protein source may be beneficial to uremic patients with glomerular filtration rate below 4 to 5 ml./minute.

Table 15-1. **40 g. Protein Diet**

Foods Allowed	Amount	Foods Forbidden
Milk	1 to 2 cups daily	Cream, dishes containing milk or cream
Eggs	2 eggs may be substituted for 2 oz. of meat.	Dishes containing eggs
Meat, fish, or poultry	2 oz. daily	In excess of 2 oz.
Cheese	2 oz. may be substituted for 2 oz. of meat.	Dishes containing cheese
Potatoes	2 servings daily	In excess of 2 servings
Vegetables	3 servings, other than potatoes	In excess of 3 servings
Fruits	As desired	
Cereal and bread	4 servings daily	In excess of 4 servings
Beverages	As desired	Dishes containing milk or cream
Desserts	Fruits used as desired; milk dessert may be substituted by omitting milk proportionately. Jello may be used in place of 1 serving of bread	Other than those specified
Fat	Butter, oil, salad dressing as desired	
Miscellaneous	All seasonings and flavorings, hard candies	Nuts, peanut butter

Note: This diet is inadequate in calcium, phosphorus, thiamine, riboflavin, niacin, and folic acid. If a higher caloric diet is required, carbohydrates in fruit, fruit juices, jelly, and hard candy may provide additional calories.

1. The long-term effects of such diets on nutritional status and uremic toxicity have not yet been well documented.

L. The optimal daily calorie intake for patients with chronic renal failure is not well defined, but at least 35 Cal./day is recommended.

M. There is not adequate information on vitamin requirements for patients with advanced uremia.

1. It is recommended, however, that such patients receive preparations providing 5 mg./day of pyridoxine HCl, 1.0 mg./day of folic acid, and the recommended daily allowances of the other water-soluble vitamins.

2. Because serum levels of vitamin A are usually elevated in uremia, it is not recommended to give supplements of this vitamin.

II. Adult Patients Treated With Dialysis

A. Patients reaching dialysis therapy are often protein depleted and have been ingesting inadequate quantities of protein and calories. They require careful attention regarding their dietary therapy.

B. About 30 to 40% of the amino acids lost during hemodialysis are essential. Therefore, the need for high quality proteins is increased.

C. Patients treated with hemodialysis twice weekly, utilizing the Kiil, Klung, or twin-coil dialyzers, are maintained in neutral or positive nitrogen balance with protein intake of 0.75 g./kg./day of which 0.63 g./kg. is of high biological value.

D. Detailed and controlled data on protein requirements of dialysis patients treated thrice weekly for 6 to 8 hours per treatment are not available.

1. It is recommended, however, that protein intake should vary from 65 to 85 g./day depending on body size.

2. At least half of the protein should be of high biological value.

E. Patients treated with chronic peritoneal dialysis require greater protein intake than those maintained with hemodialysis.

1. This is mainly due to the greater loss of amino acids and protein during peritoneal dialysis.

2. These patients may require 80 to 100 g. of protein per day.

F. Calorie intake should be optimal because protein is degraded as a source of energy when the calorie intake is inadequate.

1. At least 35 Cal./kg./day should be provided to the patient treated with dialysis.

2. The diet should be supplemented with special high-calorie, low-protein and low-mineral foods available commercially.

G. Blood levels of folic acid, pyridoxine, and ascorbic acids are often decreased in patients treated with chronic dialysis.

1. A daily supplement of 1 mg. of folic acid, 10 mg./day of pyridoxine HCl, and

Table 15-2. **Suggested Meal Plan for 40 g. Protein Diet**

Breakfast	Lunch	Dinner
Fruit or juice	Vegetable plate	Juice
1 cereal with 1/2 cup of milk	1 slice of bread	2 oz. meat, fish, or poultry
1 slice of toast	Butter or margarine	1 potato or substitute
Butter or margarine	Fruit	Vegetable
Coffee or tea	Coffee or tea	Salad
Sugar—jelly	Sugar	1 slice of bread
		Fruit
		4 oz. milk
		Coffee or tea
		Sugar
	Mid-afternoon	Note: Part of dinner may be
	Fruit	taken as night snack.

100 mg. of ascorbic acid should prevent deficiencies of these vitamins.

2. Patients treated with chronic dialysis should also receive vitamin preparations that provide the daily requirements for niacin, riboflavin, thiamine, biotin, pantothenic acid, and vitamin B_{12}.

H. Patients undergoing maintenance dialysis, in whom dietary intake is not carefully supervised, frequently ingest too little protein and particularly inadequate calories.

1. Water, sodium, and potassium intake is often excessive.

2. Ad libitum diets should, therefore, be discouraged.

3. Dietary intake should be carefully monitored, and dietary adherence should be encouraged.

III. Infants and Children Treated with Dialysis

A. Retarded growth is common in children with renal failure and persists even in those treated with hemodialysis.

B. Growth retardation in major part is due to inadequate protein and calorie intake.

C. Pediatricians recommend a diet containing 1.5 g. of protein/kg./day for preadolescent children on a diet that provides 8 to 12% of the total calories from protein for children of any size.

1. At least 70% of the ingested protein should be of high quality.

D. The calorie intake should be 150 Cal./kg./day for children under 3 years of age and 100 Cal./kg. for prepubertal children who are more than 3 years old.

PROBLEMS RELATED TO HYPERLIPIDEMIA

I. Patients with chronic uremia and those treated with dialysis, frequently have a Type-IV hyperlipidemia with elevated serum levels of triglycerides.

II. More than 50% of deaths in the dialysis patients are due to cardiovascular diseases. The hypertriglyceridemia may contribute to this phenomenon.

III. Diets in which the carbohydrate content is lowered to provide 35% of the calories, and fat content is increased to supply 55% of the calories, with a polyunsaturated to saturated fatty acid ratio of 2.0, have been shown to lower fasting- and postprandial serum triglycerides in uremic and dialysis patients.

A. The efficacy of the above diets in controlling the accelerated atherogenesis in these patients has not been sufficiently documented.

SODIUM AND WATER INTAKE

I. Characteristics of Sodium and Water Excretion by the Failing Kidney

A. Sodium balance is usually maintained in patients with chronic renal failure when they ingest a usual salt intake.

1. This is due to the decreased sodium reabsorption per nephron.

B. With advanced renal failure (glomerular filtration rate below 15 ml./minute), the ability of the patient to conserve sodium during dietary sodium restriction is impaired.

C. The obligatory loss of sodium in the urine may cause salt depletion and contraction of extracellular fluid volume if sodium intake does not equal the urinary loss.

D. Similarly, the ability to excrete sodium loads is limited, and sodium retention, edema, hypertension, and congestive heart failure may develop with ingestion of large quantities of salt.

E. Patients with advanced renal failure excrete large amounts of solutes and cannot concentrate their urine.

1. These two abnormalities dictate obligatory losses of water.

2. Failure to ingest adequate amounts of water results in water dehydration.

3. Also, the ability to excrete water loads is limited.

4. The intake of large quantities of fluids, therefore, causes water retention, dilution of body fluids, and hyponatremia.

II. Sodium and Water Requirements and How to Monitor Intake

A. Most patients will maintain sodium and water balance on an intake of 2 to 8 g. of salt per day and 1.5 to 3.0 L. of water per day.

1. It should be emphasized, however, that the requirements for sodium and water vary from one patient to another.

2. Not infrequently, therefore, an individual approach is needed.

B. The simplest way to monitor adequacy of salt intake is to observe the body weight carefully.

1. Inadequate salt intake is associated with loss of weight.

2. With excessive salt ingestion, the patient's weight increases.

C. A more accurate way is to determine the lower (floor) and upper (ceiling) limits of the kidney to excrete sodium. This is done as follows:

1. The patient is prescribed a diet containing 1 g. of salt a day for 5 days.

2. On the fourth and fifth day, 24-hour urine collections are obtained for determinations of sodium excretion that will represent the obligatory rate of sodium loss.

3. The patient is then instructed to ingest 8 g. of salt a day for 5 days.

4. The 24-hour urinary excretion of sodium is determined on the fourth and fifth day to estimate the upper limit of the ability of the kidney to excrete sodium.

5. The optimal amount of sodium intake for the particular patient can then be determined.

D. It must be recognized that the sodium needs may change with further deterioration of renal function, and, therefore, continuous follow-up and surveillance of the patient is needed.

E. The water requirement of the patients with advanced renal failure ranges between 1.5 and 3.0 L./day.

1. The thirst mechanism is usually adequate to regulate the water needs of the patient.

2. Under steady state conditions, urinary output usually provides a good guide for the daily water intake, which should equal urine volume plus 500 ml. of insensible water loss.

POTASSIUM PHOSPHATE, CALCIUM, AND MAGNESIUM REQUIREMENTS

I. Potassium Intake

A. Hyperkalemia is not a common finding in patients with chronic renal failure. This is due to adaptive changes in the function of the remaining nephrons leading to increased potassium secretion.

B. Hyperkalemia in patients with chronic renal failure may be due to

1. Severe oliguria

2. Catabolic states such as infection, trauma, surgery, or steroid administration

3. Selective hypoaldosteronism

4. Excessive dietary intake of potassium

C. Excessive dietary intake of potassium is probably the most common cause of hyperkalemia in patients with renal failure. Diets containing large amounts of potassium should be avoided.

D. Daily intake of potassium should not exceed 70 mEq./day. A protein-restricted diet (40 g./day) usually provides about 50 to 60 mEq. of potassium per day.

II. Phosphate Intake

A. Phosphate retention occurs with each decrement in renal function.

1. Hyperphosphatemia, however, does not become apparent until the glomerular filtrate rate falls below 20 ml./minute due to the increased secretion of parathyroid

hormone that reduces tubular reabsorption of phosphate and allows excess phosphate to be excreted in the urine.

B. Marked hyperphosphatemia is harmful because

1. It enhances soft tissue calcification.

2. It indirectly stimulates parathyroid gland activity.

C. Control of serum phosphorus concentration toward normal is an important part of the management of patients with chronic renal failure and those treated with hemodialysis.

D. The control of serum phosphorus levels is achieved by restriction of phosphate intake, which could be partially achieved by excluding dairy foods from the diet.

E. The usual intake of phosphorus by a normal adult in the U.S. varies between 1.0 and 1.8 g./day.

F. With the elimination or restriction of dairy products and a rigid adherence to 40 g. of protein/day, the dietary intake of phosphorus can be reduced to between 600 and 900 mg./day. This may not be low enough, however, to control serum phosphorus.

G. The use of phosphate binders that render phosphate unabsorbable by the intestine is frequently needed to achieve adequate control of the hyperphosphatemia.

1. The most frequently used compounds are Alu-cap, Amphojel, and Basaljel concentrate.

2. The latter is tasteless, and only a small volume is necessary per dose. Hence, the patient can more readily follow the prescribed regimen.

3. Therapy may be started with two to three tablets of Amphojel or capsules of Alu-cap or 5 to 10 ml. of Basaljel with each meal.

4. The goal of therapy with phosphate binders is to reduce the levels of serum phosphorus to, or near, normal levels of 4.0 to 5.0 mg./100 ml.

5. Phosphate binders containing magnesium salts should be avoided.

III. Calcium Intake

A. There are at least three reasons why oral supplements of calcium should be considered for patients with chronic renal failure and those treated with hemodialysis.

1. Intestinal absorption of calcium is impaired in uremia.

2. The diets prescribed to uremic patients usually have reduced amounts of dairy products and, therefore, a low quantity of calcium.

3. These patients frequently are hypocalcemic.

B. Calcium supplements in the amount of 1 to 2 g. of elemental calcium per day may be given. Greater quantities may be used if needed.

1. Elemental calcium constitutes 40% of calcium carbohydrate, 12% of calcium lactate, and 8% of calcium gluconate.

2. Calcium chloride should be avoided in uremic patients because of its acidifying properties.

3. Calcium carbonate is inexpensive, tasteless, and relatively well tolerated.

4. A proprietary preparation, Titralac, provides 0.42 g. of calcium carbonate and 0.18 g. of glycine per tablet (e.g., 160 mg. of elemental calcium per tablet).

5. Neo-calglucon syrup is another preparation well accepted by patients, but it is costly. Each 4 ml. contains 92 mg. of calcium ion.

C. It is advisable that therapy with calcium supplements should not be initiated before the level of serum phosphorus is reduced to, or near, normal.

D. Frequent monitoring of the levels of serum calcium is important because hypercalcemia may develop.

IV. Magnesium Intake

A. The kidney is the main organ responsible for the maintenance of the level of serum magnesium within normal limits.

B. Distinct hypermagnesemia is not infrequently present in patients with advanced chronic renal failure (e.g., greater than 2.5 mEq./L.).

C. Patients with uremia should avoid excessive dietary intake of magnesium, the use of phosphate binders containing magnesium, or enemas with magnesium salts. Dangerous hypermagnesemia may develop otherwise.

VITAMIN D REQUIREMENTS

I. Vitamin D must undergo a two-step metabolic transformation, first, in the liver to 25-hydroxycholecalciferol and, subsequently, in the kidney to form the active metabolite 1,25-dihydroxycholecalciferol.

II. Patients with chronic renal failure and reduced renal functioning mass are unable to produce adequate amounts of 1,25-dihydroxycholecalciferol and, hence, have vitamin D deficiency.

III. Vitamin D deficiency is responsible directly and indirectly for the various manifestations of deranged divalent ion metabolism in uremia.

IV. Currently, the forms of vitamin D that are available for clinical use include vitamin D_2 (ergocalciferol), vitamin D_3 (cholecalciferol), and dihydrotachysterol (DHT). The metabolites of vitamin D, 25(OH)D_3 and 1,25(OH)$_2D_3$, have been synthesized and will be available for clinical use in the near future.

V. When therapy with vitamin D is required, the initial dose of vitamin D_2 is 0.625 to 1.25 mg.(25,000 to 50,000 I.U.)/day, and the initial dose of DHT is 0.125 to 0.250 mg./day.

A. Identification of a definite therapeutic effect of vitamin D is often difficult.

B. Indications of a response to vitamin D include

1. Radiographic evidence of improvement in bone disease

2. A decrease in the blood levels of alkaline phosphatase

3. An increase in the concentration of calcium or phosphorus

C. When there is clearly no response to therapy, the dose of vitamin D may be increased, but the daily dose should not be raised by more than 1.25 mg. (50,000 I.U.) every 4 to 8 weeks.

ACUTE RENAL FAILURE

I. Definition

A. Acute renal failure is a syndrome characterized by abrupt impairment or cessation of renal function manifested by oliguria or anuria.

1. The disease is frequently reversible.

2. This syndrome is commonly referred to as acute tubular necrosis.

B. The illness may follow nephrotoxic or ischemic injuries to the kidneys.

C. Several mechanisms may underlie the oliguria. They include

1. Reduction in glomerular filtration rate per nephron, due to preglomerular vasoconstriction or a decrease in afferent arteriolar pressure

2. Excessive filtrate reabsorption through damaged tubular epithelium

3. Tubular obstruction by casts

II. Clinical Characteristics

A. The clinical course is characterized by two stages—an oliguric phase and a diuretic phase.

B. Oliguric Phase

1. The oliguric phase usually lasts 7 to 12 days, but may persist up to 7 weeks.

2. During this phase, the patient is uremic and displays abnormalities in fluid and electrolyte homeostasis.

3. These may include hyperkalemia, hypermagnesemia, hyperphosphatemia, hyponatremia, hypocalcemia, and acidosis.

4. The urinary output ranges between 50 and 400 ml./day.

C. Diuretic Phase

1. During the diuretic phase, urinary output increases gradually and pro-

gressively, and may reach several liters per day.

2. The signs and symptoms of uremia subside gradually.

3. The patient usually recovers within 15 to 25 days after the onset of the diuretic phase.

III. Dietary Therapy

A. Fluid intake should equal urinary output and other extrarenal losses of water plus 400 ml./day.

1. This takes into consideration insensible water loss and endogenous water production.

2. It is better to err by giving too little water than by giving too much.

3. Adequate water intake by these patients is judged by normal blood levels of sodium and daily weight loss of 0.2 to 0.5 kg.

B. Salt intake may range between 3 and 5 g./day unless congestive heart failure or hypertension is present. Under such circumstances, salt intake should not exceed 1 g./day.

C. Potassium intake should be restricted because its excretion is decreased.

D. Nutrition should provide basal protein and calorie requirements.

1. Pure carbohydrate diets have been replaced by protein of high biological value and large amounts of carbohydrates in the form of glucose, candy, jellies, or Karo syrup mixtures.

2. The patient may receive 40 g. of protein/day with glucose supplements of 100 to 200 g./day.

E. Because most patients with acute renal failure are treated with dialysis, fluid, salt, and protein intake can be liberalized, depending on the frequency of the dialysis treatment.

F. Patients who are unable to eat may be fed with intravenous infusions of mixtures of hypertonic glucose and amino acids.

TOTAL PARENTERAL NUTRITION IN PATIENTS WITH KIDNEY DISEASE

I. Indications

A. Patients with acute or chronic renal failure may sustain intercurrent illnesses that render them unable to eat normally.

1. Under these circumstances, encouraging dietary intake, administration of liquid diets through tubes or enterostomies, or elemental diets often may be used to provide good nutrition.

2. Not infrequently, patients are unable to receive nourishment through the alimentary tract.

3. Parenteral nutrition then must be employed.

B. In acute renal failure, the use of total parenteral nutrition (TPN) has been associated with greater anabolism and enhanced recovery of renal function, although survival may not be improved. Hyperkalemia, hyperphosphatemia, and hypermagnesemia may also be better controlled.

C. In chronic renal failure, marked wasting may be ameliorated, and prolonged convalescence is often shortened with TPN.

II. Method of Administration

A. For most conditions, patients should receive at least 35 Cal./kg./day and close to 3000 Cal./day if possible.

B. Severe catabolic conditions, such as burns, may be associated with energy requirements of 6000 Cal./day or more.

C. The two major sources of energy intake, glucose and fat emulsions, provide special hazards for the uremic patient.

1. Insulin resistance and glucose intolerance may lead to hyperglycemia with glucose infusions.

2. Decreased capability to clear triglycerides normally can promote hypertriglyceridemia with infusions of fat emulsions.

3. Patients must be monitored closely for these complications.

D. The optimal mixtures of amino acids for TPN are not clearly established.

1. It is probably preferable to use solutions of free L-amino acids rather than protein hydrolysates.

2. The infusion of 12 to 30 g./day of essential amino acids is associated with lower urea production.

3. Essential amino acids solutions should contain histidine, which is considered essential for both normal and uremic persons.

4. Solutions providing 40 to 80 g./day of mixtures of essential and nonessential amino acids may promote greater anabolism despite the formation of more urea.

E. The volume of the infusate should be limited because of oliguria.

1. More energy per milliliter of infusate can be produced by using 70% glucose solutions. When the latter are mixed with equal volumes of amino acids, a final glucose concentration of 35 g./100 ml. will be attained.

2. Solutions containing 10% fat emulsions provide slightly fewer calories per milliliter of water than does a 35% glucose solution. A 20% lipid emulsion provides the most calories per milliliter of water but is presently unavailable in the U.S.

3. The volume of the infusate may be reduced if the patient is able to ingest small quantities of carbohydrate and fats that provide part of his calorie needs.

F. In the uremic patient whose serum electrolyte concentrations are normal and relatively constant, infusion therapy is started with approximately the following quantities of nutrients: sodium, 50 mEq./L.; potassium, 35 mEq./L.; phosphate, 20 mEq./day; magnesium, 8 mEq./day; and calcium, 10 mEq./day.

1. When the concentration of an electrolyte is elevated, it may be prudent not to administer it at the onset of TPN.

2. However, patients must be monitored extremely carefully as the marked anabolism that often occurs with initiation of TPN may cause serum potassium, phosphorus, or magnesium levels to fall precipitously.

G. The infusate should contain pyridoxine hydrochloride, 10 mg./day; folic acid, 1.0 mg./day; vitamin C, 100 mg./day; vitamin K, 7.5 mg./day; and the minimum daily requirement of the other water-soluble vitamins.

H. TPN solutions are usually hypertonic and must, therefore, be infused into a high-flow vein to avoid vascular inflammation and thrombosis. The infusates are usually delivered through a catheter inserted into the superior vena cava through the subclavian vein.

1. TPN solutions may be infused into the blood access sites for hemodialysis such as arteriovenous fistulas or shunts using a Y adapter.

2. The use of the same vascular access for both TPN and hemodialysis may reduce the longevity of such access sites.

3. These routes are best used, therefore, when the patient does not require dialysis therapy for a long time.

III. Other Uses for Amino Acids in Dialysis Patients

A. In acutely or chronically uremic patients who are eating poorly and who otherwise are not receiving parenteral nutrition, one may infuse 42 g. of essential and nonessential amino acids and 175 to 200 g. of glucose into the venous lines of the dialyzer.

1. This procedure provides an intravenous nutritional supplement with each dialysis with very little risk or discomfort to the patient.

2. Addition of minerals is usually not necessary because the dialysate contains many electrolytes.

B. One hazard of the above procedure is

reactive hypoglycemia after cessation of the infusion. This may be prevented by the following procedures:

    1. Infuse the solution at a constant rate throughout the dialysis treatment.

    2. Do not stop the infusion before dialysis is completed.

    3. Use 175 to 200 g./L. of dextrose rather than the more usual 250 g.

    4. Feed the patient a carbohydrate source (e.g., two slices of bread) 20 to 30 minutes before the end of the infusion.

    5. Reactive hypoglycemia can be avoided by administering amino acids with low quantities of glucose (5 to 10%) and fat emulsions. However, infusion of lipids possibly may decrease the efficiency of dialysis.

    C. Others recommend the infusion of 17 g. of essential amino acids including histidine and some carbohydrate during the last 90 minutes of each hemodialysis therapy.

    1. This treatment has been suggested for use in the management of usual dialysis patients.

    2. In these patients, the concentrations of various serum proteins increase after several months of such therapy.

SUGGESTED READINGS

Bergström, J., Fürst, P., and Norée, L.O.: Treatment of chronic uremic patients with protein-poor diet and oral supply of essential amino acids (I. Nitrogen balance studies). Clin. Nephrol., *3:*187, 1975.

Berlyne, G.M., and Shaw, A.B.: Giordano-Giovannetti diet in terminal renal failure. Lancet, *2:*7, 1965.

Giordano, C.: Use of exogenous and endogenous urea for protein synthesis in normal and uremic subjects. J. Lab. Clin. Med., *62:*231, 1963.

Giovannetti, S., and Maggiore, Q.: A low-nitrogen diet with proteins of high biological value for severe uraemia. Lancet, *1:*1000, 1964.

Kopple, J.D.: Dietary requirements. *In* Massry, S.G., and Sellers, A.L. (eds.): Clinical Aspects of Uremia and Dialysis. Springfield, Charles C Thomas, 1976.

Kopple, J.D., and Blumenkrantz, M.J.: Nutritional therapy of the urologic patient. Urol. Clin. North Am., *3:*403, 1976.

Kopple, J.D., and Coburn, J.W.: Metabolic studies of low protein diets in uremia (I. Nitrogen and potassium). Medicine, *52:*583, 1973.

Massry, S.G., and Coburn, J.W.: Divalent ion metabolism and renal osteodystrophy. *In* Massry, S.G., and Sellers, A.L. (eds.): Clinical Aspects of Uremia and Dialysis. Springfield, Charles C Thomas, 1976.

Norée, L.O., and Bergström, J.: Treatment of chronic uremic patients with protein-poor diet and oral supply of essential amino acids (II. Clinical results of long-term treatment). Clin. Nephrol., *3:* 195, 1975.

Walser, M.: Ketoacids in the treatment in uremia. Clin. Nephrol., *3:*180, 1975.

16. NEW CONCEPTS OF THE DIET THERAPY OF DIABETES MELLITUS

Harold S. Cole, M.D.
Rafael Camerini-Davalos, M.D., D.Sc.

Diet therapy is of major importance in the control of diabetes mellitus. A consistent calorie, carbohydrate, fat, and protein intake removes at least one variable in the regulation of blood sugar. The new exchange lists for the planning of diabetic diets have added some spice and variety and relieved the rigidity and monotony of former prescriptions (see Appendix 16-A).

Good control of juvenile (insulin-dependent) diabetes cannot be obtained with insulin alone. Dietary restrictions are essential factors in its management. Many patients with maturity onset diabetes may be controlled by diet alone without the addition of insulin or oral hypoglycemic agents.

Because previous studies have shown that more than 50% of diabetic patients fail to follow their prescribed diets, restrictions are minimal in those who are not obese and who have had reasonable eating habits. Scales have been abandoned in favor of common household measuring devices—the cup, tablespoon, slices, and ruler. Eventually, visual measurement is sufficent. The inclusion of between-meal snacks and desserts allows for more flexibility.

I. Aims of the Diabetic Diet

A. To help normalize the carbohydrate dysmetabolism

B. To supply adequate amounts of all nutrients—carbohydrates, fats, proteins, vitamins, and minerals

C. To maintain blood lipids within the normal range

D. To be readily accepted and to provide foods similar to those offered to the remainder of the family

E. To normalize body weight
1. Obese diabetics must lose weight. This is paramount, whether the patient is a child or adult.
2. Normal weight adults must maintain their weight and energy potential.
3. Diabetic children must consume sufficient calories for adequate nutrition and normal weight gain and growth.

F. To improve the patient's feeling of well-being

G. To permit normal activity

H. To satisfy the tastes and the ethnic and religious standards of diabetic patients[3]

II. New Concepts of Diet Therapy

A. Much investigation has been done in recent years particularly on dietary control of blood lipids.

B. The new theories emphasize relatively high-carbohydrate, low-fat diets as well as restricting refined sugar intake. High-fiber carbohydrates are increased.
1. The basal or control diets contain 45% carbohydrate, 40% fat, and 15% protein.
2. The new diets that were studied contained at least 60% of total calories as carbohydrates, with fat content lowered to about 25%, while protein intake remained at 15%.
3. The data suggest that a high-carbohydrate diet actually increases the sensitivity of peripheral tissues to both endogenous and exogenous insulin. The glucose tolerance also improves, and lower levels of serum insulin are observed.
4. The control of diabetes and insulin secretory capacity appear to be maintained despite the increase in carbohydrate intake. In addition, the liberalization of carbohydrates might facilitate the reduction of saturated fat and cholesterol in the diabetic diet.

5. Diets in which 70% or more of calories are derived from refined carbohydrates have been shown to elevate serum triglycerides in insulin-treated diabetics. These low-fat diets have also been shown to decrease plasma cholesterol in both controls and insulin-treated diabetics.

6. It has been suggested that fiber retards and reduces the digestion of starch by amylase and that fiber-depleted plant food might promote obesity.

a. One study concluded that a very low-fat and high-carbohydrate diet, administered as fiber-rich foods, resulted in a greater decrease of both serum triglycerides and cholesterol than did the diet of refined carbohydrates.

b. Excellent high-fiber carbohydrate foods include baked beans, rice, whole wheat bread, blackberries, and blueberries (see Table 13-1).

c. Patients who consume a high-fiber diet have been reported to experience a fall in blood glucose. This may result in a decreased requirement for insulin or for oral hypoglycemic drugs.

III. Requirements of the Diabetic Diet

A. An updated *Exchange Lists for Meal Planning,* published jointly by the American Diabetes Association and the American Dietetic Association, has recently been completed.

1. This guide book emphasizes that it should be used with the help of a physician, nurse, or dietician.

2. The updated exchange lists are based on a concern for total calories and for modification of fat intake.

3. The list of milk exchanges is subdivided into non-fat-, low-fat-, and whole milk groups.

4. Starchy vegetables are included with bread exchanges.

5. The meat list has the three categories of lean-, medium-fat-, and high-fat meats and other protein-rich foods.

6. Fat exchanges clearly show which kind of fat is contained in foods—saturated or polyunsaturated.

B. The caloric requirements of the diabetic will depend on certain patient-related factors.

1. Age: Child, adolescent, adult, or geriatric patient

2. Weight: The obese diabetic requires a nutritionally adequate diet which is restricted in calories. The underweight patient will receive a high-calorie diet.

3. Physiological situation: Pregnancy and growth increase the calorie requirements.

4. Activity, as related to weight, determines the caloric needs of the diabetic patient (see Table 16-1).

a. Patients who are sedentary and overweight require only 15 to 20 Cal./kg./day.

b. Those who are of normal weight but pursue sedentary occupations require 30 Cal./kg./day.

c. Underweight diabetics require 45

Table 16-1. **Caloric Requirement of Adults, Related to Activity**
(Cal./kg./day)

	Marked Activity	Moderate Activity	Sedentary	Bed Rest
Underweight (< 20% of ideal weight)	45–50	40	35	20–25
Ideal Weight	40	35	30	15–20
Overweight (> 20% of ideal weight)	35	30	15–20	15

(Cole, H., and Camerini-Davalos, R.: Current concepts in clinical nutrition. Med. Clin. North Am. *54:*1577, 1970) to 50 Cal./kg./day when they are markedly active.

IV. Children's Diets

A. Children's diets are based upon age and nutritional status.

1. In general, children require 1000 Cal./day at 1 year of age plus 100 Cal. for each additional year. Thus a 6-year-old child receives 1500 Cal., and an 11-year-old child receives 2000 Cal.

2. Several hundred Cal. are either added or subtracted from the diet, if the child is respectively underweight or obese.

B. Adequate provision must be made for growth, activity, and maintenance of body weight.

1. During peak growth periods, adolescent boys require from 3100 to 3600 Cal./day, and adolescent girls require from 2400 to 2700 Cal./day.

V. Diets in Pregnancy

A. Pregnant diabetics should gain weight at a regular and even rate.

1. A total gain during pregnancy of 20 to 28 lbs. is optimal and a reasonable objective.

2. This could be achieved by a total gain of 1.5 lbs. in the first 10 weeks and subsequently an average of 0.8 lbs. per week.

B. Pregnant diabetics should eat 200 to 300 Cal./day in addition to the calorie intake necessary for maintaining body weight.

1. This will suffice for meeting the energy needs of pregnancy.

2. The caloric content must not be less than 36 Cal./kg. of pregnant body weight.

C. Protein needs are met by adding 10 to 20 g. of protein per day to the maintenance level of 1 g./kg. of ideal weight.

1. By giving 1.3 g./kg./day, the protein requirements generally will be fulfilled.

VI. Partition of Calories

A. Carbohydrate Requirements

1. A difference of opinion exists as to the optimal proportion of carbohydrate and fat prescribed for the diabetic.

2. Since the average American diet consists of about 50% carbohydrate, this amount or even a little more is acceptable.

3. When calorie restriction is required, the amount of fat may be decreased to allow for additional carbohydrate.

4. The carbohydrate necessary in the daily diet is calculated by dividing the total daily calorie requirement by 10 (see Table 16-2).

Table 16-2. **Examples of Calculation of Caloric Requirements and Partition of Diabetic Diet**

Male
Ideal weight, 150 lb.
Actual weight, 154 lb. (70 kg.)
Activity, marked
70 kg. $\times$ 40 cal. = 2800 cal.
2800/10 = 280 g. carbohydrate
280/2 = 140 g. fat
280/2 = 140 g. protein

Female
Ideal weight, 108 lb.
Actual weight, 110 lb. (50 kg.)
Activity, sedentary
50 kg. $\times$ 30 cal. = 1500 cal.
1500/10 = 150 g. carbohydrate
150/2 = 75 g. fat
150/2 = 75 g. protein

a. An 11-year-old child, for example, who requires 2000 Cal. needs 200 g. of carbohydrate per day.

b. A 60 kg. adult who performs marked activity will require 2400 Cal. per day (60 kg. $\times$ 40 Cal./kg.). The 2400 divided by 10 gives 240 g. of carbohydrate per day, approximately 40% of the total daily calories.

5. Amounts of carbohydrates greater than 300 g./day may be too much for the metabolic capacity of the diabetic and may result in marked glucosuria.

B. Protein Requirements

1. Children under 3 years of age require 2.5 g. of protein per kg., and older children require 2 g./kg./day.

2. The protein allowance for healthy adults is at least 1 g./kg. of body weight.

3. The diabetic patient may require an additional supplement of up to 0.5 g./kg./day to counteract losses from gluconeogenesis and ketogenesis associated with impaired glucose utilization.

4. The daily number of grams of protein needed can be easily obtained by dividing the carbohydrate requirement (in grams) in half (see Table 16–2). This result approximates 20% of the total calories.

C. Fat Requirements

1. The average amount of fat in the American diet ranges between 35 and 40%.

2. Diabetic diets should limit their total fat calories to this amount or less.

3. The recommended polyunsaturated-saturated fat ratio is 2.5:1.

4. Supplementation of a low-saturated-fat diet with increased amounts of polyunsaturated fats not only makes it more palatable and interesting but may lower serum cholesterol (see Chap. 10).

5. The grams of fat in the diet are calculated exactly as is the protein content — the grams of carbohydrate per day divided in half (see Table 16–2). The result is the number of grams of fat required.

a. This amount approximates 40% of the total calories.

b. This amount is a maximum which can easily be reduced.

D. Vitamins and Minerals

1. The American Diabetes Association Exchange Diet, prescribed with the above caloric requirements and partitions, contains sufficient vitamins and minerals for the well controlled diabetic.

2. Poorly controlled diabetics or those with infections, polyuria, or ketoacidosis may require vitamin supplementation, especially of the water-soluble vitamins (high B complex and vitamin C).

E. Alcohol

1. Moderate amounts of alcohol may be added to the diabetic diet.

2. The relatively high caloric value of alcohol must be considered in the formulation of the diet.

3. Beer contains 45 Cal./100 ml.; red, white, and rosé wines and champagne average about 80 Cal./100 ml.; dessert wines such as sweet sherry and port have about 150 Cal./100 ml.; and the distilled spirits such as whiskey, brandy, gin, and vodka contain about 240 Cal./100 ml.

F. Converting the Diet Prescription into Meals

1. The foods in the diabetic diet are commonly available and are generally the same as for individuals without diabetes.

2. The foods should be measured after

Table 16-3. **Criteria of Adherence to Diet**

Free Diet*	Poor*	Fair	Good	Excellent
Patients who admitted eating everything, including sweets and pastries	Avoidance of sweets and pastries, but otherwise diet variable and, in general, unrestricted	Estimation of quantities of food with avoidance of sweets and pastries and excesses of carbohydrate-rich food, but frequent dietary indiscretions	Generally careful adherence to diet with weighing or measuring food not less than once a month, but with occasional dietary indiscretions	Careful adherence with weighing or measuring of food not less than once a week and almost never a dietary indiscretion

*Patients who had taken free diets or whose adherence was classified as poor were considered as having failed to follow a diet.

cooking. A standard 8 oz. measuring cup, a measuring teaspoon, and a tablespoon are all that are needed.

3. Meats should be baked, broiled, roasted, or boiled. Foods should not be fried unless fat allowed in the meal is used.

4. The following foods should be prohibited in the diet: sugar, candy, honey, jam, jelly, marmalade, syrup, pie, cake, cookies, pastries, condensed milk (containing added sugar), soft drinks (except diet soft drinks), and candy-coated gum.

5. Fried, scalloped, or creamed foods, beer, wine, or other alcoholic beverages should be avoided.

6. In using diabetic exchange lists, foods in the same list are interchangeable (e.g., one bread-type food for another bread-type food, but not for meat or for fruits).

VII. Adherence to Diet

A. Dietary management is accepted to be of cardinal importance in the control of diabetes. Criteria for ascertaining adherence to the diet are listed in Table 16–3.

B. An attempt to improve patient compliance is essential to avoid the complications which result in poorly controlled diabetes.

1. Motivation is a very important factor in diet compliance. The personality of the physician and the zeal with which the diet is advocated by him are important in motivating patients.

2. Behavior modification by interested psychologists has proved successful in selected cases.

3. Small group sessions led by a nutritionist or physician or, occasionally, even one-to-one sessions, might be required.

4. Frequent follow-up visits by the patient have proved fruitful. These should be at 2-week intervals for the first 2 months and then once a month for the balance of the first year.

5. Feedback—keeping the patients informed as to results of their progress, laboratory results, and physical examination findings—maintains their interest.

C. Of primary importance is that in the preparation of diabetic diets, the dietary habits and food preferences of the individual, his religious and ethnic background, and his social and economic status be taken into account to ensure compliance.

D. The diet should be measured with common household measures—cups, slices, tablespoons, ounces—and it should be neither rigid nor weighed. Deviations in small amounts occurring sporadically usually are not of significance.

E. Family involvement—the participation of parents of diabetic children and the spouses of diabetics—can be an important asset in motivating adherence to diets.

Appendix 16-A. **Diabetes Exchange List**

List 1 foods allowed as desired (need not be measured)

Seasonings: Cinnamon, celery salt, garlic, garlic salt, lemon, mustard, mint, nutmeg, parsley, pepper, saccharin and other sugarless sweeteners, spices, vanilla, and vinegar.

Other Foods: Coffee or tea (without sugar or cream), fat-free broth, bouillon, unflavored gelatin, rennet tablets, sour or dill pickles, cranberries (without sugar), rhubarb (without sugar).

Vegetables: Group A—insignificant carbohydrate or calories. You may eat as much as desired of raw vegetable. If cooked vegetable is eaten, limit amount to 1 cup.

Asparagus	Lettuce
Broccoli	Mushrooms
Brussels sprouts	Okra
Cabbage	Peppers, green
Cauliflower	or red
Celery	Radishes
Chicory	Sauerkraut
Cucumbers	String beans
Eggplant	Summer squash
Escarole	Tomatoes
Greens: beet, chard, collard,	Water cress
dandelion, kale, mustard,	
spinach, turnip	

List 2 vegetable exchanges

Each portion supplies approximately 7 g. of carbohydrate and 2 g. of protein, or 36 calories.

Vegetables: Group B—One serving equals 1/2 cup, or 100 g.

Beets	Pumpkin
Carrots	Rutabagas
Onions	Squash, winter
Peas, green	Turnips

List 3 fruit exchanges

(fresh, dried, or canned without sugar or syrup) Each portion supplies approximately 10 g. of carbohydrate, or 40 calories.

	household measurement	weight of portion
Apple	1 small (2″ diam.)	80 g.
Applesauce	1/2 cup	100 g.
Apricots, fresh	2 med.	100 g.
Apricots, dried	4 halves	20 g.
Banana	1/2 small	50 g.
Berries	1 cup	150 g.
Blueberries	2/3 cup	100 g.
Cantaloupe	1/4 (6″ diam.)	200 g.
Cherries	10 large	75 g.
Dates	2	15 g.
Figs, fresh	2 large	50 g.
Figs, dried	1 small	15 g.
Grapefruit	1/2 small	125 g.
Grapefruit juice	1/2 cup	100 g.
Grapes	12	75 g.
Grape juice	1/4 cup	60 g.
Honeydew melon	1/8 (7″)	150 g.
Mango	1/2 small	70 g.
Orange	1 small	100 g.
Orange juice	1/2 cup	100 g.
Papaya	1/3 med.	100 g.
Peach	1 med.	100 g.
Pear	1 small	100 g.
Pineapple	1/2 cup	80 g.
Pineapple juice	1/2 cup	80 g.
Plums	2 med.	100 g.
Prunes, dried	2	25 g.
Raisins	2 tbsp.	15 g.
Tangerine	1 large	100 g.
Watermelon	1 cup	175 g.

List 4 bread exchanges

Each portion supplies approximately 15 g. of carbohydrate and 2 g. of protein, or 68 calories.

	household measurement	weight of portion
Bread	1 slice	25 g.
Biscuit, roll	1 (2″ diam.)	35 g.
Muffin	1 (2″ diam.)	35 g.
Cornbread	1 1/2″ cube	35 g.
Flour	2 1/2 tbsp.	20 g.
Cereal, cooked	1/2 cup	100 g.
Cereal, dry (flakes or puffed)	3/4 cup	20 g.
Rice or grits, cooked	1/2 cup	100 g.
Spaghetti, noodles, etc.	1/2 cup	100 g.
Crackers, graham	2	20 g.
Crackers, oyster	20 (1/2 cup)	20 g.
Crackers, saltine	5	20 g.
Crackers, soda	3	20 g.
Crackers, round	6–8	20 g.
Vegetables Beans (lima, navy, etc.), dry, cooked	1/2 cup	90 g.
Peas (split peas, etc.) dry, cooked	1/2 cup	90 g.
Baked beans, no pork	1/4 cup	50 g.
Corn	1/3 cup	80 g.
Parsnips	2/3 cup	125 g.
Potato, white, baked or boiled	1 (2″ diam.)	100 g.
Potatoes, white, mashed	1/2 cup	100 g.
Potatoes, sweet, or yams	1/4 cup	50 g.
Sponge cake, plain	1 1/2″ cube	25 g.
Ice cream (Omit 2 fat exchanges)	1/2 cup	70 g.

List 5 meat exchanges

Each portion supplies approximately 7 g. of protein and 5 g. of fat, or 73 calories. (30 g. equal 1 oz.)

	household measurement	weight of portion
Meat and poultry (beef, lamb, pork, liver, chicken, etc.) (med. fat)	1-oz. slice (4″ × 2″ × 1/4″)	30 g.
Cold cuts	1 1/2-oz. slice (4 1/2″ sq. 1/8″ thick)	45 g.
Frankfurter	1 (8–9 per lb.)	50 g.
Codfish, mackerel, etc.	1 slice (2″ × 2″ × 1″)	30 g.
Salmon, tuna, crab	1/4 cup	30 g.
Oysters, shrimp, clams	5 small	45 g.
Sardines	3 med.	30 g.
Cheese, cheddar, American	1 slice (3 1/2″ × 1 1/2″ × 1/4″)	30 g.
Cheese, cottage	1/4 cup	45 g.
Egg	1	50 g.
Peanut butter.	2 tbsp.	30 g.

Limit peanut butter to one exchange per day unless carbohydrate is allowed for in diet plan.

List 6 fat exchanges

Each portion supplies approximately 5 g. of fat, or 45 calories.

	household measurement	weight of portion
Butter or margarine . .	1 tsp.	5 g.
Bacon, crisp	1 slice	10 g.
Cream, light, 20% . . .	2 tbsp.	30 g.
Cream, heavy, 40% . .	1 tbsp.	15 g.
Cream cheese	1 tbsp.	15 g.
French dressing	1 tbsp.	15 g.
Mayonnaise	1 tsp.	5 g.
Oil or cooking fat. . . .	1 tsp.	5 g.
Nuts	6 small	10 g.
Olives	5 small	50 g.
Avocado	1/8 (4″ diam.) . .	25 g.

List 7 milk exchanges

Each portion supplies approximately 12 g. of carbohydrate and 8 g. of protein; the fat content and total calories vary with the type of milk. (One fat exchange equals 5 g. of fat.)

	measurement	fat exchanges	calories
Milk			
Buttermilk	1 cup . . .	—	80
Evaporated, undiluted	1/2 cup .	2	170
Nonfat dry milk mixed according to directions on box	1 cup . . .	—	80
Nonfat dry milk powder	1/4 cup .	—	80
Skim	1 cup . . .	—	80
2% butterfat	1 cup . . .	1	125
Whole	1 cup . . .	2	170
Yogurt, plain, made with skim milk . . .	1 cup . . .	1	125

Miscellaneous foods

The following foods may be used in your diet if you wish. They must be figured into the daily diet plan, with the food exchanges allowed as indicated.

	measurement	exchanges
Chili sauce	1 tbsp. . . .	1 List 2 vegetable
Fish sticks, frozen . . .	3 sticks . . .	1 bread, 2 meat
Fruit-flavored gelatin .	1/4 cup . . .	1 bread

Ginger ale	7 oz.	. . . .	1 bread
Ice cream, vanilla, chocolate, strawberry	1/2 cup	. . .	1 bread, 2 fat
Low-calorie dressing, French or Italian . .	1 tbsp.	. . . .	—†
Potato chips	10 large or 15 small	. .	1 bread, 2 fat
Sherbet	1/2 cup	. . .	2 bread
Vanilla wafers	6	. . . . . .	1 bread
Waffle, frozen	1 (5 1/2″)	.	1 bread

†The fat and calorie content do not have to be counted if the amount is limited to 1 tablespoonful.

(This exchange list is based on the recommendations of the American Diabetes Association and The American Dietetic Association in co-operation with the Diabetes Branch, U.S. Public Health Service, Department of Health, Education, and Welfare)

SUGGESTED READINGS

Albrink, M.J., Davidson, P.C., and Newman, R.: Lipid-lowering effect of a high-carbohydrate, high-fiber diet. Diabetes, *25*:324, 1976.

American Diabetes Association, Inc., The American Diatetic Association: Exchange Lists for Meal Planning—A Helpful Guide for a Healthier You. 1976.

Brunzell, J.D., Lerner, R.L., Hazard, W.R., Porte, D., and Bierman, E.L.: Improved glucose tolerance with high-carbohydrate feeding in mild diabetes. New Engl. J. Med., *284:*521, 1971.

Brunzell, J.D., Lerner, R.L., Porte, D., and Bierman, E.L.: Effect of a fat-free high-carbohydrate diet on diabetic subjects with fasting hyperglycemia. Diabetes, *23:*138, 1974.

Trowell, H.C.: Dietary-fiber hypothesis of the etiology of diabetes mellitus. Diabetes, *24:*762, 1975.

Tunbridge, R.E.: Sociomedical aspects of diabetes mellitus. Lancet, *2:*893, 1953.

Weinsier, R.L., Seeman, A., Herrera, M.G., Simmons, J.J., and Collins, M.E.: Diet therapy of diabetes —description of a successful methodologic approach to gaining diet adherence. Diabetes, *23:* 669, 1974.

Weinsier, R.L., Seeman, A., Herrera, M.H., Assal, J.P., Soeldner, J.S., and Gleason, R.E.: High- and low-carbohydrate diets in diabetes mellitus: Study of effects on diabetic control, insulin secretion and blood lipids. Ann. Intern. Med., *80:*332, 1974.

17. TREATMENT OF OBESITY

Seymour L. Halpern, M.D.

BASIC PRINCIPLES

I. Obesity should be classified with other metabolic disorders, such as diabetes and gout.

A. It is similarly characterized by multiple biochemical disturbances.

B. These include increased insulin resistance, glucose intolerance, changes in fatty acid metabolism, and alterations in other hormonal and enzymatic processes and in cell physiology.

II. Obesity is the most common form of disturbed nutrition seen in the U.S.

A. The incidence increases in middle-aged persons.

B. Approximately one-third of the adult population is overweight (20% or more over ideal weight).

III. The harmful effects produced by obesity per se, as well as its adverse effects on other associated conditions such as hypertension and cardiovascular disease and the fact that all clinical and actuarial studies indicate its undesirable effect on morbidity and mortality, render this a serious medical disorder.

A. It may be an acute or chronic condition.

B. Overweight persons who reduce and stay reduced have been shown to statistically increase their chance of living a longer and healthier life.

C. Actuarial tables demonstrate that morbidity and mortality statistics in the U.S. would be significantly and favorably altered if all physicians, both primary care and specialists, accorded the appropriate medical attention to treating obesity.

D. The physician must treat obesity as seriously as he does any other disease. Whether or not obesity is the primary reason for the patient consulting the physician, he should devote the necessary attention to correcting it.

IV. As far back as 1893, Sir William Osler observed in his *Textbook of Medicine* that there were three important factors to be considered in obesity, namely, overeating, lack of exercise, and excessive intake of alcoholic beverages. Today these three factors still are of prime clinical importance.

V. It should be stressed at the outset that obesity can be successfully treated.

A. The frequent failures reported are due to treating this disorder in a haphazard manner.

B. Many of the major illnesses that are successfully treated today would demonstrate an equally poor recovery record if they were treated in the same casual manner as is obesity.

OBESITY AS A HEALTH HAZARD

I. Obesity is a health hazard to persons of all ages but more so to males than to females.

A. It is a major contributing factor to premature death among males.

1. In persons under age 40, obesity probably correlates more than any other factor with the incidence of fatal myocardial infarction in males.

2. In persons over age 40, it plays a significant role in coronary artery disease, not only in itself, but because it is an etiological factor in producing hypertension and hyperlipidemia.

3. Hypertension and hyperlipidemia also have been demonstrated to be materially associated with atherosclerosis and myocardial infarction.

B. Successful weight reduction not only eliminates the role of obesity in coronary artery disease, but it improves hypertension and hyperlipidemia.

C. Weight reduction is probably the most important factor in correcting Type-IV hyperlipoproteinemia (hypertriglyceridemia), the most prevalent hyperlipidemia, and is essential in the treatment of Type-IIb and Type-III hyperlipoproteinemias.

II. Virtually all patients who manifest diabetes mellitus after the age of 40 are obese at the time of the discovery of the diabetes.

A. These patients may have normal or even excess insulin, but a high degree of resistance to insulin is present.

B. Successful weight reduction reverses this insulin resistance, improves the diabetes, and may even eliminate the necessity for using insulin or oral hypoglycemic medication.

III. In persons of all ages, mortality rates are higher among the obese than those of normal weight.

A. It is common knowledge, as well as a statistical fact, that the lean person, who subsists on a well-balanced diet, is the one most likely to live to be 80 or 90 years old and also to do so in a gracious manner.

B. Several studies have shown that untreated massively obese persons (over 200% of normal weight) rarely live to be 50 years old.

IV. Overweight persons who reduce experience practically the same mortality as those of normal weight.

A. Similarly, mortality rates of people who reduce are consistently below those who remain overweight.

B. Mortality, as an example, particularly from cardiovascular disease and diabetes, decreased considerably in many parts of Europe during World War II when food supplies were drastically reduced. This trend was reversed when food became more abundant.

V. The recent reduction in mortality rates from cardiovascular diseases may be in part attributed to people's weight consciousness during the past decade.

VI. Orthopaedic problems, peripheral vascular disorders (venous and arterial), and most other disease states, with the exception of tuberculosis, are unfavorably influenced by obesity.

VII. It has been suggested recently that overnutrition may contribute to the development of certain cancers in humans such as cancer of the colon and the breast.

VIII. Obesity is a social, occupational, and educational liability.

A. All other factors being equal, the best jobs go to persons of normal weight.

B. In professional school admissions, the obese person frequently is discriminated against in favor of the slender and normal weight person.

DEFINITIONS

I. Overweight refers to the state of having a weight higher than that indicated by tables of desirable weights according to height and frame, which have been developed by the Society of Actuaries and life insurance carriers (see Table 17-1).

II. Obesity refers to a condition of excess fat in the body.

A. In general, excluding edematous patients, persons who are 20 lbs. or more overweight are overfat or obese as well.

1. Exceptions to this rule are muscular athletes.

2. Persons who are overweight because of their muscularity can be easily distinguished at physical examination from those who are overweight because of excess adipose tissue.

B. Complicated examinations usually are not necessary to determine the presence of obesity.

1. Measuring the person's height and weight and performing the usual comprehensive physical examination, which includes inspection and palpation, will make evident the existence of this abnormal nutritional state.

C. There are various sophisticated ways

of determining the presence of obesity, but none have proved more beneficial for routine office practice than the height-weight-frame tables. Certain measurements such as those obtained by using skin fold calipers, highly popularized recently, have not proven to be more reliable indicators.

D. Whatever the etiology of obesity, the cause of obesity is always an imbalance of caloric intake in food and caloric expenditure by the body.

1. When an obese person loses weight on a well-balanced diet the cell mass (lean body mass) remains essentially unchanged.

2. There is some loss of extracellular fluid.

3. Virtually all the weight lost is fat.

Table 17-1. **Desirable Weights in Pounds, According to Frame (In Indoor Clothing)**

	Height (with shoes on) 1-inch heels		*Small Frame*	*Medium Frame*	*Large Frame*
	Feet	*Inches*			
Men of Ages 25 and Over	5	2	112–120	118–129	126–141
	5	3	115–123	121–133	129–144
	5	4	118–126	124–136	132–148
	5	5	121–129	127–139	135–152
	5	6	124–133	130–143	138–156
	5	7	128–137	134–147	142–161
	5	8	132–141	138–152	147–166
	5	9	136–145	142–156	151–170
	5	10	140–150	146–160	155–174
	5	11	144–154	150–165	159–179
	6	0	148–158	154–170	164–184
	6	1	152–162	158–175	168–189
	6	2	156–167	162–180	173–194
	6	3	160–171	167–185	178–199
	6	4	164–175	172–190	182–204

	Height (with shoes on) 2-inch heels		*Small Frame*	*Medium Frame*	*Large Frame*
	Feet	*Inches*			
Women of Ages 25 and Over	4	10	92– 98	96–107	104–119
	4	11	94–101	98–110	106–122
	5	0	96–104	101–113	109–125
	5	1	99–107	104–116	112–128
	5	2	102–110	107–119	115–131
	5	3	105–113	110–122	118–134
	5	4	108–116	113–126	121–138
	5	5	111–119	116–130	125–142
	5	6	114–123	120–135	129–146
	5	7	118–127	124–139	133–150
	5	8	122–131	128–143	137–154
	5	9	126–135	132–147	141–158
	5	10	130–140	136–151	145–163
	5	11	134–144	140–155	149–168
	6	0	138–148	144–159	153–173

For women between 18 and 25, subtract 1 pound for each year under 25.

(This table was prepared by the Metropolitan Life Insurance Company. It was derived primarily from data of the Build and Blood Pressure Study, 1959, published by the Society of Actuaries.)

4. The reverse is true when an person with normal tissue composition gains excess weight.

ETIOLOGY

I. Genetic

A. Genetic factors, though poorly understood, may play a role in the production of morbid obesity.

B. There is some evidence to indicate that there may be a slight difference even among healthy people in the ability to handle calories.

C. Genetic factors probably are responsible for the fairly automatic control of body weight, even when no thought whatsoever is being given to the amount of food ingested. Most people have little variation in their body weight over a period of years.

D. It is evident that regulating factors must be present within the body that help match the caloric intake with the output in most circumstances, for even a very slight deviation from the actual needs over a period of time can cause a significant change in body weight.

II. Pathologic Mechanisms

A. A small percentage of persons, probably under 5%, are obese because of pathologic or physiologic disorders. These may involve the thyroid, pituitary, adrenal, or other endocrine glands.

B. The obesity produced by endocrine disorders often can be ascertained from a comprehensive history and physical examination. Laboratory examinations to confirm the diagnosis, should be made, however.

III. Lack of Nutritional Knowledge

A. For several decades after the discovery of the important role of vitamins, nutrition education during the school years and thereafter was devoted principally to insuring adequate vitamin intake.

B. Education relative to the caloric value of foods and the relationship of the quality of food to its calories was thoroughly lacking (e.g., protective vs. energy vs. empty calorie foods).

C. Lack of nutritional knowledge leads to unwise selection of foods, especially during middle life when caloric needs are decreasing, and is a major factor in middle age obesity.

IV. Modern Life-style

A. The conveniences produced by our technological explosion with its resulting mechanization and adverse effects on the energy equation (e.g., significantly decreased caloric output) have been a major factor in the increased incidence of obesity in America and other highly developed nations.

1. Modern transportation, especially the automobile and elevator, results in less walking. Few people will walk up and down stairs when they can ride an elevator instead.

2. Washing machines, dryers, dishwashers, and other household devices materially decrease the homemaker's caloric output.

B. Automation has reduced the energy expended in many other occupations too.

V. Pregnancy

A. There seems to be a constant swing of the pendulum from those physicians who deplore gain in weight during pregnancy to those who extol it.

B. The present consensus is that an optimal weight gain for a woman during pregnancy is 22 to 24 lbs. (10 to 11 kg.) The maximum weight gain in a normal pregancy should be 26 lbs. (12 kg.).

C. It is important for the obstetrician to stress that in the postpartum period a woman should return as rapidly as possible to her normal weight.

VI. Obesity in Childhood

A. Overweight children produce an excess of adipose cells, which they bear as an oppressive health factor for the remainder of their lives.

B. There still are too many parents who believe that a fat child is a healthy child.

C. Obesity in infancy is almost always due to overfeeding.

1. It is less likely to occur in breast-fed infants than in those who are bottle-fed.

2. A breast-fed baby will stop suckling when its normal demands are satisfied.

3. In bottle-fed infants, the entire formula is usually fed even if it is not required by the baby because most mothers dislike discarding the leftover formula.

4. Early forced feeding of solid foods because of peer pressure from other mothers also may contribute to excessive caloric intake.

D. Obese children are three times more likely to become obese adults than normal-weight children.

VII. Adolescence

A. The large consumption of junk foods by adolescents often results in an excess caloric intake that leads to over-weight.

B. This is especially true of adolescents who are not athletically inclined and who, therefore, do not engage in significant exercise and active recreation.

C. The relatively sedentary adolescent can easily be victimized by the teenage diet and can become an adult who has to fight off life-long obesity.

VIII. Social-Cultural Factors in Adult Life

A. Many people associate hearty eating with success, especially first and second generation Americans.

B. This increase in caloric consump-

tion frequently comes at a time in life when calorie expenditure is decreased because success also is accompanied by the acquisition of convenience equipment and by leisure time spent in sedentary types of recreation.

IX. Psychiatric Factors

A. Psychiatric obesity refers to obesity produced by increased food intake as a result of emotional or psychological disturbances.

1. These may be deep-seated and may require active psychiatric therapy.

2. But many persons who become obese due to less severe emotional problems can be aided by the newer techniques of behavior modification.

B. Conversely, obesity per se can lead to perverse behavior characteristics which can perpetuate obesity, and a vicious cycle ensues.

X. Iatrogenic Obesity

A. Iatrogenic obesity results from poorly conceived therapeutic diets.

B. These may be prescribed by physicians for conditions such as convalescence from illness, injury, or surgery.

C. This situation is to be deplored. It is a consequence of the inadequate nutrition education of the medical student and house officer, as well as a lack of awareness by many practicing physicians of the patient's diet habits and of the potential disabilities produced by obesity.

CLASSIFICATION

Obesity, like anemia has been called an abnormal sign rather than a disease process per se. Analagous to diabetes, it is a disease process which affects multiple systems. Like diabetes, obesity can be classified principally into two categories, namely, juvenile obesity and adult-onset obesity.

I. Juvenile Obesity (Hyperplastic Obesity)

A. In juvenile obesity, there is a marked increase in the amount of adipose tissue cells—hyperplastic obesity.

1. Too many calories ingested in infancy and early childhood leads to an overproduction of fat cells.

2. This occurs most rapidly in the first few years of life.

3. At first, there is hyperplasia (an increased number of fat cells), and, later, there is hypertrophy (enlargement of the fat cells).

4. Until growth and development are completed, hyperplasia continues as long as there is caloric excess.

5. Just as growth ceases at some point during adolescence, the formation of fat cells also ceases.

6. From then on, excess calories contribute only to further hypertrophy of adipose tissue cells.

7. Fat cells, once they are developed, unfortunately, do not disappear.

8. The size of the fat cell can vary, but the number remains the same.

B. For this reason, fat children are inclined to be fat adults.

1. As many as 80% of obese children will become obese adults.

C. Thus dietary control of obesity must start early in life.

II. Maturity Onset Obesity (Hypertrophic Obesity)

A. In hypertrophic obesity, the total number of fat cells is not altered, but the size of the individual cells is greatly enlarged.

1. Hypertrophic obesity generally is not as severe as hyperplastic obesity.

2. A distended adipose cell displays physical, biochemical, and physiological intracellular abnormalities.

B. The totality of numerous and enlarged adipose cells leads to further physiologic, biochemical, and anatomical aberrations in individual organs and whole organ systems.

C. Obesity can produce physical and emotional aberrations and has family disruptive potentials similar to alcoholism.

TREATMENT

Prevention is the best form of treatment. Adjusting caloric content of the diet to the needs of the person at all stages in life is the only way to prevent abnormal weight gain. Because it is more difficult to treat obesity of the hyperplastic variety than the hypertrophic form, prevention and treatment of obesity must start almost at birth.

I. Physician Motivation

A. Motivation is as essential on the part of the physician as it is for the patient. Frequently patients who are highly motivated will go to the physician specifically for the purpose of weight reduction, only to become discouraged by the physician's lack of concern.

B. There is a statistically significant difference in the results achieved in the treatment of obesity between those patients who receive instructions in their therapeutic diet and regular dietary counselling by a physician or physician extender and those patients with the same degree of obesity and motivation who receive similar diets but little dietary counselling or follow-up.

C. An awareness of the hazards of obesity is a prerequisite for the physician to detect and initiate treatment of obesity in patients who present themselves with other medical disorders as well as among those undergoing a periodic health examination.

D. The motivated physician who makes measurement of weight, height, and body build an important part of every new patient's visit will have a high degree of success in detecting obesity and initiating treatment at an optimal phase.

II. Patient Motivation

A. Patient motivation is essential for successful weight reduction.

1. The motivating factor can be health-related or based on social or cultural reasons.

2. In all cases, there must be a motivating force that is personally meaningful to the patient.

B. A goal should be set at the very first visit.

1. A graph should be plotted for the patient to visualize his progress on future visits.

2. Successful achievement of a goal should be commended.

3. Failure to lose the desired amount of weight should be treated by examining the cause, reinforcing motivating factors, and optimistic encouragement but not by chastising or by accusing the patient of cheating.

III. Diet

A. Diet remains the cornerstone of therapy for all forms of obesity.

1. Dietary treatment involves lowering the caloric intake below that of the caloric expenditure.

2. Total caloric intake is less important than caloric intake in relation to caloric requirements.

3. The degree of this differential will determine the rate at which weight loss takes place.

B. Unless the individual is excessively overweight, it is normally sufficient to lose at a rate of 2 to 2½ lbs. each week. Smaller weight losses may be desirable for some people.

C. The exact amount of dietary calories required is determined by the caloric deficit necessary to achieve a 3500 cal. deficit/lb./week.

1. For example, a patient who requires 2500 cal. daily for weight maintenance theoretically should lose 2 lbs./week

on a 1500 cal. diet if the energy output remains stable.

D. Small weekly weight losses frequently can be achieved by utilizing a prudent diet in which all portions are decreased and highly concentrated caloric foods omitted, but exact caloric calculations are not made (see Table 17–2 and Table 17–3).

1. Reduction of alcohol intake is an important element of a prudent diet.

2. Omitting 2 to 3 cocktails or highballs a day, everything else in the diet remaining unchanged, can add up to a 3500-cal. deficit, or 1 lb./week.

E. A graphic flow sheet is valuable in following week-to-week weight loss. Predicted values can be made of anticipated weight loss.

F. The patient should be cautioned that artificial factors can influence the actual weight loss in any one week.

1. In the premenstrual phase for example, many women gain between 2 and 5 lbs.

2. The inadvertant dietary consumption of too much salt can also influence the amount of fluid retention in some persons.

3. Women, especially, tend to retain fluid in hot weather and after standing for a long period of time.

4. In these instances, transient fluid retention may be greater than the fat loss and the scale may show no weight reduction even though the patient has been dieting conscientiously and "inches" have been lost.

G. The physician should take the time to discuss with the patient diet and all other factors which can influence weight. The physician should avoid severely reprimanding the patient if anticipated weight loss is not achieved on a specific visit.

H. Patients should be recommended not to weigh themselves more than once a week.

1. Weight should be measured at the same time of the day and with approximately the same clothes, either in the physician's office or at home.

2. Daily small fluctuations of weight induced by normal physiologic processes can cause emotional trauma to such an extent that the patient trying to lose weight might abandon the dietary regimen all together.

I. Continuous counselling and encouragement is essential for the patient.

1. It should be emphasized on the first visit that, although the patient may require as little as 800 or 900 cal./day to achieve effective and steady weight reduction, this intake usually can be doubled for weight maintenance.

2. Assuring the patient that he will not become a dietary invalid, but eventually will be able to enjoy most foods with only prudent restriction, enhances the patient's incentive to achieve the weight goal quickly.

Table 17-2. **Foods Allowed and Foods Forbidden on a Weight-Reduction Diet**

Foods Allowed	Amount	Foods Not Allowed
Meat and Fish Group	3–4 oz. twice a day	
Lean roast meat		Pork
Chicken		Bacon
Turkey		Goose
Lean fish		Duck
Shellfish, prepared without fat		Fat fish (tuna and salmon)
Dairy Group		
Egg, boiled or poached	1 per day	Whole milk
Milk (skim or buttermilk)	1½ pints daily	Cream
Cottage cheese (dry)	4 oz. daily	Butter
		Oleomargarine
		Cheese (other than cottage)
Vegetable and Fruit Group	Unlimited	Any not specified in allowed foods.
Asparagus		
Green beans		
Beets		
Broccoli		
Brussel sprouts		
Cabbage		
Celery		
Carrots		
Dandelion greens		
Lettuce		
Mushrooms		
Greens		
Cucumber		
Eggplant		
Endive		
Leeks		
Onions		
Okra		
Radishes		
Sauerkraut		
Sea kale		
Sorrel		
Spinach		
Squash, summer		
Squash, yellow		

(Continued)

Table 17-2. **Foods Allowed and Foods Forbidden on a Weight-Reduction Diet** *(Continued)*

Foods Allowed	Amount	Foods Not Allowed
Vegetable and Fruit Group (Continued)		
Turnips		
Swiss chard		
Tomato		
Watercress		
Fresh fruit	2 servings daily	Sweetened fruit
Citrus fruit	1 serving daily	Dried fruit
Bread and Cereal Group		
Bread (enriched or whole wheat)	1 slice daily	Cakes
		Pastries
Miscellaneous		
Spices and condiments	In moderation	Gravies
Lemon	Unlimited	Sauces
Vinegar	Unlimited	Dressings
Saccharin or sucaryl	As needed for sweetening, in moderation	Olives
		Pickles
Tea	Unlimited	Nuts and nut butter
Coffee	Unlimited	Carbonated beverages
Clear broth or bouillon	Unlimited	Alcoholic beverages

Table 17-3. **Sample Menus For A Weight-Reduction Diet**

Breakfast

4 oz. orange juice
1 soft boiled egg
1 thin slice whole wheat toast
6 oz. skim milk
Coffee (no cream)

Lunch

Clear bouillon
3 oz. sliced chicken
¾ cup spinach
Sliced tomato and lettuce
Fresh fruit
Tea with lemon

Dinner

3 1/2 oz. veal
1/2 cup string beans
1/2 cup summer squash
Tossed greens with vinegar
Strawberries
6 oz. skim milk
Black coffee

Breakfast

1/2 grapefruit
1 poached egg
1 slice rye toast
6 oz. skim milk
Coffee (no cream)

Lunch

2 tablespoons cottage cheese with olives
1/2 cup shredded cole slaw (cabbage) (use vinegar and salt to season)
3 stalks asparagus on 1/2 slice whole wheat toast
1 small sliced orange
Tea with lemon

Dinner

3 1/2 oz. roast chicken
1/2 cup cooked carrots
1 small broiled tomato
Salad—2 large lettuce leaves with sliced cucumber
2 halves canned pears (no syrup)
6 oz. skim milk
Black coffee

Special Instructions

1. Eat only small portions of allowed foods. For example, 4 oz. of orange juice = 50 calories; 8 oz. = 100 calories (calorically equivalent to cola drinks).

2. Avoid all trimmings. Mayonnaise, standard salad dressings, gravies, and sauces, for example, are all very high in calories, frequently higher than the foods they are placed on.

3. No between-meal snacks. If unavoidable, due to excessive hunger, snacks should consist of fresh, raw vegetables, such as tomatoes, cucumbers, lettuce, carrots, and celery. These are all very low in calories, and all require chewing.

3. It should be emphasized, though, that they no longer can eat freely.

4. Instruction in caloric balancing when the stage of weight maintenance is reached, will permit patients to incorporate most of their favorite foods into the diet.

J. Very rapid weight loss should be discouraged. I have found that patients who lose 5 or more pounds per week, even those who are tremendously overweight, eventually break the diet.

K. Meals should be balanced and properly spaced.

L. It is important for the patient to eat a good breakfast.

1. This should supply from one-fourth to one-third of the total daily calorie needs.

2. Persons who eat breakfast tend to resist the temptation to snack between meals.

3. A high-protein breakfast tends to depress the appetite, while a high-sugar breakfast or no breakfast may stimulate the appetite.

4. It can be explained to the patient that because breakfast usually follows a 12- to 16-hour period of starvation, it is important to supply energy to the body.

5. An orange juice, donut, and coffee breakfast can lead to inappropriate insulin secretion with mid-morning hypoglycemia, fatigue, and a desire to snack.

M. Bizarre and fad diets are to be decried.

1. They are not only unsound physiologically, but they may have adverse effects on health.

2. They cannot form the basis of a permanent diet.

3. When bizarre diets are finally discontinued, as they always are, the patient returns to his former eating habits and obesity.

4. Diet education and the induction of permanent new eating habits can only be achieved during the active weight-loss phase with a diet that is based on sound nutrition principles.

N. Starvation and semi-starvation are indicated only for a small proportion of excessively obese patients (more than 100% over the desirable weight) for whom other dietary methods have failed.

1. Starvation is preferable to surgery.

2. Starvation is not without danger and should be short-term.

3. Weight lost during starvation frequently represents loss of lean body mass, while weight lost on a well-balanced diet represents almost exclusively reduction in adipose tissue.

4. Treatment of obesity by total starvation should be done in a hospital with daily medical supervision.

5. As soon as possible, a low-calorie nutritious diet should be commenced.

O. High-fiber, low-calorie diets are currently being prescribed by some physicians.

1. It is easier to ingest many more calories when eating high-sugar foods, such as candy and cake, than when consuming unrefined carbohydrates (e.g., fruits such as apples).

2. Fibrous foods take a long time to chew, are relatively low in calories, and give a feeling of satiety, while refined carbohydrates frequently have an opposite effect.

P. Chemically defined elemental diets and very low-carbohydrate or carbohydrate-free diets produce an initial large weight loss because of loss of sodium and water from the body.

1. This can be gratifying to the patient.

2. However, further weight loss is dependent on the calorie content of the diet.

3. Such diets can never serve as the basis for long-term weight control and diet reeducation.

4. Furthermore, very low-carbohydrate diets frequently produce ketosis which can be harmful to the body.

5. Elemental diets composed of protein hydrolysates and related compounds can produce hypokalemia and other chemical aberrations, cardiac arrhythmias, and even death.

IV. Exercise

A. Exercise is an important part of a weight control program because of the obvious increased expenditure of calories.

1. Exercise also helps to keep tissues firm and is an aid to the circulation and the digestive tract.

2. Exercise has to be active on the part of the patient, and not passive.

B. Too much emphasis has been placed on exercise for weight reduction as a result of the intense advertising by so-called reducing salons and related enterprises.

1. It should be emphasized that there is no such tissue as cellulite.

2. Fat on the buttocks, thighs, and other selected areas is the same as fat elsewhere.

3. There is no injection or exercise which can selectively reduce fat in thigh areas.

C. It is easy to ingest more calories than are expended if appetite is stimulated by the exercise, and if a diet is not carefully adhered to.

1. It takes far too much activity to burn up energy calories to achieve a significant weight loss.

a. For example, 12 minutes of running, 18 minutes of swimming, or 25 minutes of bicycling are required to burn up the

Table 17-4. **Amount of Exercise Required to Burn Off a Given Number of Calories**

Food	Minutes of Activity			
	Walking (3.5 mph) 5.2 cal./minute	*Bike Riding* 8.2 cal./minute	*Swimming* 11.2 cal./minute	*Running* 19.4 cal./minute
Apple, large	19	12	9	5
Bacon, 2 strips	18	12	9	5
Banana, small	17	11	8	4
Beer, 1 glass	22	14	10	6
Bread and butter	15	10	7	4
Cake, 2 layer, 1/12	68	43	32	18
Carbonated beverage, 1 glass	20	13	9	5
Carrot, raw	8	5	4	2
Cereal, dry 1/2 cup with milk and sugar	38	24	18	10
Chicken, fried 1/2 breast	45	28	21	12
Club sandwich	113	72	53	30
Cookie, plain	3	2	1	1
Egg, fried	21	13	10	6
Ham, 2 slices	32	20	15	9
Hamburger sandwich	77	49	36	21
Ice Cream, 1/6 quart	37	24	17	10
Malted milk shake	97	61	45	26
Martini (Manhattan, Daiquiri, etc)	40	25	18	12
Milk, 1 glass	32	20	15	9
Milk, skim, 1 glass	16	10	7	4
Orange juice, 1 glass	23	15	11	6
Pancake with syrup	24	15	11	6
Peach, medium	9	6	4	2
Pie, apple, or other fruit	77	49	36	21
Pizza, cheese, 1/8	35	22	16	9
Pork chop, loin	60	38	28	16
Shrimp, french-fried	35	22	16	9
Spahgetti, 1 serving	76	48	35	20
Steak, T-bone	45	29	21	12
Strawberry shortcake	77	49	36	21

calories in one martini. Twice this amount of exercise is needed to burn up the calories in one fast-food hamburger.

2. Exercise, even vigorous exercise, does not permit the person who has problems with weight to eat freely (see Table 17-4 and Table 17-5).

D. Exercise as part of one's life-style is useful to prevent weight gain and to maintain weight loss.

1. It has been emphasized frequently by detractors of exercise that it takes 35 miles to walk off a pound.

2. It is clear, however, that by briskly walking 1 mile every day, one can prevent the gain of weight of 1 lb. every 35 days or greater than 10 lbs. a year.

3. Thus, over a period of many years, habitual active exercise can be of critical importance in maintaining normal weight.

E. Treatment of obesity involves both physician and patient motivation. Although diet remains the core of any treatment regimen, an exercise program should be combined with the diet. Together, they

Table 17-5. **Caloric Values of Snack Foods**

Sandwiches	Calories
Hamburger	450
Swiss cheese	400
American cheese	400
Bacon and tomato with mayonnaise	550
without mayonnaise	500
Roast beef	300
Ham	350
Cream cheese	400
Fruits	
3 cooked prunes	75
1 small banana	92
25 medium grapes	89
1 medium apple	90
1 glass orange juice	100
Nuts	
Peanuts (1 oz. bag)	200
Pecan nuts (1 oz.)	250
Almonds (dried kernels, 1 oz.)	200
Chocolate bar with 2 nuts	300
Desserts	
Ice cream, all flavors (4 oz. serving)	250
Milkshakes (4 oz. serving)	250
Sundaes with flavor and whipped cream	500
Ice cream soda (10 oz.)	300
Apple pie (1 serving of other fruit pie)	450
Layer cake (1 serving)	400
Beverages	
Flavored sodas, such as cream, raspberry, cherry, (8 oz. without ice cream)	100
Cola drinks (8 oz.)	100
Malted milk flavored with ice cream (8 oz.)	375
Ginger ale (8 oz.)	75
Tea and coffee with cream and sugar (1 tsp.)	65
Alcoholic Beverages	
Beer (8 oz.)	100
Mixed drinks, highball, manhattan, martini, daiquiri	200
Scotch, rye, bourbon (1 oz.)	75

make the ideal couple for both preventing and treating obesity.

V. Drug Therapy

A. The basis of treatment of obesity is always diet. The adjunctive use of medication, however, should not be dismissed.

B. There are many people who have developed a habit of excessive eating in whom the temporary use of an anorexiant agent can facilitate the reprogramming of the patient's "appestat" and the retraining of eating patterns.

1. It should be explained to the patient that anorexiants are used solely as an initial adjunct to therapy, and that, as soon as possible, such supportive measures should be decreased and then discontinued.

2. Amphetamines should be avoided, and anorexiants which are not subject to abuse should be utilized.

C. The use of thyroid is indicated if there is evidence of hypometabolism. The smallest amount of thyroid that can be used should be determined.

1. Myxedematous patients are extremely sensitive to thyroid extract and should be started on as little as ¼ or ½ gr.

2. It is not necessary to have an excessively low, myxedematous level of T_3 and T_4. (In doing the measurement of T_4, the influence of anovulatory drugs and similar preparations should be considered.)

3. Patients with a borderline low T_4 who have other signs and symptoms of hypometabolism may respond favorably to small doses of thyroid, because these patients often experience a metabolic drop in response to severe caloric reduction.

4. In many instances, family members of patients with manifestations of hypometabolism and a T_4 that is borderline low will have a T_4 in the middle or upper range indicating that genetically the patient should have a higher T_4.

5. The response to a low-calorie diet in these patients thus may be enhanced by adding thyroid to the regimen.

6. Thyroid or other hormone therapy should not be administered to patients if there is no evidence of an abnormality.

7. Giving large amounts of thyroid to a patient who does not need it can suppress the patient's own thyroid, and iatrogenic hypothyroidism is induced.

D. Human chorionic gonadotropin hormone (HCG) has not been shown to have any physiologic action that could aid in weight reduction.

1. Claims that it aids in "selective" weight reduction have not been substantiated.

2. The 500 cal. diet usually prescribed concurrently is the basis of any favorable results reported.

E. A maintenance vitamin supplement may be indicated if there is evidence in the diet history of possible substandard nutrition because of self-planned, fad, or ill-conceived diets.

VI. Psychotherapy

A. Group Therapy

1. Organizations such as TOPS (Take Off Pounds Sensibly), Weight Watchers, and Obesity Anonymous may at times reinforce motivation.

2. The diets proposed by most of these groups are diets based on established concepts and as such are acceptable.

3. There are no sound follow-up data available.

4. It is suggested that long-term results might not be satisfactory.

5. Group therapy has not been proved superior to individual therapy.

B. Behavior Modification

1. This is being used more frequently for people who are excessively obese, often pathologically so, and this is preferable to surgical therapy.

2. The basis for this type of therapy is that obese persons have been found to be more responsive to external stimuli than normal or lean people are.

a. For example, the time of day acts

as a stimulus for hunger rather than normal physiological factors.

3. The reported results of behavior modification are encouraging.

C. Hypnosis

1. Hypnosis has been utilized to temporarily curb the appetite in a few selected compulsive eaters.

2. It is of temporary value only.

VII. Acupuncture

A. There is no evidence that acupuncture or related forms of treatment have any beneficial effect on obesity.

B. It may serve as a temporary form of psychotherapy and probably should be classified as such.

C. Long-term results are poor unless there is concurrent diet education with the establishment of new eating habits.

VIII. Surgery

A. Surgical correction of obesity with a form of jejunoileal bypass should be a last resort measure.

B. It is indicated only in excessively obese patients, in whom all other measures have failed.

C. These short-circuiting procedures eliminate a large segment of the absorption surface of the small intestine.

1. Much of the food eaten, therefore, will not be absorbed.

D. In theory, surgery permits weight reduction despite continued excess calorie intake.

E. Many biochemical aberrations have been produced following this procedure.

1. Liver pathology, kidney stones, and other serious complications have been reported, which occasionally have proven fatal.

F. The patient has a long period of postoperative convalescence which may result in a critical interruption of employment or education.

FACTORS IN SUCCESSFUL WEIGHT REDUCTION

I have always believed that one of the principal attributes of humans is their educability. If a physician treats obese patients with respect and empathy, he can take advantage of the patient's motivation and educability and can institute and maintain a successful weight reduction program. Prognosis is influenced by various factors, which are summarized below.

I. Age

A. Both the age at onset, as well as the actual age of the patient, are important in determining and predicting success.

1. Because persons who have developed obesity in childhood have a plethora of adipose tissue cells, adults with a history of childhood obesity are much more difficult to treat.

2. These patients must be instructed that they are similar to persons with diabetes and other medical disorders who must follow some dietary program for the remainder of their lives.

B. When both the patient and the physician were highly motivated, young adults who were excessively obese have been known to achieve a weight lower than that of their adolescent years.

C. Patients who become obese in middle life usually can return to their standard weight without difficulty.

1. As a rule of thumb, most persons would be close to their desirable weight if they had maintained the weight they had had in their early 20s.

II. Duration

A. The duration of obesity is a factor in success.

B. Even though long-standing obesity may be more difficult to correct than one of recent onset, it should be emphasized that it is always of value to improve one's dietary habits.

C. It is never too late to treat obesity because the medical benefits of weight loss will be achieved whatever the duration of the obesity.

D. "I have been fat all of my life" should not be a deterring factor.

III. Sex

A. Motivating factors for losing weight may be different in males and females.

B. In both sexes, the potential for achieving a state of health and of optimal physical, mental, and emotional well-being can be utilized as a goal.

C. Properly presented, health factors act as a powerful motivating factor, especially with males.

D. In the case of women, appeals to the ego and to various social considerations may be needed.

E. Today, economic factors, such as the ability to advance in their chosen profession, can be a prime consideration to both men and women.

IV. Marital Status

A. In the past, it was stated that single and divorced persons frequently are better candidates for weight reduction.

B. Currently, the consensus is that this is no longer the case.

C. Married persons lose weight with equal success.

D. The increased attention, love, and respect that is invariably displayed by the spouse after successful weight reduction can help act as a permanent motivating force for maintaining weight control.

V. Degree of Obesity

A. The degree of obesity only influences the length of time needed to achieve weight control.

B. A high degree of obesity is not a de-terrent to successful weight reduction if practical goals are set.

1. For a person who is 150 lbs. over-weight, for example, it may suffice to lose 100 to 125 lbs., a goal that can be realisti-cally achieved without becoming a her-culean task.

2. Initial weight loss in such a patient will be rapid because of fluid loss from the body and because of the large discrepancy between the calories needed to maintain the overweight status and the patient's actual needs.

C. The week-to-week weight loss will be determined not only by the difference between the calories ingested and the theoretical needs for the person's normal weight, but also by the caloric intake as compared with the calories required for the overweight state.

D. As one approaches normal weight, this difference becomes smaller, and the diet must be adhered to strictly.

E. It is at this time that communication between the patient and the physician becomes critical to achieving successful weight reduction.

VI. Emotional Adjustment

A. Emotional maladjustment in the patient should be ascertained at the initial visit, and corrective measures, drugs or psychotherapy, should be instituted along with diet.

B. Obesity may be a manifestation of depression.

C. Contrariwise, at times, very obese patients may become depressed when they lose weight very rapidly.

D. The more emotionally stable the person is, the easier it is to accomplish weight loss.

VII. Economic Factors

A. People in low socio-economic groups may have a greater tendency to be obese because they eat low-cost, starchy, high-calorie foods.

B. Furthermore, they may not have the same motivating social factors as the well-to-do.

C. Nevertheless, socio-economic status should not be an element in successful weight reduction if a proper motivating factor is present.

D. The diets prescribed should be nutritionally adequate, varied in content, and, although limited in calories, should be based on the normal diet, taking into account not only personal, religious, and ethnic considerations, but also socio-economic factors.

1. This is the only approach that will lead to correct eating habits, no matter what the socio-economic status of the patient.

E. If patients who attend clinics do not do as well as those visiting a private nutrition specialist, it is because the amount of time, attention, communication, and instruction differs with the two groups.

SUGGESTED READINGS

Bray, G., and Gallagher, T. F., Jr.: Regulatory obesity in man. Clin. Res., *18:*537, 1970.

Council on Foods and Nutrition: A critique of low-carbohydrate ketogenic weight reduction regimens: a review of Dr. Atkin's diet revolution. J.A.M.A., *224:*114, 1973.

Halpern, S. L.(ed.): Symposium on obesity. Med. Clin. North Am., *48*, 1964.

Hirsch, J., and Knittle, J.: Cellularity of obese and non-obese human adipose tissue, Fed. Proc., *29:*1516, 1970.

Kiell, N. (ed.): The Psychology of Obesity. Springfield, Illinois, Charles C Thomas, 1973.

Mayer, J.: Overweight. Englewood Cliffs, Prentice-Hall, 1968.

Salans, L. B., and Wise, J. K.: Metabolic studies on human obesity, Med. Clin. North Am., *54:*1533, 1970.

Schacter, A., and Gross, L.: Manipulative time and eating behavior. J. Pers. Soc. Psychol., *10:*98, 1968.

Weil, W. B., Jr.: Current controversies in childhood obesity, J. Pediatr., *91:*2, 1977.

Yallow, R. S., Glick, S. M., Roth, J., and Berson, S. A.: Plasma insulin and growth hormone levels in obesity and diabetes. Ann. N.Y. Acad. Sci., *131:*357, 1965.

Yang, M., and Van Itallie, T. B.: Composition of weight lost during short term weight reduction, J. Clin. Invest., *58:*722, 1976.

18. NUTRITION IN CANCER

Athanasios Theologides, M.D., Ph.D.

Nutrition can be adversely affected by the development, progression, and treatment of cancer. Although some of these effects may be induced by the patient himself, the major ones are the result of the disease, the therapy, and the complications.

I. Patient-Induced Nutritional Deficiency

A. Patients with cancer frequently search their nutritional history for dietary factors supposedly etiologic in the genesis of their disease.

B. Subsequently, they may change their diets in an effort to control the cancer and to improve their general health.

C. The changes may be both of omission or decreased intake of certain foods and of consumption of large quantities of various nutrients, vitamins, and minerals.

D. Such changes may produce an imbalanced diet, and massive doses of vitamins, minerals, and other nutrients may have some toxic effects.

II. Disease-Induced Malnutrition

A. Usually, it is the disease and the treatment and their complications that lead to malnutrition and tissue wasting in the patient with cancer. These do so by causing

1. Decreased food ingestion
2. Impaired digestion and absorption
3. External loss of nutrients
4. Competition for nutrients between the tumor and the host, which results in nutritional deficiencies in the patient.
5. Inappropriately elevated energy expenditure of the host

III. Effects of Malnutrition

A. Malnutrition and debilitation affect tolerance to treatment and prognosis.

B. Patients with Hodgkin's disease and certain other tumors who have weight loss as part of the initial presentation of their tumor have a worse prognosis than the ones without weight loss.

C. Malnourished cancer patients do not tolerate surgery, radiotherapy, and chemotherapy as well as those in a better nutritional state do because

1. Tissue function and repair is affected.
2. Humoral and cellular immunocompetence is impaired.
3. There are alterations in the metabolism of administered drugs due to changes in the patient's hepatic microsomal enzyme activity.

IV. Management

A. The physician should direct the nutritional management. The patient should strive to maintain an adequate intake of proteins, carbohydrates, lipids, vitamins, minerals, and calories in general, in order to achieve the desired goal of minimizing weight loss and forestalling or correcting nutritional imbalances and deficiencies.

ETIOLOGY AND PREVENTION OF MALNUTRITION

I. Decreased Food Ingestion

A. Anorexia is the primary reason for a decreased consumption of food. Early satiety also is a factor.

1. The cancer itself is the main contributory factor in the genesis of the anorexia.

2. Usually it is only the control of the disease with surgery, radiotherapy, or chemotherapy that causes significant improvement in appetite.

3. There are no drugs that can stimulate appetite in the anorectic cancer patient, although pharmacologic doses of adrenocorticosteroids, given for other reasons, may result in a transient increase in appetite.

B. Patients with cancer frequently complain that the food does not smell or taste the same anymore or that they cannot stand the smell or taste of certain foods.

1. Because olfaction and gustation are the major senses that influence acceptance or rejection of food, any alterations in sensitivity and hedonic perception may modify interest in food.

2. It is not known to what extent these olfactory sensory changes contribute to a decreased food intake or how to improve the hedonic effect of food odor.

3. Changes in taste sense may be induced by cancer and therapy.

a. Elevation of the taste threshold for sucrose and lowering of the taste threshold for bitter taste have been observed.

b. The lowered threshold for bitter taste might be responsible for a patient's dislike of meat.

c. But while the patient may dislike beef or pork, he or she may still accept poultry and fish.

d. However, even if an aversion to the latter gradually develops, adequate protein intake can be maintained with eggs and dairy products.

4. If the patient complains of changes in taste and smell sensations, then he or she should be the advisor and guide for seasoning and the aroma of food and should experiment with different flavors and odors.

C. A common symptom in patients with cancer is an early satiety or easy filling.

1. The patient feels hungry at the beginning of the meal, but after a few bites and the consumption of a small quantity of food, he feels full.

2. The pathogenesis of this symptom remains unclear in most instances, except in cases in which the capacity of the stomach is decreased due to intragastric or extragastric tumor.

3. The only helpful advice to the patient is to eat many small meals containing food of high caloric and nutritional value.

4. There are many ways to add calories to foods without increasing significantly the total volume.

D. After the diagnosis of cancer, psychological and emotional disturbances, such as depression, anger, anxiety, and grief, may curtail the appetite.

1. In this case, psychotherapy, emotional support, and drugs for anxiety and depression may have a beneficial effect on food consumption.

2. Control of pain and insomnia, also, may occasionally increase appetite.

E. A drop in food intake may also be caused by interference with ingestion by a cancer that is strategically located in the oropharyngeal area, the esophagus, the stomach, or the small intestine, as well as by surgical, radiotherapeutic, and chemotherapeutic management of the cancer.

F. Surgery such as partial or total glossectomy or mandibulectomy may hinder mastication and deglutition. Esophagectomy or gastrectomy may also affect food intake.

1. Irradiation to the head-neck region may induce xerostomia, dental deterioration, oropharyngitis, and esophagitis, with difficulties in chewing and painful swallowing.

2. Chemotherapy may cause stomatitis, pharyngitis, and esophagitis with a sticking sensation or pain on swallowing.

3. Moreover, a superimposed Candida infection will aggravate the mucositis.

4. For patients with stomatitis, rinsing the mouth with a local anesthetic, such as

lidocaine hydrochloride (Xylocaine Viscous), and administration of pain medication before meals may alleviate the discomfort with chewing and swallowing.

5. For those with oral mucositis, warm saline irrigation of the mouth is helpful, and when oral moniliasis is present, nystatin should be administered.

G. In patients with xerostomia, it may be helpful to lubricate the mouth with synthetic salivas during and after eating and to use other common lubricants such as gravy, butter, margarine, and milk during meals. Beer and bouillon have been noted to help, also.

1. Occasionally, cold food may be better tolerated than warm, although most patients with stomatitis prefer their food at room temperature.

2. Highly seasoned and acid spicy foods, which are poorly tolerated in stomatitis, should be avoided. Food should be soft or even liquified, especially for patients with dentures.

H. Radiotherapy and chemotherapy frequently cause nausea and vomiting.

1. These may be minimized by the use of antiemetics and by avoiding liquids with meals.

2. If the patient experiences nausea, discomfort, or pain during or after eating, he or she may become conditioned to avoid eating.

3. Frequently, this conditioned aversion may persist even after the causative factor has been removed or alleviated and may even require behavior modification therapy comparable to that used in anorexia nervosa.

4. The basic principle involves positive reinforcement of food intake and negative reinforcement of food rejection.

5. Hypnosis has been used in an effort to overcome conditioned aversion to food.

I. In patients with severe anorexia from extensive hepatic involvement with cancer and in those with severe hepatotoxicity from prolonged use of certain antineoplastic agents like methotrexate, the appetite may be best in the morning and may become worse as the day advances.

1. These patients should be advised to eat a big breakfast and, in general, to consume more food in the morning hours and to eat small frequent meals in the afternoon and evening hours.

II. Impaired Digestion and Absorption

Because indigestion and malabsorption are common complications in cancer, an important clinical consideration is the ability of the patient with cancer to digest and to effectively absorb the ingested food.

A. Cancer of the stomach may cause digestive disturbances.

B. Extensive replacement of the pancreas with tumor and involvement of the pancreatic duct, the common bile duct, and the biliary tree in general may affect secretion of pancreatic juice and bile.

1. This interferes with food digestion and absorption, especially of fat and fat-soluble substances.

2. Pancreatic extracts given with meals, or even more frequently, may control the malabsorption.

3. Occasionally, sodium bicarbonate supplements may be helpful.

C. Some degree of impaired small intestinal function with malabsorption may develop in patients with malignant neoplastic disease, even when the malignant process exists outside of the alimentary tract.

1. A partial villose atrophy of the jejunal mucosa may be observed in such patients.

2. Tumors may secrete a variety of potent pharmacologic substances that cause increased intestinal motility and diarrhea and result in malabsorption.

3. The best known of such clinical entities are the carcinoid and Zollinger-Ellison syndromes.

4. Moreover, malabsorption of various nutrients may result from infiltration of

the small intestine with lymphoma or solid tumor and from significant mesenteric lymphadenopathy and lymphedema of the intestinal wall.

5. Ascites also may disturb intestinal function and absorption. In such cases, the control of the cancer or the ascites will improve the absorptive capacity of the intestine.

D. Malabsorption may further result from alimentary tract surgery.

1. Esophageal resection with vagotomy may cause steatorrhea.

2. Gastrectomy is often followed by postgastrectomy malabsorption syndromes.

3. Resection of jejunum or ileum may result in inadequate absorption of certain nutrients depending on the area removed.

4. Gastrocolic or enterocolic fistulas may be responsible for nutrients bypassing large segments of the small intestine.

a. In these cases, the steatorrhea of the short-bowel syndrome can sometimes be circumvented by the use of medium-chain triglycerides, which are taken up directly into the portal venous system.

b. An elemental diet may provide readily absorbed amino acids and simple sugars to patients with a short bowel and fistulas.

5. In patients with a blind loop syndrome created by gastrointestinal surgery, broad spectrum antibiotics may favorably influence absorption of certain substances by suppressing abnormal growth of certain bacteria in the intestinal flora.

E. Irradiation to the abdomen and pelvis may cause a direct acute or late enteritis in the irradiated segment.

1. Histologic findings of the mucosa in postirradiation enteritis are somewhat comparable to those seen in malabsorption enteritis from other causes.

2. Diets that are low in gluten, lactose, fat, roughage, and residue may be tolerated better, especially by children (see Chap. 12 for examples of these diets).

3. Radiotherapy also may have an indirect anatomic effect on the bowel through endarteritis or small intestinal vessels.

4. The resulting direct and indirect anatomic complications such as mucosal atrophy and flattened villi, fibrosis, stenosis, necrosis, ulcerations, hemorrhage, obstruction, and fistula formation may alter the intestinal physiology.

F. Most antineoplastic agents damage the rapidly proliferating epithelium, causing ulcerations of the bowel mucosa and infections which adversely affect intestinal function.

1. Clinically, this is usually manifested as diarrhea, which should be controlled to minimize malabsorption.

2. With diarrhea, potassium loss should be anticipated and prevented, or potassium deficiencies should be corrected.

3. During a period of severe intestinal toxicity, elemental diets may be absorbed better than regular food.

III. External Loss of Nutrients

In addition to losses in the gastrointestinal tract because of impaired absorption, the patient with cancer may have other external nutrient losses.

A. Protein and probably lipids are lost in protein-losing enteropathy with lymphomas and solid tumors involving the small intestine.

B. Albumin may be lost in the urine in a nephrotic syndrome of a variety of etiologies that may occur with cancer and repeated therapeutic removal of malignant effusions.

C. These losses may be minimized with control of the tumor.

D. With cancer replacing most of the pancreas, glucosuria may be observed, but the total loss of glucose is not of great consequence.

E. The diabetes mellitus that follows pancreatic resection, however, should be controlled carefully with insulin and a properly balanced diet.

IV. Tumor-Host Competition

Competition for nutrients between the host and a more aggressive partner, the tumor, could result in nutritional deficiencies in the host.

A. For example, an increased uptake of folic acid by the tumor, leading to a deficit of that particular vitamin in the patient, is observed frequently.

B. Theoretically, an adequate nutrient supply should be capable of replenishing the metabolic pool and of providing for the needs of the host and even of a large tumor, so the host will not be deprived.

1. This is the case in pregnancy, in which the woman thrives in the presence of a rapidly growing fetus.

C. In cancer patients, however, even forced external feeding and parenteral hyperalimentation can only transiently reverse the tissue wasting of the host. Therefore, it appears that the cancerous cachexia is not simply the result of starvation of the host (with the tumor trapping the nutrients) but is a more complex problem with major alterations in the host's metabolism.

V. Increased Energy Expenditure

The increased caloric expenditure at the basal state, occurring in most cancer patients, does not appear to be due to the quantity of malignant tissue present, but rather to a systemic effect on the host.

A. The cancer itself, by causing a disturbance in the host's adaptive mechanisms for energy conservation, normally used when the food consumption falls, induces the host to maintain a higher basal metabolic rate.

B. Furthermore, concomitant infections with fever and other complications may also contribute to a higher basal metabolic rate.

C. In the presence of a hypermetabolic state and decreased caloric intake, the patient ends up utilizing his or her own adi-

pose tissue and muscle mass as a source of metabolic fuel.

D. To lower the energy expenditure, one should try to control the cancer and to correct the complications.

NUTRITIONAL EVALUATION

The patient with cancer, after the initial examination, should have periodic nutritional evaluations throughout the course of the disease. This can be done with the usual clinical approaches of dietary and clinical history, physical examination, and with simple anthropometric measurements. Rarely, some sophisticated tests may be needed, and, frequently, a therapeutic trial may establish whether a vitamin or nutrient deficiency exists.

I. Clinical Studies

A. The nutritional history should include a description of eating habits, meal composition, and food composition with an estimate of average daily caloric and protein intake.

1. Any recent changes should be evaluated.

2. Part of the clinical history should be a careful review of the function of the gastrointestinal system, especially in respect to indigestion, a change in bowel movements, and volume and consistency of feces.

B. The body weight-height index initially is an objective criterion of the patient's nutritional status.

1. A subsequent weight loss is taken as evidence of a negative caloric balance.

2. However, this is not a very dependable index because as the disease progresses, patients with cancer develop a tendency to retain intracellular and extracellular fluid.

3. Their increased total body water may mask a wasting of fat and muscle, giving a false assurance.

C. Other simple anthropometric measurements include the determination of arm circumference and of skin fold thickness.

1. Arm circumference, reflecting muscle mass, is usually measured in the mid-upper arm, but the same arm must be measured every time.

2. Skin fold thickness, representing fat stores, is measured with special calipers in the skin over the triceps muscle or the scapula.

3. A periodic recording of these parameters can be very useful for the nutritional follow-up. With the body weight, they provide a better picture of a change in the nutritional status.

II. Laboratory Studies

A. The hematocrit and serum albumin are simple laboratory values with nutritional relevance.

1. Serum albumin, along with transferrin and total iron-binding capacity (TIBC), reflects the visceral protein status.

B. More sophisticated studies to evaluate nutrition may include nitrogen balance, 24-hour urine creatinine excretion, and a creatinine-height index that will reflect the body lean muscle mass.

C. Analysis of the feces is useful in determining malabsorption of protein or fat.

D. Biochemical tests for various vitamins and enzymes in the serum, urine, and red blood cells are useful when they are available.

E. Because the immunocompetence of the host is affected by malnutrition and debilitation, a periodic evaluation of the cellular immune system by estimating total lymphocyte count and delayed cutaneous hypersensitivity to common antigens (P.P.D., SKSD, mumps, Thichophyton's and Candida) is also helpful in following the nutritional status of the patient.

NUTRITIONAL MANAGEMENT

I. General Principles

A. The nutritional needs in cancer vary so much from person to person and in the same person from time to time during the course of the disease and with different treatments, that it is totally unrealistic to provide a simplified nutritional formula for the patient with cancer.

1. Instead, the nutritional program should be totally individualized and periodically readjusted to meet the patient's specific changing nutritional needs and dietary and eating peculiarities. In this respect, the contribution of the clinical dietitian cannot be overemphasized.

B. Because there usually are some nutritional problems from the time of the original diagnosis of a visceral cancer, the nutritional management should be coordinated with the overall therapeutic plan from the beginning. The specific nutritional recommendation will depend on the nutritional state of the patient, the type of cancer, the anticipated therapy, and the prognosis.

C. After the development of cancer, the nutritional needs may be higher than they were when the person was healthy.

1. If a minimum of 30 to 35 Cal./kg. with 1.0 g. of protein/kg. body weight was adequate for that person to maintain weight when afebrile, with normal metabolic rate and limited activity, then after the development of cancer, he or she may need more calories, protein, vitamins, and minerals in order to maintain a nutrition and energy balance.

2. With progression of the disease and with various therapies, the needs for specific nutrients, minerals, and vitamins may change.

D. When curative surgery is anticipated, a short period of nutritional rehabilitation, replenishment of deficiencies, and correction of water, electrolyte, and acid-base imbalances may be advisable.

E. Following curative surgery, the management should be directed toward restoring the patient's nutritional health to the pre-illness level with increased protein and calorie intake, adequate carbohydrates, fat, vitamins, and minerals, along with exercise and other physical therapy when needed. Adverse nutritional implications from complications or after-effects of surgery, should be prevented when possible or managed as outlined in Chapter 11.

F. During radiotherapy, in an effort to maintain their weight, patients should be prevented from resorting to a deficient and imbalanced diet because of anorexia and nausea. After curative radiotherapy, a nutritional rehabilitation, if needed, can be achieved with a gradual increase of food intake of a balanced, easily digestible, and absorbable diet.

G. The major nutritional problems appear in patients with recurrent, unresectable, radioresistant, or disseminated cancer who are treated with aggressive chemotherapy. In this group of patients, one or more of the previously described mechanisms may cause a negative caloric balance, eventually resulting in the complete syndrome of cancerous cachexia.

H. the gastrointestinal tract is functioning properly in the patient with advanced cancer who is receiving chemotherapy, gastrointestinal feeding is preferable to parenteral nutrition. This enteral feeding can be accomplished through oral alimentation or through a nasogastric, esophagogastric, gastric, or jejunal feeding tube.

I. For the oral feeding, the value of common food, modified in texture and consistency, blenderized, and liquefied, and the importance of frequent small feedings of food high in caloric and nutritional value have been emphasized earlier (see p. 259).

1. Because it is digested faster, a diet of low fat content should be implemented.

2. A regimen of nibbling rather than of widely spaced large meals is very important, especially in the presence of early satiety.

J. For tube feeding, either the common family food, blenderized and liquefied, or commercial preparations can be used.

1. A very thin pliable nasogastric tube should be inserted, which can be tolerated well, sometimes for weeks.

2. The risk of a feeding gastrostomy done well is minimal, while a jejunostomy, although technically a little more difficult, has the advantage that it obviates the problem of gastric reflux.

3. Because a bolus might cause diarrhea and, occasionally, manifestations of a dumping syndrome, the feeding should be given slowly through the tube.

4. For the passage of thicker preparations through a thin tube, a mechanical pump is more dependable than gravity flow to drip-feed.

5. In patients receiving hyperosmolar and high-protein feedings, the water balance should be evaluated and corrected daily. Without sufficient water, the kidneys may be unable to clear metabolic products, resulting in hyperosmolar loading.

6. If there is no glucose in the urine, a specific gravity higher than 1.020 should alert one to give the patient more water.

K. After chemotherapeutic control of the cancer, the restoration of wasted tissues is a slow process, but correction of vitamin and mineral deficiencies can often be accomplished rapidly. With reactivation of the disease, a new constellation of nutritional challenges appear, and a revised nutritional approach may be needed.

L. When the decision is reached to provide only a symptomatic management of the patient with the advanced untreatable cancer, extra attention to type and preparation of food may offer one of the few remaining pleasures in life as well as provide some nutritional support.

II. Elemental Diets

A. The commercially available elemental or defined diets contain mixtures of pure amino acids or protein hydrolysates, simple carbohydrates, small quantities of essential fatty acids, and other triglycerides, minerals, and vitamins.

1. The powder or concentrated forms can be diluted in water, soft drinks, or milk.

2. For patients with lactase deficiency, the formulas containing milk products and milk as a diluent should be avoided.

3. See tables in Chapter 12 and Chapter 20 for details of nutritional formulas.

B. The elemental diets have properties that are potentially useful in the nutritional support of the cancer patient.

1. They can be nutritionally balanced and complete dietary formulations.

2. They have a high nutritional value, relatively flexible composition, and complete water solubility.

3. They are easily digestible and readily absorbable.

C. Elemental diets also may have several undesirable effects and potential complications.

1. In most cases, these are described on the package by the manufacturer.

2. Fortunately, the occurrence of major complications is uncommon (see Chap. 20).

D. In the nutritional management of the patient with advanced cancer, the elemental diet can be used either as a sole source of nutritional support or as a nutritional supplement between meals.

1. Because it is bulk-free and is absorbed directly across a relatively short segment of the small intestine without the requirements for intestinal or pancreatic secretions, the main indications for its use are malfunction of the gastrointestinal tract, short bowel, and intestinal fistulas.

2. Such a diet may protect the patient from losing weight due to malabsorption resulting from radiotherapy- or chemotherapy-induced enteritis.

E. As a supplement between meals, elemental diets can provide additional calories and nutrients to the anorectic, cachectic cancer patient.

1. Three packages of elemental diet taken between meals may increase caloric intake by approximately 900 Cal. daily.

2. Slow sipping is important to prevent bloating, nausea and, hyperosmolar diarrhea.

3. Because of the unpalatability of elemental diets and the flavor fatigue, it is very difficult to convince patients to continue using them for more than a few days.

4. Only the appreciation of their importance in contributing calories and nutrients can assure patients' acceptance and cooperation for longer periods.

F. When the elemental diet is given as the sole source of total nutritional support, it is very difficult to voluntarily consume the required volume orally.

1. In such cases, a small pliable nasogastric tube should be inserted to secure total control of the caloric and fluid intake.

2. This hypertonic elemental diet should be given through a tube at a constant rate for a given 24-hour period rather than as intermittent boluses. A pump with a controllable speed for continuous administration is preferable to the unpredictable gravity dripping from a plastic bag reservoir.

3. Because most elemental diets are hyperosmolar, tube feeding should begin with diluted solutions in small volumes per hour, then increase in concentration and volume gradually so as to reach the required caloric and fluid intake in 5 to 6 days.

4. Because there is usually some fluid retention during the administration of the elemental diet, occasional monitoring of the patients' fluid and electrolyte balance and urine specific gravity is imperative.

5. Patients on nasogastric tube feeding have a potential risk of aspiration, which should be guarded against.

G. When the reasons and indications for elemental diet alimentation are no longer present, the patient should return gradually to common food oral feeding.

III. Total Parenteral Nutrition

A. Total parenteral nutrition (TPN) plays an important role in the nutritional management of selected patients with advanced cancer.

1. It can provide all the nutritional requirements for prolonged periods during and after the administration of effective chemotherapy, which is very toxic to gastrointestinal tract.

2. The technique involves insertion of a catheter into a central vein (usually subclavian) and infusion of concentrated nutrient preparations in quantities and composition individualized for the patient.

3. With this approach, nutrition may be improved and maintained in a malnourished, debilitated cancer patient.

4. This assures better tolerance of antineoplastic therapy.

5. TPN should not be used merely to prolong survival of patients who are at the end stage of their disease.

B. The patients selected for TPN should have a cancer that is potentially controllable with surgery or radiotherapy and responsive to available chemotherapy.

1. They also should be unable to meet their nutritional requirements through enteral feeding, because they are unable to ingest adequate food or because their gastrointestinal tract is incapable of adequately digesting and absorbing nutrients.

2. Of these patients, those who weigh 5 kg. or more below the ideal body weight and who have a serum albumin concentration of less than 3 g./100 ml. are candidates for TPN.

3. The goal should be to provide adequate nutrition before and during treatment and to maintain and increase the body weight, enabling better tolerance of the treatment and a faster recovery.

4. Hopefully, with tumor regression and recovery from the adverse effects of chemotherapy and radiotherapy, appetite will return, the gastrointestinal tract will function properly, and the weight that was gained will be maintained with oral intake.

C. TPN usually requires a team of a physician, nurse, pharmacist, and dietician to prepare the nutritional fluids, insert the central catheter, guarantee sterility, and supervise safe administration.

1. Close clinical observation and biochemical monitoring is imperative to prevent or correct various metabolic complications that may occur with TPN, and meticulous care is needed to keep the incidence of catheter-related infections very low (see also Chap. 11 and Chap. 20).

D. A 10% fat emulsion (Intralipid) given intravenously in a peripheral vein concomitantly with glucose and free amino acid solutions represents another approach to short-term parenteral alimentation.

1. It can be used also in cancer patients who have an inadequate or imbalanced oral food intake to provide essential fatty acids, triglycerides, amino acids, lipids, and glucose.

2. This combination of free amino acids, lipids, glucose, electrolytes, other minerals, and vitamins is a simple approach to parenteral nutrition through a peripheral vein, and it is useful for short-term nutritional maintenance.

3. There are potential local and systemic complications, the Intralipid cannot be mixed with other intravenous fluids, and no electrolyte solutions or drugs can be added to the preparation.

4. Administration of Intralipid and amino acids with sugar should be through a separate I.V. needle or through a shared needle or catheter with a Y-connector at the needle hub or catheter end.

IV. With improved surgical techniques, more aggressive radiotherapy, more effective chemotherapy, and prevention and control of complications of the disease and of the treatment, a greater number of patients with cancer may live longer.

A. Maintenance of a good nutritional state permits more effective use of, and greater tolerance to, radiotherapy and chemotherapy.

B. Good nutritional management of these patients may contribute to a longer survival and may improve the quality of their life.

SUGGESTED READINGS

Butterworth, C.E., and Blackburn, G.L.: Hospital malnutrition. Nutr. Today, *10* (March/April):8, 1975.

Copeland, E.M., MacFadyen, B.V., Jr., Lanzotti, V.J., and Dudrick, S.J.: Intravenous hyperalimentation as an adjunct to cancer chemotherapy. Am. J. Surg., *129*:167, 1975.

DeWys, W.D., and Walters, K.: Abnormalities of taste sensation in cancer patients. Cancer, *36*:1888, 1975.

Hegedus, S., and Pelham, M.: Dietetics in a cancer hospital. J. Am. Diet. Assoc., *67*:235, 1975.

Recommended Dietary Allowances. ed. 8. Washington, D.C., Academy of Sciences, 1974.

Russell, R.I.: Progress report. Elemental diets. Gut, *16;*68, 1975.

Schein, P.S., MacDonald, J.S., Waters, C., and Haidak, D.: Nutritional complications of cancer and its treatment. Semin. Oncology, *2*:337, 1975.

Shils, M.E.: Nutrition and neoplasia. *In* Goodhart, R.S., and Shils, M.E. (eds.): Modern Nutrition in Health and Disease: Dietotherapy. ed. 5. Philadelphia, Lea and Febiger, 1973.

Theologides, A.: The anorexia-cachexia syndrome. A new hypothesis. Ann. N.Y. Acad. Sci., *230*:14, 1974.

Theologides, A.: Nutritional management of the patient with advanced cancer. Postgrad. Med., *61*: 97, 1977.

19. MINERALS IN MEDICAL PRACTICE

Robert D. Lindeman, M.D.

I. The ultimate goal of the physician interested in mineral nutrition is to assure his patients an optimal intake of all essential minerals and prevent overexposure (toxicity) to both essential and nonessential minerals.

A. Although it has been assumed in the past that the average diet in this country provides an adequate intake of each of the essential trace elements, marginal deficiencies have been found even in persons on an "adequate" diet.

B. Recommended daily requirements for a number of essential minerals have recently been made (see Table 19-1).

C. Deficiencies rarely exist in such a severe form that they are easily recognized clinically, and marginal deficiencies commonly develop and are not detected. The frequency and the severity of the deficiencies and excesses of the essential minerals are now being defined in specific physiologic (pregnancy and stress), pharmacologic (drug therapies), and disease states (gastrointestinal disorders with malabsorption, renal diseases with impairment in mineral conservation or excretion, and endocrine disturbances).

D. Evidence has been accumulated to support such interesting hypotheses as:

1. Chromium deficiency may be important in the development of adult onset diabetes mellitus.

2. Vanadium and chromium deficiency may be important in the development of atherosclerosis.

3. Cadmium excess may be important in the development of hypertension.

E. Virtually all of the 92 naturally occurring elements have been identified in human tissues. Four bulk cations (sodium, potassium, calcium, and magnesium) and eleven trace minerals (iron, zinc, copper, manganese, seleium, molybdenum, chromium, cobalt, nickel, vanadium, and silicon) have been identified as essential to health. Only recently have the last three trace elements been added to the list of biologically active, essential trace minerals. Others (e.g., tin, titanium, and aluminum) will very likely be added in the future.

F. The following criteria are necessary to establish a trace mineral as essential:

1. The mineral must be biologically ubiquitous, in other words, the supply must

Table 19-1. **U.S. Recommended Daily Allowances for Dietary Intakes of Minerals**

Minerals	Recommended Daily Allowances for Adults and Children > 4 yr.
Calcium	1000 mg.
Phosphorus	1000 mg.
Iodine	150 μg.
Iron	18 mg.
Magnesium	400 mg.
Zinc	15 mg.
Copper	2 mg.

Requirements for calcium, phosphorus, and magnesium are increased 20 to 30% in pregnant and lactating females. Other minerals recognized as essential but with no established RDA are sodium, potassium, chromium, manganese, molybdenum, nickel, selenium, silicon, tin, and vanadium.

(Federal Register *41*:46172, October 19, 1976)

be adequate to provide a uniform exposure for all living organisms.

2. The chemical nature must be compatible with some physiologic function.

3. The mineral must pass the placental barrier and be present in newborn infants.

4. The concentration must remain fairly constant in serum and tissues.

5. Homeostatic mechanisms to control concentrations must be demonstrated.

6. The mineral must be of low toxicity in oral doses.

7. Biological effects must be demonstrated by deficiencies of the mineral.

G. The following list shows the approximate quantities in the body of each of the essential trace minerals.

Approximate Quantities of Bulk and Trace Metals in a 70 kg. Man

Calcium	1000 g.	Cadmium	30 mg.
Potassium	140 g.	Vanadium	20 mg.
Sodium	110 g.	Tin	17 mg.
Magnesium	20 g.	Selenium	13 mg.
Iron	4200 mg.	Manganese	12 mg.
Zinc	2300 mg.	Nickel	10 mg.
Strontium	320 mg.	Molybdenum	9 mg.
Lead	120 mg.	Chromium	1.7 mg.
Copper	72 mg.	Cobalt	1.5 mg.
Aluminum	61 mg.		

H. The best $(+++)$, good $(++)$, fair $(+)$, and poor $(-)$ food sources for minerals are shown in Table 19-2.

I. Three additional, nonessential, trace minerals (lead, mercury, and cadmium) now are known to accumulate acutely and chronically and to produce toxic manifestations.

J. Many other trace minerals found in human tissue have not been established as biologically essential and only rarely accumulate sufficiently to produce clinically recognizable toxicity. Large amounts of barium, boron, rubidium, and strontium, for example, can be found in the human body. The distribution of strontium and barium is similar to that of calcium, and the distribution of rubidium is similar to that of potassium. This suggests that these cations may be interchangeable in the body.

K. Those substances common to all organic materials (carbon, nitrogen, and oxygen) are present in limitless quantities and, therefore, should not be responsible for isolated deficiencies or toxicity.

SODIUM

I. General Considerations

A. Sodium is the major extracellular cation, and its availability in the body controls intravascular and extracellular fluid volume.

B. The normal serum sodium concentration ranges from 135 to 148 mEq./L.

C. Much of the evaluation of sodium balance in the body is derived from clinical assessments rather than from laboratory values.

D. The concentration of sodium in the serum is not necessarily an indication of total body sodium. For example, a low serum sodium may be seen with a deficient or an excess of total body sodium, depending on the extracellular fluid volume.

E. Total body sodium can be estimated by multiplying serum sodium concentration by an estimate of extracellular fluid volume (recognizing that a small amount of sodium may be found in the bone cells).

F. Estimates of the volume of body fluid are important data, but often they are difficult to determine.

G. Figure 19-1 shows the potential combinations of serum sodium concentrations and extracellular fluid volumes.

II. Hyponatremia

A. A low serum sodium concentration may result from loss of sodium in excess of osmotically obligated water (primary salt depletion), retention of water in excess of sodium (water intoxication, dilutional hyponatremia, syndrome of inappropriate ADH), or a combination of both.

B. It may also result from displacement of plasma water with large molecular weight solute (lipids and proteins) or addition to the extracellular fluid volume (ECFV) of an uncharged solute (glucose) that moves water from the intracellular to the extracellular spaces thereby diluting the sodium and increasing urinary sodium losses.

III. Hyponatremia With Contracted ECFV (Primary Salt Depletion)

A. Etiology

1. In patients with clinical evidence of volume depletion (weight loss, thirst, orthostatic hypotension, and decreased skin turgor and sweating), continued loss of sodium with retention of water due to persistent secretion of ADH leads to hyponatremia.

2. If the urinary sodium concentration is less than 10 mEq./L., one can suspect decreased salt intake, excessive sweating, or gastrointestinal salt losses.

3. If the urinary sodium excretion is greater than 10 mEq./L., inappropriate renal losses of sodium and water should be suspected as the cause of the hypovolemia.

4. The excessive use of diuretics, adrenal or pituitary insufficiency, and intrinsic renal disease (salt-losing nephritis, advanced renal failure, or renal tubular acidosis) need to be considered as possible etiologies.

5. In severe vomiting with metabolic alkalosis and bicarbonate wasting, urinary sodium concentrations also may be elevated despite hypovolemia and hyponatremia.

B. Manifestations

1. Hyponatremia with either decreased or increased ECFV may result in central nervous system symptomatology that may range from anxiety, agitation, and confusion to convulsions and coma.

C. Treatment

1. Treatment is with isotonic or hypertonic saline.

2. Management of the patient when one is unclear whether he is dealing with

   a. Primary salt depletion (contracted ECFV), or

   b. A dilutional hyponatremia, or

   c. Syndrome of inappropriate ADH

Table 19-2. **Mineral Content of Six Food Sources**

Minerals	Meats	Seafood	Dairy Products	Vegetables	Fruits	Grains and Cereals
Sodium	+ +	+ +	+	−	−	+
Potassium	+ +	+ +	+	+	+ + +	+
Calcium	−	+	+ + +	+	−	+
Phosphorus	+ +	+ +	+ + +	−	−	+
Magnesium	+	+	+	+	+	+ +
Iron	+ + +	+	−	−	−	−
Zinc	+ + +	+ +	+	+	−	+ +
Copper	+ + +	+	+	+	+	+
Manganese	−	−	−	+ + +	+ +	+ + +
Selenium	+ + +	+ +	+	−	−	+
Molydenum	+	−	−	+	+	+ + +
Cobalt	+	+ + +	−	−	−	+
Chromium	+ +	+	+ +	−	−	+
Vanadium	−	+	+	+ + +	−	+ +
Silicon	−	−	−	+	−	+ + +
Iodine	−	+ + +	+	+	−	+

+ + + = Best sources
+ + = Good sources
+ = Fair sources
− = Poor sources

SERUM SODIUM CONCENTRATION		EXTRACELLULAR FLUID VOLUME		
		LOW	NORMAL	HIGH
LOW		DEHYDRATION (Primary Salt Loss) Na^+ Loss $\gg H_2O$ Loss	PSEUDOHYPONATREMIA Hyperglycemia Hyperlipemia Hyperproteinemia	DILUTIONAL HYPONATREMIA Congestive heart failure Cirrhosis Nephrotic syndrome INAPPROPRIATE ADH WATER INTOXICATION H_2O Retention $> Na^+$ Retention
NORMAL		DEHYDRATION Na^+ Loss $= H_2O$ Loss	NORMAL	UNCOMPLICATED EDEMA H_2O Retention $= Na^+$ Retention
HIGH		DEHYDRATION (Primary Water Loss) H_2O Loss $> Na^+$ Loss	HYPERALDOSTERONISM HYPERCORTISONISM	STEROID EXCESS SALT INTOXICATION Na^+ Retention $> H_2O$ Retention

Fig. 19-1. Salt and water disturbances.

(expanded ECFV)—and this differential can be difficult—is discussed on p. 272.

IV. Hyponatremia With Normal ECFV (Pseudohyponatremia)

A. *Etiology*

1. A decrease in serum sodium concentrations does not always indicate a decrease in the osmolality of body fluids.

2. In cases of hyperglycemia, the main cause of the hyponatremia is the glucose-related increase in osmolality in the extracellular fluid followed by a movement of water from the intracellular to extracellular fluid compartments and a subsequent renal loss of excessive extracellular fluid and electrolytes.

3. The serum sodium concentration in hyperlipemia and hyperproteinemia is diminished because of the volume occupied by the lipids or proteins. If the lipids or proteins are removed from the plasma, the sodium concentration in the remaining plasma water is then found to be normal.

B. *Manifestations:* Patients are asymptomatic.

C. *Treatment:* No treatment is needed for these entities.

V. Hyponatremia With Expanded ECFV

A. *Etiology*

1. *Entities Responsible for Hyponatremia With Expanded ECFV*

    a. Dilutional hyponatremia

    b. Syndrome of inappropriate antidiuretic hormone (SIADH)

    c. Water intoxication

2. *Dilutional Hyponatremia*

    a. Impairment in water excretion occurs commonly in situations in which urinary salt excretion also is severely impaired.

    b. Patients with advanced cardiac, hepatic, and renal diseases with gross edema are severely limited in their ability to eliminate both salt and water in the urine (dilutional hyponatremia). Unless receiving diuretics, they exhibit marked sodium retention (urine sodium concentrations < 10 mEq./L.).

3. Syndrome of Inappropriate Antidiuretic Hormone (SIADH)

a. A diagnosis of SIADH can be made only when other causes of hyponatremia have been eliminated. The following criteria must be met:

(1) The extracellular fluid osmolality and sodium concentration must be decreased.

(2) The urine must be hypertonic to serum.

(3) Sodium excretion in the urine continues to exceed 10 mEq./L. despite hyponatremia.

(4) Adrenal, renal, cardiac, and hepatic functions must be normal.

(5) The hyponatremia must be corrected by water restriction.

b. A persistently high level of circulating ADH is considered inappropriate when neither hyperosmolality of the serum nor volume depletion, the usual stimuli to ADH release, is present.

c. Inability to excrete water leads to volume expansion that, by multiple renal mechanisms, leads to increased urinary salt loss.

d. The syndrome of inappropriate ADH secretion is seen most frequently in patients with pulmonary neoplasms, most notably oat cell carcinoma, but it may be seen associated with other malignancies and pulmonary diseases, cerebral disorders (trauma, infection, tumor, C.V.A.), drug therapy (thiazides, sulfonylureas, antitumor agents), myxedema, and porphyria.

4. Water Intoxication

a. It is difficult, if not impossible, for a normal person to drink enough water to develop symptoms of hyponatremia (water intoxication). Vomiting prevents this from happening.

b. Patients with schizophrenia, on the other hand, appear to be capable of drinking sufficient water to become symptomatic.

B. Manifestations: The central nervous system manifestations are described on p. 270.

C. Treatment

1. The universal practice of sharply restricting salt intake but not restricting fluid intake in edematous patients is probably appropriate in most patients with heart failure, cirrhosis, nephrotic syndrome, or renal insufficiency.

2. A restricted sodium intake can be accomplished by

a. Avoiding salt in preparation of food and subsequent seasoning at the table

b. Using unsalted butter

c. Avoiding canned vegetables

d. Omitting food with a high sodium content (e.g., cured meats or fish, ham, salt pork, corned or chipped beef, salted nuts, potato chips, crackers, broths, and spices)

e. Moderating the intake of meats, fish, and milk because these foods are moderately high in salt content

3. Once a dilutional hyponatremia begins to develop, however, it also may be necessary to restrict water intake.

a. Diuretic therapy is indicated with salt and water retention.

b. Furosemide has the advantage over the thiazides in that it will eliminate the ability to concentrate the urine thereby allowing greater loss of water with salt removed.

4. Additional therapy should be aimed at the underlying disease (e.g., administration of digitalis to patients with heart failure).

5. In non-edematous patients, it is frequently difficult to distinguish between salt depletion hyponatremia in renal salt-wasting disorders and SIADH.

a. Serum osmolality and sodium concentrations are low. Urine osmolalities hypertonic and sodium excretions are variable but are often fairly large.

b. In salt depletion states, volume depletion appropriately stimulates ADH; in SIADH, the increased ADH levels are often unexplained.

c. Blood urea nitrogen concentrations tend to be elevated in salt depletion.

They are often normal or subnormal in SIADH.

6. Monitoring the central venous pressure may be necessary if one remains unsure clinically which entity he is dealing with.

a. If the CVP is less than 4 cm.H_2O, isotonic or hypertonic saline can be infused until the CVP increases above 8 cm.H_2O.

b. If the CVP is high initially, then fluid restriction is the appropriate treatment.

c. If the patient has left-sided heart failure, as many older patients do, a Swann-Ganz catheter will provide added safety.

7. If overhydration should develop with pulmonary edema, furosemide can be given. In 1973, a method of using furosemide with replacement of urinary electrolytes for patients with SIADH was introduced. This can result in adequate correction in 6 hours.

8. Treatment of water intoxication is water restriction.

VI. Hypernatremia

A. Etiology

1. Hypernatremia most frequently occurs in persons who, because of their inability to communicate, are unable to obtain sufficient water to replace losses.

a. Simple dehydration may result from inadequate intake of fluids in unconscious or neglected persons with nervous system or mental diseases when they refuse fluids or become unable to ingest them, or in persons with obstructive lesions of the upper gastrointestinal tract.

b. An occasional patient with neurological disease may have an impaired thirst mechanism which makes him susceptible to dehydration (e.g., surgical intervention in patients with aneurysms of the circle of Willis may result in damage to the thirst center).

(1) These patients, unless required to ingest a measured quantity of fluids daily, are prone to develop progressive dehydration and hypernatremia.

c. Stroke patients who are fed high-protein formula diets by nasogastric feeding tubes without adequate water also may develop simple dehydration. The increased solute load increases fluid losses in the feces and urine.

2. Simple dehydration also may result from excessive loss of water from the kidneys.

a. Renal losses are most marked in patients with diabetes insipidus, but loss of concentrating ability due to hypercalcemia, hypokalemia, or advanced renal disease also may be a cause of dehydration.

b. Patients with increased urinary solute, most notably those with uncontrolled diabetes mellitus, lose water in excess of sodium (non-ketotic hyperosmolar coma).

c. Pituitary diabetes insipidus may be neoplastic, traumatic, post-operative, infectious, granulomatous, vascular, or hereditary in origin.

d. Nephrogenic diabetes insipidus is an uncommon disease, but may occur as an acquired lesion due to amyloidosis, potassium deficiency, or interstitial disease.

3. Hypernatremia with normal or expanded ECFV may be seen in patients with excessive circulating corticosteroids (Cushing's syndrome) or aldosterone.

4. Hypernatremia (salt intoxication) may result from ingestion of large, hypertonic quantities of sodium chloride or bicarbonate.

B. Manifestations

1. Thirst is the earliest symptom of water loss.

2. In patients with impaired thirst or inability to obtain sufficient water, desiccation may be manifested as fever, flushing, loss of sweating, and dryness of the tongue and mucous membranes.

3. A tachycardia develops, and personality changes occur.

4. With severe dehydration, hallucinations, delirium, manic behavior, convul-

sions, and coma may develop. Similar psychiatric disturbances are seen in salt intoxication, in which many punctate cerebral hemorrhages develop.

C. Treatment: Treatment is aimed at replacing water orally or parenterally with 5% dextrose and water. Preventive measures need to be considered for susceptible persons.

POTASSIUM

I. General Considerations

A. Potassium is the primary intracellular cation.

1. Only about 2% of total body potassium is contained in the extracellular fluid compartment.

2. Therefore, the serum concentration of potassium may fail to reflect accurately total body potassium stores.

B. A potassium flux into cells occurs with cell growth, with intracellular nitrogen and glucose deposition, and with increases in extracellular pH.

C. Potassium leaves the cell with cell destruction, glucose utilization and decreases in extracellular pH.

D. In interpreting any given serum potassium concentration, consideration must be given to these factors affecting the ratio of intracellular to extracellular concentration because a steep concentration gradient must be maintained.

E. A dramatic example is provided by the patient with diabetic ketoacidosis who, prior to treatment, had high serum potassium levels, but with rehydration, correction of the acidosis, and treatment of the hyperglycemia with insulin shows a dramatic decrease in serum potassium concentrations as the cation moves intracellularly.

II. Hypokalemia

A. Etiology

1. Potassium depletion may result from inadequate intake, excessive gastrointestinal losses (diarrhea, bowel, and biliary fistulas), and excessive urinary loss of adrenal (hyperaldosteronism, hypercortisolism) and renal (renal tubular acidosis, salt-losing nephritis) origin.

2. Diuretic therapy remains the most frequent cause of hypokalemia.

a. The potassium-wasting effects of the thiazide and loop diuretics (furosemide, ethacrynic acid) are directly related to the increase in sodium load delivered to the distal sodium-potassium exchange site.

b. Therefore, there appears to be no advantage of one over the other in preventing potassium depletion while accomplishing a desired natriuresis.

3. Other drugs that produce hypokalemia

a. Licorice extract, used in management of ulcers, as an additive to alcoholic drinks and as a flavoring for drugs, contains glycyrrhizic acid, a substance structurally and chemically similar to aldosterone

b. Medications that contain a large amount of unreasorbable anion (penicillin, carbenicillin)

c. Acetylsalicylic acid

B. Manifestations

1. Hypokalemia usually presents with severe muscle weakness and tenderness with morphologic muscle changes which may range to frank necrosis.

2. Similar myocardial muscle damage produces EKG changes and arrythmias especially in digitalized patients.

3. The effect on the kidney is to produce polyuria (loss of concentrating ability) presumably due to renal tubular damage.

4. Neuropsychiatric manifestations may range from a depressive reaction (weakness, lethargy, apathy, fatigue, depression, anorexia, and constipation) to an acute brain syndrome (memory impairment, disorientation, and confusion).

5. Decreased intestinal motility ranging to paralytic ileus, impaired carbohydrate tolerance, and impaired growth are other manifestations of hypokalemia.

C. Treatment

1. Because an alkalosis (chloride depletion) usually accompanies hypokalemia, replacement should be with potassium chloride rather than potassium acetate, citrate, or lactate.

2. The exception would be the patient with renal tubular acidosis.

3. Intravenous repletion in severely depleted persons may be necessary but can be hazardous.

4. Rates over 40 mEq./hour or concentrations in excess of 40 mEq./L. should be used only with electrocardiographic monitoring.

5. The use of foods rich in potassium is the best way to replace potassium.

   a. Often an associated need to limit sodium intake is present, which limits the choice of foods available to accomplish this aim.

   b. Bananas, oranges, and grapefruit (whole or juice) are the best sources of potassium.

   c. Other fruits (melons, dates, prunes, and raisins) and vegetables (beans, greens, and potatoes) also are good sources.

   d. Meats, dairy products, and tomato juice have a high potassium content, but they also have a high sodium concentration.

6. When additional replacement is indicated, the potassium should be dispensed separately from the thiazides as the chloride salt in liquid form or in uncoated tablets taken with meals.

   a. Whether or not the newest slow release supplements (KCl imbedded in a wax matrix) also will produce the small bowel ulcerations previously seen with the enteric-coated thiazide-KCl combination will require further observation.

III. Hyperkalemia

A. Etiology

1. Because the distal nephron has such a large capacity for secreting potassium even in advanced renal failure, hyperkalemia develops only when some additional factor is present.

2. These include

   a. Oliguria (acute renal failure)

   b. Excessive potassium load (tissue catabolism, protein or potassium supplementation, administration of potassium penicillin G)

   c. Severe acidosis

   d. Spironolactone or triamterene diuretic therapy

   e. Deficiency of endogenous steroid (aldosterone, glucocorticoid)

B. Manifestations

1. Life-threatening hyperkalemia can develop with few symptoms.

2. Weakness and anxiety may be complaints.

3. The electrocardiographic progression of peaked T waves, loss of P waves, and widening of the QRS complex may be used to monitor the potential threat of hyperkalemia.

4. Any time the serum potassium exceeds 7.0 mEq./L., a true medical emergency exists because fatal arrythmia becomes a potential threat.

C. Treatment

1. Therapy should be initiated once serum potassium concentrations exceed 5.5 mEq./L. or earlier if progressive hyperkalemia can be anticipated.

2. Acute treatment is with glucose, insulin, and bicarbonate (to shift potassium intracellularly) and with sodium and calcium salts (physiologic antagonists).

   a. For each 500 ml. of 10% glucose that is infused, 15 units of regular insulin (one unit per 3 to 4 g. glucose) and one ampule of sodium bicarbonate (44 mEq.) may be added.

   b. The infusion must be continued until other measures are used to permanently remove potassium from the body.

3. Sodium polystyrene sulfonate (Kayexalate) resins are used to remove excess potassium from the body permanently.

   a. If complete exchange is accomplished, each gram of resin exchanges more than 2 mEq. of sodium for each 1 mEq. of potassium (other cations exchanged onto the resin account for the other 1 mEq.).

 b. This means that if 20 g. of Kayexalate is given orally three times daily, more than 120 mEq. of sodium (7 g. sodium chloride) is added to the daily intake, and this often produces problems with salt and water retention.

 c. To prevent constipation and fecal impaction and to increase salt loss through the bowel, 30 ml. of 50 to 70% sorbitol can be given with each 20 g. dose of Kayexalate.

 d. If oral intake cannot be tolerated, 60 g. of resin in 200 ml. of tap water or diluted sorbitol solution (50 ml. of 70% sorbitol plus 150 ml. tap water) can be given as a retention enema and repeated as often as necessary (up to once every hour) to obtain the desired decrease in serum potassium concentration.

 4. Florinef Acetate Tablets (fludrocortisone acetate) can be used to correct mineralocorticoid deficiency.

 5. Dialysis can be used when all else fails.

CALCIUM

I. General Considerations

 A. Serum calcium exists in three states, ionized (40 to 50%), protein-bound, primarily to albumin (40 to 50%), and complexed with organic anions such as citrate (5 to 10%).

 B. Only the ionized portion of serum calcium is physiologically active.

 C. The degree of protein binding is dependent upon the concentration of serum proteins (albumin) and the pH with the calcium binding increasing as the pH increases.

 D. Since one measures total serum ·calcium in the clinical laboratory, these factors must be kept in mind when one evaluates a serum calcium concentration.

 E. The serum concentration normally ranges between 4 and 5 mEq./L. so that only 70 mEq. of the 64,000 mEq. in the body (0.1 to 0.2%) is in the extracellular fluid.

 F. Another 20 mEq. of calcium (concentration 1 to 2 mEq./L.) is located intracellularly, where it plays an important role in mediating muscle contraction. The remainder is located in bone with only 320 mEq. (0.5%) in exchangeable form.

II. Calcium Equilibrium

 A. Only 100 to 200 mg. of the 1 g. or more of calcium ingested daily is absorbed from the intestine into the circulation.

 1. Dairy products (milk and milk products) are the principal sources of dietary calcium.

 2. Some calcium is present in leafy green vegetables, fish, and certain cereals.

 3. Meats are poor sources of calcium.

 B. The amount of calcium that is absorbed daily from the intestine must be excreted in the urine daily to maintain calcium balance.

 C. The serum and extracellular fluid calcium are in constant dynamic equilibrium with the bone that it bathes so that, normally, bone accretion matches bone resorption.

 D. A finely tuned endocrine system acts to control intestinal absorption, bone exchange, and renal excretion of calcium (and phosphorus).

 E. The long-term maintenance of total body calcium, specifically serum calcium, is dependent upon intestinal absorption of available dietary calcium under the control of the vitamin-D system.

 F. If intestinal absorption of calcium is inadequate, serum calcium concentrations fall, and this stimulates parathormone release from the parathyroids and suppresses thyrocalcitonin release from the thyroid gland.

 G. Parathormone stimulates mobilization of calcium from bone.

1. This hormone also increases urinary excretion of phosphate and increases renal tubular reabsorption of calcium.

2. Parathormone also enhances the effects of vitamin D on intestinal calcium absorption helping to increase serum calcium concentration.

H. Thyrocalcitonin, which is stimulated by an increase in serum calcium concentration, has biological effects inverse to those of parathormone.

III. Hypocalcemia

A. Etiology

1. Hypocalcemia is seen in patients with vitamin D deficiency. This can be caused by

a. Nutritional deficiency

b. Malabsorption (gastrectomy, sprue, chronic pancreatitis, chronic cathartic use)

c. Abnormal metabolism of vitamin D (vitamin D-resistant rickets, renal insufficiency, hepatic dysfunction)

2. Other etiological mechanisms are

a. Hypoparathyroidism

b. Psuedohypoparathyroidism (renal unresponsiveness to parahormone)

c. Hyperphosphatemia related to phosphate loading or renal insufficiency

d. Calcitonin-producing tumors (medullary carcinoma of the thyroid)

e. Acute pancreatitis

B. Manifestations

1. Tetany and generalized seizures are the major findings in acute hypocalcemia.

2. Cardiac arrest also can develop.

3. Chronic hypocalcemia leads to development of bone demineralization with bone pain and compression fractures.

C. Treatment

1. Correction of symptomatic hypocalcemia can be accomplished with calcium gluconate (10-ml. ampule of 10% solution provides 1 g. of calcium gluconate or 90 mg. of elemental calcium) given intravenously.

a. Intravenous administration of calcium gluconate should not exceed 50 mg. per minute or a total of 2 g. without checking serum calcium concentrations especially in patients receiving digitalis preparations.

2. Oral calcium gluconate (1-g. tablets) or lactate (300-mg. tablets) may be used in treating mild or latent hypocalcemic tetany. Up to 8 g. of oral calcium gluconate daily is well tolerated.

3. Caution must be used when correcting a coexisting acidosis with sodium bicarbonate as the ratio of ionzied to protein-bound calcium decreases as *p*H increases, sometimes precipitating symptomatic calcium deficiency.

4. Vitamin D supplements increase serum calcium by enhancing intestinal absorption of calcium, by increasing calcium reabsorption from bone, and by increasing urinary phosphate excretion.

5. A number of synthetic preparations have been advocated as effective therapy.

a. Ergocalciferal (vitamin D_2) 1.25 mg. or dihydrotachysterol 0.125 mg. up to three times daily can be used as initial therapy and monitored with serum calcium concentrations to determine maintenance therapy.

IV. Hypercalcemia

A. Etiology

Hypercalcemia can be caused by

1. Increased parathormone activity (primary or tertiary hyperparathyroidism, or parathormone-producing tumors)

2. Enhanced vitamin D activity (vitamin D intoxication, sarcoidosis, tuberculosis)

3. Enhanced bone reabsorption due to metastatic tumors involving bone

4. Multiple myeloma

5. Immobilization

6. Thyrotoxicosis

7. Milk-alkali syndrome

8. Thiazide therapy

9. Adrenal insufficiency

B. Manifestations

1. Patients with hypercalcemia develop the following problems:

a. Neurologic—drowsiness, lethargy, stupor, muscle weakness, fatigue, decreased reflexes

b. Gastrointestinal—anorexia, nausea, vomiting, constipation, ileus

c. Renal—polyuria, nocturia, nephrocalcinosis, renal stones, azotemia

d. Cardiovascular—conduction defects, bradycardia, hypertension, potentiation of digitalis effect

e. Pruritus

f. Eye abnormalities—band keratopathy and metastatic calcifications in the sclera

C. Treatment

1. The initial therapy in patients with hypercalcemia should be rehydration with normal saline. This usually decreases serum calcium concentrations by hemodilution and increases urine calcium excretion.

2. Furosemide and ethacrynic acid will increase urinary calcium excretion.

a. The thiazides, in contrast, decrease urine calcium excretion and should be avoided.

3. A 40-mg. dose of prednisone daily for 7 to 10 days will correct the hypercalcemia (by decreasing vitamin D-mediated calcium absorption from the intestine) in most cases of sarcoidosis, multiple myeloma, and vitamin D intoxication and about half the cases of non-osseous malignancy including the peptide-secreting tumors.

a. Prednisone is less effective when there is extensive bone invasion with tumor and is only rarely effective in hyperparathyroidism.

4. Inorganic phosphate can be administered intravenously as a buffered 0.1% molar solution (0.081 mole disodium and 0.019 mole monopotassium phosphate).

a. Orally, 2 g. of phosphate as sodium- or potassium phosphate daily represents initial management for most patients with chronic hypercalcemia.

b. Commercial preparations that contain this quantity are available in liquid (Phospho-Soda, 3 teaspoons daily), powder (Neutra-Phos, 2 teaspoons daily), and capsule (Neutra-Phos, 8 capsules daily) forms.

5. Mithramycin appears to be the drug of choice in treating the hypercalcemia of metastatic malignancy.

a. Initial treatment consists of daily doses of 25 μg./kg. body weight.

b. This anti-tumor agent can produce bone marrow suppression and other side effects, so close monitoring of patients is necessary.

c. Good responses are observed within 48 hours (two doses) in almost all patients, and the dosage needs to be individualized after the first few days.

6. Other agents and techniques which have been used to treat hypercalcemia include isotonic sodium sulfate, ethylenediaminotetraacetic acid (EDTA), peritoneal dialysis and hemodialysis, and indomethacin.

MAGNESIUM

I. General Considerations

A. The human body contains about 20 g. (2200 mEq.) of magnesium.

B. Only about 20 mEq. or 1% of this is in the extracellular fluid producing a serum concentration of 1.4 to 2.0 mEq./L.

C. Normally 20 to 25% of the serum magnesium is protein bound, 10 to 15% is complexed with organic anion, and 65 to 70% is present as free or ionized magnesium.

D. Only the free or ionized form of magnesium is physiologically active.

E. Approximately 35 to 40% of all magnesium (800 mEq.) is present intracellulary (concentration 26 mEq./L) making it the second most prevalent cation inside the cell.

F. The remaining 60 to 65% (1400 mEq. is present in bone with about 400 mEq. in exchangeable form with extracellular fluids.

G. Magnesium, in addition to serving as an important element in the structure of bone, serves as an activator of many enzyme systems, most notably those involved in the generation of energy (e.g., transfer of phosphate from adenosine triphosphate to adenosine diphosphate). Oxidative phosphorylation in mitochondria and protein synthesis also are dependent on magnesium.

II. Hypomagnesemia

A. Etiology

1. Low serum magnesium concentrations are seen most frequently in patients with gastrointestinal disorders (diarrhea and malabsorption) or alcoholism.

2. They also may be seen in patients with certain endocrine problems (hyperparathyroidism, hyperaldosteronism), fluid and electrolyte disturbances (diabetic ketoacidosis, hypercalcemia), excessive diuretic therapy, renal tubular disease, and acute pancreatitis.

B. Manifestations

1. Neurologic manifestations are the most prominent findings in patients with low serum magnesium concentrations.

2. These included marked anxiety, hyperirritability, disorientation, confusion, hallucinations, seizures, hyperreflexia with positive Babinski signs, and tremor.

3. Patients also may develop tetany with a positive Chvostek's sign, negative Trousseau's sign, and absence of muscle cramps.

4. Other findings include tachycardia, hypertension, arrythmias, vasomotor changes, profuse sweating, and muscle weakness.

C. Treatment

1. The daily requirement for magnesium is 300 to 400 mg. with about 100 mg. of this absorbed from the intestine and ultimately excreted in the urine.

2. Theoretically, 100 mg. (8 mEq.) of magnesium or 1 g. of magnesium sulfate

given parenterally daily should provide a positive magnesium balance.

3. If the patient is able to eat, magnesium is universally present in most foods. No foods are exceptionally good sources.

a. Chocolate, nuts, fruits, vegetables (greens, beans, and potatoes), and cereals (wheat and corn) generally are better sources than meats, seafoods, and dairy products.

4. Symptomatic magnesium deficiency can be treated with intravenous, intramuscular, or oral magnesium sulfate.

a. The rate of intravenous infusion should not exceed 150 mg./minute (equivalent to 1.5 ml. of a 10% solution).

b. Magnesium sulfate is available in 10% (20-ml. ampule) and 50% (2-ml. ampule) concentrations.

c. Intramuscular magnesium sulfate, although painful on administration, can be given in dosages of 2 g. (4 ml. of a 50% solution) every 4 to 6 hours during the first day and tapered thereafter.

d. Oral magnesium sulfate can be given safely in doses up to 8 g. daily. It is, however, a strong cathartic and, therefore, of limited value as replacement therapy in symptomatic magnesium deficiency.

IV. Hypermagnesemia

A. Etiology

1. High serum magnesium concentrations are seen primarily in patients with renal failure treated with magnesium-containing antacids (Gelusil, Maalox, and other brands) and cathartics (milk of magnesia).

B. Manifestations

1. Lethargy, hyporeflexia, and respiratory depression are seen in patients with high serum magnesium concentrations.

C. Treatment

1. Although usually no treatment other than stopping exogenous magnesium is necessary, calcium gluconate or

Calcium Gluceptate can be used as a physiologic antagonist in treating respiratory depression.

IRON

I. General Considerations

A. Sixty to 70% of the body iron is found in hemoglobin and myoglobin.

B. Approximately 20% is held in storage in a labile form (ferritin, hemosiderin) in the liver, spleen, bone marrow, and other tissues, in which it can be utilized for the regeneration of hemoglobin in case of blood loss.

C. The remaining 10% of iron is firmly fixed in the tissues with small amounts incorporated in the heme-containing mitochrondrial enzymes, the flavin-iron enzymes such as succinic dehydrogenase, and red cell catalase.

D. The normal dietary intake is in the range of 12 to 15 mg./day.

1. Only 0.5 to 1.5 mg. of the dietary iron is absorbed. (This is slightly higher in children and menstruating women.)

2. In some poorly defined way, the iron content in the body regulates iron absorption from the intestine.

3. Only the ferrous ion is absorbed.

E. Once in the circulation, very little iron is lost through the intestine (biliary excretion), skin, and kidney.

F. Because 20 to 25 mg. of hemoglobin iron is liberated from catabolized red cells daily, effective mechanisms must be present to conserve and reutilize this iron.

G. The serum iron concentration normally ranges between 65 and 175 μg./100 ml.

II. Iron Deficiency

A. Etiology

1. Blood loss from any origin (gastrointestinal tract, menstruation) can produce an iron deficiency anemia.

2. An inadequate intake of iron alone leads to anemia primarily in infants on a milk diet.

3. A high dietary phosphate interferes with iron absorption.

B. Manifestations

1. A hypochromic, microcytic anemia (hemoglobin concentration less than 12 g./100 ml.) and decreased serum iron concentrations are the principal findings in iron deficiency.

2. Because serum iron concentrations, along with iron-binding capacities (normally 250 to 410 μg./100 ml.), also are decreased in infections, malignancies, and other forms of stress, bone marrow stains for hemosiderin (Prussian blue reaction) also can be utilized to identify depleted iron stores.

3. Patients with iron deficiency anemia develop glossitis, cheilosis, dysphagia, fingernail changes, gastric atrophy, and paresthesias.

C. Treatment

1. Diet

a. Red meats, especially liver, are the best dietary sources of iron.

b. Leafy green vegetables, such as spinach, and eggs and dried fruits are other good sources.

2. The usual oral iron supplement is ferrous sulfate (0.3 g. tablets three times daily).

3. Imferon (50 mg. of elemental iron per ml.) can be given intramuscularly to patients unable to tolerate oral iron. The dosage is dependent on the severity of the anemia and the weight of the patient.

III. Iron Excess

A. Etiology

1. Hemochromatosis

a. An excessive amount of iron is absorbed from the intestine in patients with hemochromatosis, an inherited inborn error of metabolism, leading to chronic iron excesses in vital organs.

2. Excess Intake

a. Hemochromatosis (iron deposition with tissue damage) or hemosiderosis (iron deposition without tissue damage) can develop in adults after long-term ingestion of excessive iron.

b. It also can occur in young children who are fed excessive iron supplements.

B. Manifestations

1. Hemochromatosis is characterized by development of cirrhosis, skin pigmentation (bronzing), cardiomegaly with congestive failure, and diabetes mellitus.

2. It can be identified by the iron deposits in the bone marrow and tissues.

3. High serum iron concentrations and saturation of the iron-binding protein, transferrin, are present.

C. Treatment

1. The therapy in hemochromatosis is aimed at removing excess iron from the body.

2. Phlebotomies of 500 ml. weekly will accomplish this with the time required dependent on the excess iron stores in the body.

3. If excess intake is the cause, this should be stopped.

ZINC

I. General Considerations

A. Zinc is the metal component or activator of many enzymes (carbonic anhydrase, alkaline phosphatase, the dehydrogenases, and the carboxypeptidases).

B. Its availability governs the tissue concentrations and activities of certain zinc metalloenzymes and the rate of synthesis of the nucleic acids and protein, thereby importantly influencing tissue growth and reparative processes.

C. Most of the zinc in the serum is bound to protein (two-thirds loosely to albumin or prealbumin and one-third tightly to an α-2 macroglobulin).

D. Only 2 to 5% of the total serum zinc is present as free ultrafilterable zinc.

E. The normal mean serum concentration is 100 μg./100 ml. (normal range 70 to 130 μg./100 ml.).

II. Zinc Deficiency

A. Etiology

1. Induced acute and chronic zinc deficiencies are well documented in animals and humans.

2. It is unclear whether the low serum zinc concentrations observed in patients with a variety of clinical disorders such as cirrhosis and other hepatic diseases, nephrotic syndrome, renal insufficiency, malabsorption, acute and chronic infectious diseases, and hematological disorders such as sickle cell anemia are indicative of a true clinical or subclinical zinc deficiency or merely reflect a decrease in zinc-binding proteins, which also are reduced in these conditions.

3. The correlation of serum zinc concentrations with decreased serum albumin concentrations is poor so that this, with other evidence, suggests another protein with a molecular weight similar to albumin (possibly prealbumin) may be the major zinc-binding protein.

4. On the other hand, many of the acute and chronic manifestations of zinc deficiency are commonly observed in patients with conditions associated with low serum albumin and zinc-binding problems.

5. A number of dwarfed adolescent males on low dietary zinc intakes have been identified as zinc deficient with the manifestations listed below. These patients showed a substantial growth spurt after receiving supplemental zinc.

6. Foods high in fiber and phytate interfere with zinc absorption from the intestine.

7. Acrodermatitis enteropathica is a disease of infants characterized by erythematous and vesiculobullous dermatitis,

diarrhea and alopecia, severe growth retardation, delayed sexual maturation, and frequent infections. It is an inherited (autosomal recessive) partial defect in intestinal zinc absorption that is reversed by parenteral zinc.

B. Manifestations

1. Patients with acute histidine-induced hyperzincuria and hypozincemia develop anorexia, dysfunction of taste and smell, intention tremor, ataxia, mental disturbances, and mouth ulcers.

2. Chronic zinc deficiency is characterized by growth retardation, anemia, hypogonadism, hepatosplenomegaly, and impaired wound healing.

C. Treatment

1. Most combinations of foods would provide the 15 mg. of zinc required to meet the daily RDA. More important is the amount of phytate (breads) and other agents in the diet which will bind ingested zinc and limit absorption.

2. Zinc sulfate up to 220 mg. three times daily (50 mg. elemental zinc per tablet) can be given orally for suspected zinc deficiency. It appears to be safe. The only side effect is transient nausea.

III. Zinc Excess

A. Etiology

1. Zinc is one of the least toxic trace elements when given orally.

2. Only with accidental or intentional (suicidal) ingestion of zinc salts can toxicity be produced.

3. Contamination of dialysis water stored in a galvanized tank sufficient to increase plasma zinc concentrations to 700 μg./100 ml. produced only nausea, vomiting, fever, and anemia.

B. Manifestations

1. Ingestion of large quantities of most zinc salts produces nausea, vomiting, and diarrhea.

2. If a corrosive form of zinc is ingested (zinc chloride), severe necrosis and ulceration of the gastrointestinal tract may occur.

C. Treatment

1. No treatment should be necessary as the liver through biliary secretion into the intestine can remove excess zinc effectively.

COPPER

I. General Considerations

A. Copper is the metal component of the respiratory enzyme cytochrome oxidase and is involved in metabolic and enzymatic activities as diverse as hemoglobin synthesis, bone and elastic tissue development, and the normal function of the central nervous system.

B. The normal serum copper concentration ranges from 90 to 140 μg./100 ml. but is slightly higher in women.

C. Over 90% of serum copper is bound to the α-2 globulin ceruloplasmin.

D. The remainder is loosely bound to albumin or amino acids or is free (ionized).

E. Because ceruloplasmin accounts for such a large fraction of the serum copper, changes in its concentration determine the copper concentration in serum with few exceptions.

F. The normal copper intake of humans is estimated to be 2 to 5 mg./day, an amount that is adequate to easily maintain a positive copper balance.

II. Copper Deficiency

A. Etiology

1. Copper deficiency has not been described in adult humans because almost any diet contains the several milligrams daily that is necessary to prevent a deficiency.

2. Copper deficiency has been observed in infants with chronic diarrhea or malabsorption or on a diet consisting almost exclusively of milk.

3. Menkes' kinky hair syndrome is a

sex-linked, fatal infantile disorder due to a genetic defect in the intestinal absorption and transport of copper and represents a true copper deficiency state.

4. Low serum copper concentrations have been reported in malabsorption syndrome, in protein-losing enteropathies, and in nephrotic syndrome, but it is difficult to establish that these patients have symptomatic copper deficiency.

B. Manifestations

1. A syndrome of neutropenia and iron deficiency anemia correctable by administration of copper has been encountered in infants.

2. Copper-depleted persons lose the ability to utilize stored iron with the loss of the copper enzyme ferroxidase that controls the conversion of iron from the ferrous to ferric form.

3. In Menkes' kinky hair syndrome, infants show retardation of growth, defective keratinization and pigmentation of hair, hypothermia, degenerative changes in aortic elastin, scurvy-like changes in the skeleton, and progressive mental deterioration. The progression of this syndrome cannot be prevented by the administration of oral copper.

C. Treatment

1. Copper occurs in sufficient quantity in foods. The development of a deficiency in humans consuming a usual varied diet is unlikely.

2. In patients with Menkes' syndrome, some response can be obtained with parenteral copper, but not by the oral form.

III. Copper Excess

A. Etiology

1. Copper toxicity is not common in humans. It occurs only when a deliberate attempt has been made to ingest excessive amounts of some substance such as copper sulfate.

2. It also has been seen in renal failure

patients when copper tubing has been used in their hemodialysis machines.

3. Wilson's disease is an autosomal recessive disorder with excessive copper accumulation in liver, brain, and kidney producing characteristic damage and with decreased concentrations of serum copper and its binding protein, ceruloplasmin.

4. It is currently felt that decreased biliary excretion of copper is the primary defect in Wilson's disease.

5. The high serum copper concentrations observed in pregnancy, after administration of estrogen, in infections, collagen vascular diseases, myocardial infarction, malignancies including leukemia, and cirrhosis probably are of little nutritional significance.

6. An increase in serum ceruloplasmin concentrations is responsible for the high serum copper concentrations observed in pregnancy or after estrogen administration.

B. Manifestations

1. The ingestion of more than 15 mg. of elemental copper produces nausea, vomiting, diarrhea, and intestinal cramps.

2. Larger amounts produce shock, hepatic necrosis, intravascular hemolysis, renal toxicity, coma, and death.

3. In Wilson's disease, a chronic hepatitis, neurologic disorders characterized by resting and intention tremors, choreoathetosis, dysarthria and disturbances in gait and coordination, and proximal renal tubular disease (Fanconi's syndrome) are usually seen.

4. Copper deposits in the cornea (Kayser-Fleischer rings) are useful in making the diagnosis.

C. Treatment

1. The chronic administration of penicillamine or other chelating agents can keep patients with Wilson's disease in negative copper balance and free of neurologic and hepatic disease for many years.

MANGANESE

I. General Considerations

A. Manganese can activate a large number of metal-enzyme complexes. Other metals, however, such as magnesium may substitute for manganese in most instances.

B. The normal serum concentration is 2 to 3 μg./100 ml., presumably most of this is transported in serum bound to the B-1 globulin transmanganin.

C. About 40% of the 3 to 4 mg. of manganese ingested daily is absorbed and subsequently excreted in bile and pancreatic juice.

D. Little manganese is excreted in urine.

E. A positive balance can be maintained with as little as 20 μg./day.

F. Cereal grains, leafy green vegetables, wheat germ, coffee, and tea are good sources of manganese; meat and milk are poor sources of manganese.

II. Manganese Deficiency

A. Etiology

1. Manganese deficiency does not appear to develop in humans unless a deliberate attempt is made to eliminate this mineral from the diet.

2. Because of the difficulty in measuring serum concentrations, no studies are available to determine if serum concentrations are depressed in specific diseases or disorders.

B. Manifestations

1. A single patient placed on a manganese-deficient diet on a metabolic ward developed a striking hypocholesterolemia along with weight loss, dermatitis, nausea, vomiting, and slow growth and color changes of hair and beard.

2. Animals on a deficient diet exhibit defective growth, bone abnormalities, reproductive dysfunction, central nervous system abnormalities (ataxia), and disturbances in lipid metabolism.

C. Treatment

1. A normal diet should prevent or correct any deficiency.

2. Manganese supplements are not available commercially and probably are unnecessary.

III. Manganese Excess

A. Etiology

1. Although manganese is one of the least toxic trace minerals, toxicity has been recognized in South American manganese miners after prolonged inhalation of the mineral.

B. Manifestations

1. The disease is characterized by a clinical picture similar to that found in encephalitis.

2. Clinical changes begin insidiously with anorexia, apathy, headache, impotence, and speech disturbances.

3. Eventually the clinical picture resembles parkinsonism with mask-like facial expression, monotonous voice, intention tremor, muscle rigidity, and spastic gait with exaggerated reflexes and clonus.

C. Treatment

1. Acute toxicity has been reversed with chelating agents such as EDTA and penicillamine.

2. L-dopa has been utilized to treat the chronic neurologic manifestations of manganese excess.

SELENIUM

I. General Considerations

A. Selenium is concerned with growth, muscle function, the integrity of the liver, and fertility, in ways that are poorly understood.

B. It is closely but not completely associated with vitamin E as the vitamin and mineral appear synergistic in correcting deficiency states.

C. This may be because both selenium and vitamin E function as antioxidants.

D. Seafood, meats, dairy products, and wheat grain are the best dietary sources of selenium.

E. Cooking appears to vaporize the mineral, and much of it is lost in the atmosphere.

F. The average daily intake ranges from 60 to 150 μg.

G. Selenium is lost in urine, feces, sweat, and hair in nearly equal quantities.

II. Selenium Deficiency

A. Etiology

1. Because of the difficulty in measuring serum selenium levels in humans, only a single report describing serum concentrations in various disease states using neutron activation analysis is available.

2. Patients with gastrointestinal malignancies were reported to have reduced serum concentrations, but the significance of this finding remains to be determined.

3. Birds and other ruminant animals from selenium-deficient areas (East Coast and Pacific Northwest) develop characteristic abnormalities due to a dietary deficiency. The "white muscle disease" of calves, lambs, and foals and hepatic necrosis in pigs are good examples.

B. Manifestations

1. Weight loss, listlessness, and alopecia developed in primates on a selenium-deficient diet along with a myopathy and hepatic degeneration that ultimately led to death.

2. Retarded growth, infertility, liver necrosis, muscular dystrophy, and an exudative diathesis have been reported in other animal species.

C. Treatment

1. The normal diet for humans contains sufficient selenium so that no supplements should be necessary except possibly in persons who avoid meats and dairy products.

2. The daily requirement for health maintenance remains to be determined.

III. Selenium Excess

A. Etiology

1. Selenium toxicity has never been reported in humans but it could develop from the consumption of vegetables and grains which are grown in seleniferous areas.

2. Large areas in the western U.S. east of the Rocky Mountains have seleniferous soils. Here toxicity often is observed in cattle and horses feeding on seleniferous weeds.

B. Manifestations

1. Chronic toxicity in humans is manifested by discolored and decayed teeth, chronic arthritis, loss of hair, brittle nails, edema, gastrointestinal disorders, and infertility.

2. The "blind staggers" observed in animals ingesting seleniferous weeds are characterized by weakness, lassitude, visual impairment, loss of appetite, and paralysis with respiratory failure.

C. Treatment

1. No specific therapy has been described or needed since selenium toxicity has not been reported in humans.

MOLYBDENUM

I. General Considerations

A. Molybdenum is a cofactor of xanthine and aldehyde oxidase and is a copper antagonist.

B. Grains and legumes are the primary sources of this mineral.

C. The average daily intake is 200 to 500 μg. with equal losses through urine and feces.

II. Molybdenum Deficiency

A. An increase in caries and defective growth have been attributed to a deficiency of molybdenum.

B. A deficiency state can be potentiated by a high copper intake.

C. No deficiency has been documented in humans.

D. Xanthine renal calculi have been reported in animals with molybdenum deficiency.

III. Molybdenum Excess

A. It has been suggested that the high incidence of hyperuricemia in certain parts of the world may be related to consumption of excess molybdenum from foods grown in molybdenum-rich soils.

B. No toxicity has been documented in humans.

C. A condition in cattle known as "teart" (diarrhea, anemia, hair changes) has been attributed to molybdenum toxicity or copper deficiency.

COBALT

I. General Considerations

A. Cobalt is the metal cofactor of vitamin B_{12}.

B. There also is some evidence that it may play some role in immunity.

C. About 300 μg. are absorbed daily from the diet, and most of this is excreted in the urine.

D. Seafood, meats, grains, and cereals are all good sources of cobalt.

II. Cobalt Deficiency

A. There are no reports of cobalt deficiency in animals or humans presumably because it is such a commonly available nutrient.

B. Such a small amount is needed in the body that it has not been possible to produce a deficiency even with special diets.

C. If a deficiency did exist, one would expect to see a clinical picture of pernicious anemia with hematologic and neurological manifestations due to vitamin B_{12} deficiency.

D. As little as 1 μg. of vitamin B_{12} (cobalamin) administered parenterally can cause a remission of pernicious anemia.

III. Cobalt Excess

A. Cobalt chloride orally (150 mg. daily for 7 days) has been shown to produce polycythemia in humans.

B. Quantities in excess of 500 mg./day in humans are necessary to produce toxicity.

C. Excessive cobalt in some ingredients of beer have been implicated as a possible cause of myocardiopathy.

CHROMIUM

I. General Considerations

A. Recently evidence has accumulated suggesting that chromium may play an important role in carbohydrate and lipid metabolism.

B. The metabolism of chromium is poorly understood because of the low concentrations in tissues and biological fluids and the difficulty in analysis.

C. Less than 5% of ingested chromium is absorbed, and the main route of excretion is through the kidney.

D. Vegetable oil, shortening, and margarine are the best sources of chromium; meats and dairy products also are good sources.

E. The trivalent chromium binds to transferrin and appears to be the biologically important form of the mineral.

F. Serum chromium concentrations fail to reflect body chromium nutrition and, therefore, are of little value in evaluation of deficiency states.

G. This may be because the biologically active form of trivalent chromium is an organic chromium-containing, low molecular weight material known as "glucose tolerance factor" (GTF) rather than free trivalent chromium.

II. Chromium Deficiency

A. Etiology

1. Animals fed a chromium-deficient diet develop impaired growth, severe glucose intolerance approaching frank diabetes, and an increased incidence of atheromatous lesions in the aorta.

2. In humans, it has been suggested that some elderly diabetics may be chro-

mium deficient, and efforts have been made to correct the glucose intolerance by increasing trivalent chromium intake.

B. Treatment

1. Chromium chloride ($CrCl_3 \cdot 6H_2O$), 50 μg., three times daily, has been utilized in elderly diabetics with inconclusive results.

2. Inorganic chromium is so poorly absorbed that it is difficult to replenish with this source.

3. Organic chromium, such as the GTF in brewer's yeast, may be the best source.

III. Chromium Excess

A. Ingestion of chromium produces little toxicity and is confined primarily to gastrointestinal disturbances.

NICKEL

I. General Considerations

A. Only recently has it been possible to demonstrate that nickel is an essential trace element activating certain enzymes and is firmly bound in DNA and RNA.

B. Grains and vegetables appear to be good sources for dietary nickel.

II. Nickel Deficiency

A. Patients with cirrhosis of the liver and chronic uremia have low serum nickel concentrations.

B. Whether this is indicative of a true nickel deficiency or merely reflects a decrease in nickel-binding protein (nickeloplasmin) remains undetermined.

C. Nickel deficiency has not been described in humans.

D. Animals placed on a nickel-deficient diet develop impaired reproduction, abnormalities in hair growth, and ultrastructural changes in the liver.

E. Whether or not patients with malabsorption or other disorders might become deficient also remains unclear.

III. Nickel Toxicity

A. Nickel is regarded as having extremely low toxicity.

B. The increased serum concentrations in patients with myocardial infarction, cerebrovascular accidents, and burns are probably of no nutritional significance.

VANADIUM

I. General Considerations

A. Although vanadium has long been recognized to have biological actions, it only recently has been added to the list of essential trace elements.

B. About 2 mg. of the mineral is ingested daily by the average person, and almost all of this is excreted in the stool.

C. Very little vanadium shows up in the urine.

D. Most of the vanadium is present in fat, bone, teeth, and serum very likely bound to an unidentified carrier protein.

E. The mean serum vanadium level is 42 μg./100 ml. (range 35 to 48).

F. Vegetables, especially leafy green vegetables, and grains (cereals) are the best sources of vanadium.

II. Vanadium Deficiency

A. A deficit has not been recognized in humans.

B. Administration of vanadium as the oxytartarovanate (125 mg./day) to normal persons has been reported to lower serum lipid concentrations.

C. This may be a pharmacologic rather than physiologic effect.

D. A deficit in animals produces reduced body growth, an abnormality in lipid metabolism (increased serum cholesterol and triglyceride concentrations), impaired reproduction, and epiphyseal distortion.

III. Vanadium Excess

A. Toxicity is produced only with very large excesses of the mineral. Toxicity causes gastrointestinal irritation and green tongue.

B. Inhaled vanadium dusts cause pulmonary irritation.

SILICON

I. General Considerations

A. Silicon is the newest element shown to be essential for animals. It is necessary for an early stage of bone calcification in rats and chickens.

B. Silicon appears to be involved in mucopolysaccharide metabolism of the cartilage matrix.

C. Grains and beer are good sources of silicon; meats are poor sources of silicon.

II. Silicon Deficiency

A. Animals fed silicon-deficient diets showed impaired growth and skeletal defects.

B. No deficiency has been noted to occur in humans.

III. Silicon Excess

A. Toxicity has not been described in humans.

NON-ESSENTIAL, TOXIC TRACE MINERALS (LEAD, CADMIUM, AND MERCURY)

I. General Considerations

A. Certain, apparently non-essential, trace metals are known to accumulate in tissues and biological fluids, producing acute and chronic toxicity.

B. No known biological functions are dependent upon these trace minerals, although they will interfere with the biological functions of other trace minerals by replacing them as the metal components of enzymes or vitamins.

C. The most important elements encountered clinically are lead, cadmium, and mercury, however, other metals (aluminum, tin, and nickel) also might cause toxicity or be carcinogens.

D. For example, aluminum toxicity has been reported in chronic renal failure patients ingesting large amounts of antacids which contain aluminum hydroxide. It remains unclear whether the symptoms are related to the associated hypophosphatemia or due to aluminum accumulation.

II. Lead Toxicity

A. Etiology

1. Lead is a general metabolic poison, which accumulates both acutely and chronically in humans.

2. Ingestion of lead-based paint by chewing on painted surfaces has been the major cause of toxicity in children.

3. Occupational contamination in industries using lead, such as battery factories, and ingestion of acid solutions such as cider from lead-containing vehicles are two common sources of exposure for adults.

B. Manifestations

1. Lead poisoning produces a clinical picture involving several organ systems.

a. Non-specific   gastrointestinal symptoms—anorexia, constipation, nausea, vomiting, and colicky abdominal pain

b. Central nervous system disturbances—irritability, confusion, lethargy, coma, convulsions, slowness of perform-

Table 19-3. **Abnormal Concentrations and Excretions in Children and Adults**

	Children	Adults
Serum Δ ALA	> 20 μg./100 ml.	
Urine Δ ALA	> 5 mg./24 hours	> 10 mg./24 hours
Urine coproporphyrin	> 150 μg./24 hours	> 200 μg./24 hours
Blood lead	> 40 μg./100 ml.	> 60 μg./100 ml.

ance, intelligence defects, psychomotor disturbances, and personality changes

    c. Peripheral neuropathies—weakness in heavily used muscles producing foot or wrist drop progressing to paralysis

    d. Renal tubular defects (Fanconi's syndrome)

    2. Laboratory abnormalities include anemia, basophilic stippling of red cells, lead lines in long bones, decreased Δ-aminolevulinic acid (ALA) dehydrase activity with increased serum and urine ALA activities, increased urinary coproporphyrins, and increased blood lead levels (see Table 19-3).

  C. Treatment

    1. Removal of the patient from the source of lead exposure is the first step.

    2. When blood lead levels exceed 80 μg./100 ml. or when the patient is symptomatic between 50 and 80 μg./100 ml., chelation therapy is indicated.

    3. Calcium EDTA (calcium versanate) can be given to the adult as two 500-mg. tablets, four times daily, for 10-day periods.

    4. Penicillamine, 250 to 500 mg., twice daily, can be used as an alternative in patients who develop gastrointestinal intolerance to EDTA.

    5. These dosages must be scaled down by weight in children.

III. Cadmium Toxicity

  A. Etiology

    1. Cadmium is widely present in the atmosphere, in drinking water, in cigarette smoke, and in various foods (shellfish, grains, vegetables, and coffee).

    2. It is widely used in the metal industry in plating processes and as a pigment.

    3. It is sometimes used in prosthetic dentistry so that all persons have potential exposure in varying degrees.

  B. Manifestations

    1. Symptoms of acute toxicity include nausea, vomiting, diarrhea, abdominal pains, myalgia, increased salivation followed by dry mouth, pneumonitis, pulmonary edema, hepatic necrosis, and renal cortical necrosis.

    2. Emesis prevents the retention of large excesses (10 mg. of cadmium) of ingested mineral and undoubtedly helps to decrease the frequency of severe toxicity.

    3. Chronic toxicity may present with proteinuria, emphysema, anemia, kidney stones, and bone demineralization.

    4. "Itai-Itai" disease (translated to "ouch-ouch" disease) in Japan was linked to ingestion of water downstream from a mine that had a high cadmium concentration. Many of the residents of this area developed bones so brittle that they frequently fractured them, thereby giving the entity its name.

    5. Evidence has accumulated to suggest that an increased uptake of cadmium may be an etiological factor in such diverse conditions as testicular tumors, renal dysfunction, hypertension, atherosclerosis, the chronic diseases of old age, and cancer.

  C. Treatment

    1. Attempts should be made to avoid excessive exposure.

    2. Because the metal produces toxicity by inhibiting enzymes dependent on zinc, copper, and cobalt, one therapeutic approach might be to give these metals as physiological antagonists. In animal studies, for example, administration of zinc will prevent development of the cadmium-induced testicular destruction.

    3. The use of chelating agents has not been reported for the treatment of cadmium toxicity.

IV. Mercury Toxicity

  A. Etiology

    1. Alkylated mercury compounds are much more toxic than non-alkylated mercury compounds.

    2. Environmentally, methyl mercury is the most important alkylated compound.

    3. Once inorganic mercury is released into the environment, methylation can

occur through bacterial action in such places as the sediment of waterways.

4. Methyl mercury then becomes available to the food chain, which reaches humans through edible fish or shellfish or through ingestion of animals feeding on these fish or contaminated grains.

5. It also can be picked up from chlor-alkali plants, fungicides used in the pulp and paper industry, mercury catalysts in industry, residues from the burning of fossil fuels, and medical and scientific wastes.

B. Manifestations

1. Shellfish contamination produced a cerebral palsy-like illness (mild to moderate spasticity, chorea, ataxia, coarse tremors, seizures, and severe mental retardation) in a large number of children (6%) in the area around Minnemota Bay, Japan.

2. Similar manifestations have been reported in isolated cases of mercury poisoning.

C. Treatment

1. No therapeutic agents have been reported as successful in humans, but animal studies suggest penicillamine might be useful.

HALOGENS (CHLORIDE, IODIDE, FLUORIDE, BROMIDE)

The family of anions with a single negative charge are known as the halogens.

I. Chloride

A. Consideration of the metabolism of chloride as a subject separate from that of sodium and acid-base balance probably is unnecessary as chloride is the primary matching anion for sodium and varies only with disturbances in acid-base balance.

B. Of the 2000 mEq. of chloride in the normal adult, 75% is located in the extracellular fluid.

C. The daily intake varies between 80 and 250 mEq. Most is excreted in the urine.

D. Patients with a metabolic alkalosis, generally due to loss of gastric acid (chlo-

ride content up to 150 mEq./L.), develop a low serum chloride concentration (chloride depletion) and a high serum bicarbonate concentration.

E. Correction can be accomplished with any form of chloride given orally or intravenously (e.g., sodium or potassium chloride; the bicarbonate salts are excreted in the urine to achieve the correction), ammonium chloride, or even dilute hydrochloric acid.

F. In contrast, patients with a metabolic acidosis may or may not develop hyperchloremia.

G. When the serum bicarbonate concentration falls, either the serum chloride concentration increases by absorbing chloride from the intestine or an anion gap develops.

1. When the serum sodium minus the chloride and bicarbonate concentrations exceed 12 mEq./L., an anion gap exists.

2. This may be due to retention of organic (lactate, salicylate, formate) or inorganic (phosphate, sulfate) anions.

3. Correction is aimed at the underlying cause and administration of intravenous or oral sodium bicarbonate or equivalent sodium salts.

II. Iodide

A. All body tissues and secretions contain trace amounts of iodine but the total amount in the body is estimated to be only 10 to 20 mg.

B. Three-fourths of this is concentrated in the thyroid gland. Other iodide is distributed much like chloride.

C. Inorganic iodide is converted in the thyroid to many forms of storage, inactive, and active thyroid hormone.

D. The primary function of iodine, through its presence in thyroid hormone, is to control the rate of cellular oxidation.

E. Serum total iodine concentrations are 8 to 12 μg./100 ml. with 1 to 2 μg./100 ml. being inorganic iodide.

F. The serum organic iodide concentration increases with hyperthyroidism and decreases with hypothyroidism. The inorganic fraction fails to change.

G. Iodine in foods is inorganic and is generally completely absorbed from the G.I. tract; excess iodine is excreted by the kidney.

H. While the manifestations of iodine deficiency are a deficient supply of thyroid hormone, various goitrogenic substances and biological defects also can prevent the thyroid from accumulating iodine and converting it into active thyroid hormone.

I. An enlargement of the thyroid is the result of an effort on the part of the thyroid to compensate for the inadequate production of hormone.

1. A dietary deficiency of iodine, therefore, is only one mechanism leading to production of goiter.

2. Endemic goiter occurs in persons who live where water and foods grown in the area are low in iodine (adult human requirement 100 to 200 μg./day).

3. Endemic goiter also is found where goitrogenic substances, which impair iodine uptake or conversion in the thyroid to active hormone, are prevalent.

J. Compulsory iodination of domestic salt is recognized as the most economical, convenient, and effective means of preventing goiter in such areas.

III. Fluoride

A. Fluoride ion has long been known to play a significant role in the prevention of dental caries.

B. It also has a beneficial effect in osteoporosis and other forms of bone demineralization by decreasing pain and by improving bone density and calcium balance.

C. Animal studies also indicate that fluoride may be necessary for maintenance of a normal hematocrit, fertility, and growth.

D. Although fluoride has not been clearly established as essential, it does have beneficial effects.

E. An important source of fluoride is drinking water. Many municipalities fluoridate their water to decrease the incidence of dental caries. To be effective, fluoride must be provided during the stage of enamel formation.

F. Seafood, dairy products, cereals, and other grains are good sources of fluoride.

G. The normal fluoride intake from water and food ranges from 0.5 to 4.0 mg./day. Excesses are excreted in the urine.

H. Topical dental application of stannous fluoride and even oral tablets that contain fluoride have been advocated as preventive measures in children.

I. Chronic excessive intake (20 to 100 mg./day), on the other hand, produces fluorosis with mottling, discoloration, and, eventually, pitting of dental enamel.

J. Larger amounts of fluoride can affect bones (osteosclerosis, exostoses of long bones) and joints and also can impair growth.

IV. Bromide

A. Bromide is so available in nature and in human tissues that it has been difficult to produce deficiencies.

B. Attempts have had no effect on general health, suggesting that bromine performs no essential function in the body.

C. Bromide is a central nervous system depressant that is found in many proprietary headache remedies and nerve tonics.

D. It is handled by the body much like chloride. In fact, it replaces chloride by increasing urinary chloride excretion.

E. Brominism occurs when the bromine concentration exceeds 9 mEq./L. It is characterized by drowsiness, lethargy, and dysarthria progressing to coma or mania with psychotic behavior.

PHOSPHORUS

I. General Considerations

A. Phosphorus, a constituent of all biological tissues and fluids, plays a central role in many vital physiologic processes, most notably

1. Formation of bone
2. Conservation and transfer of energy in the intermediary metabolism of carbohydrates, proteins, lipids, enzymes, and coenzymes
3. Maintenance of intracellular and extracellular hydrogen ion concentrations

B. Of the 700 g. of phosphorus in the average adult, 80% is captured in bone.

C. A normal diet contains between 800 and 1500 mg. of phosphorus per day with dairy products, eggs, and meat being the best sources.

D. About one-half to two-thirds of dietary phosphorus is absorbed.

E. The urinary excretion of phosphorous is dependent not only on dietary intake of phosphorus but on the state of parathyroid gland activity, vitamin D intake, extracellular fluid volume, and the state of tissue catabolism.

F. The normal serum phosphorus concentration is 2.5 to 4.5 mg./100 ml., being slightly higher in children.

II. Phosphorus Deficiency

A. Causes of Hypophosphatemia
1. Decreased phosphate intake
2. Increased intestinal phosphate loss
3. Intake of aluminum hydroxide gel, which forms unreabsorbable complexes with phosphate
4. Hyperparathyroidism
5. Proximal renal tubular defects
6. Serum phosphate also decreases acutely with respiratory (hyperventilation) and metabolic alkalosis.
7. With glucose, insulin, or epinephrine administration or stimulation, as phosphorus moves intracellularly, serum phosphate decreases.

B. Manifestations
1. The major manifestation of chronic phosphate depletion is bone demineralization (osteopenia).
2. However, muscle weakness also may be a significant complaint.

C. Treatment
1. A dose of 2 g. of oral phosphorus daily (as sodium or potassium phosphate) represents initial management for chronic hypophosphatemia and is available in liquid, powder, capsule, and tablet form.

III. Phosphorus Excess

A. Phosphorus accumulates in patients with renal insufficiency, hypoparathyroidism, or long-term, excessive phosphate intake.

B. Phosphate retention in renal failure may be responsible for metastatic calcification by increasing the calcium-phosphorous product.

C. This complication can be prevented by the use of antacids which contain aluminum hydroxide to bind phosphate in the intestine.

D. Effective treatment is 20 to 30 ml. of the aluminum hydroxide preparation, four times daily.

SULFUR

I. General Considerations

A. Essentially all foods ingested by humans contain large amounts of organically bound sulfur with the amino acids methionine, cystine, and cysteine contributing the bulk of the element.

B. Only a small fraction is inorganic sulfur.

C. Thiamine, biotin, and methionine are the only organic, sulfur-containing compounds that are considered essential.

D. Conversion of methionine to cysteine and cystine fulfill the requirements for these amino acids.

E. Deficiencies and excesses of elemental sulfur are not problems in human nutrition.

HYDROGEN

I. General Considerations

A. The blood *p*H is the negative logarithm of the hydrogen ion concentration and is utilized to describe the state of acid-base balance.

B. The body with its buffer systems jealously guards *p*H and maintains it within a narrow normal range (6.8 to 7.7 being compatible with life).

C. An acidosis results from an introduction of excess acid (defined as a substance capable of liberating free hydrogen ion) into the body fluids.

D. An alkalosis develops from loss of acid (introduction of a substance that can capture hydrogen ions from solution).

E. Alterations in acid-base balance are described in terms of changes in the CO_2 — bicarbonate system as these changes mirror shifts in all other buffer systems in the blood and tissues.

F. Easily quantified are the blood *p*H, total CO_2 content or bicarbonate, and P_{CO_2}.

G. The body must cope with introduction and removal of two types of acid.

1. Carbonic acid is derived from hydration of CO_2. The lungs remove volatile CO_2 generated during metabolism. Retention of CO_2 results in a respiratory acidosis; excessive loss of CO_2 results in a respiratory alkalosis. The P_{CO_2} is a direct measure of the respiratory component of any acid-base disturbance.

2. Fixed hydrogen ion and its associated anions are buffered in body fluids and excreted by way of the kidney or, in rare instances, through loss of gastric fluids. Retention of free hydrogen ion produces a metabolic acidosis; loss produces a metabolic alkalosis.

II. Acid-Base Disturbances

A. The four basic acid-base disturbances are listed in Table 19-3.

B. The body employs compensatory mechanisms to correct imposed disturbances in acid-base balance.

1. For example, in a metabolic acidosis (due to retentioin of fixed hydrogen ion), the patient respires more CO_2 (removing carbonic acid) and therefore increases blood *p*H toward normal, even though total CO_2 content falls further.

C. The normal diet contains an excess of 60 to 80 mEq. of hydrogen ion that accumulates daily and ultimately must be excreted in the urine.

1. Most of this is derived from the metabolism of ingested exogenous protein and endogenous protein catabolism, specifically the oxidation of sulfur to sulfate and of phosphorus to phosphate.

2. Small amounts of hydrogen ion also are generated from incomplete metabolism of carbohydrates (to lactic acid) and metabolism of fat.

III. Metabolic Acidosis

A. A metabolic acidosis results from

1. An excessive load of hydrogen ion (e.g., excessive tissue catabolism)

Table 19-4. **Basic Acid-Base Disturbances and the Changes in *p*H, P_{CO_2}, and Total CO_2 (or Bicarbonate) Content**

	pH	P_{CO_2}	Total CO_2 Content
Metabolic acidosis	↓	0 (↓)*	↓
Metabolic alkalosis	↑	0 (↑)*	↑
Respiratory acidosis	↓	↑	↑
Respiratory alkalosis	↑	↓	↓

*With compensatory changes.

2. An inability of the kidneys to remove acid generated (renal failure, renal tubular acidosis)

3. Frequently, both can be implicated.

B. The hydrogen ion load can be decreased by a low-protein, highcarbohydrate diet (as is used in renal failure).

C. Ingestion or infusion of sodium bicarbonate or other organic salts metabolized to bicarbonate provide a more rapid correction.

D. Shohl's solution (a mixture of citric acid and sodium citrate) provides a palatable oral replacement therapy.

IV. Metabolic Alkalosis

A. A metabolic alkalosis occurs primarily when excessive gastric acid is lost from the stomach.

B. Correction can be achieved with any form of chloride replacement as described on p. 290.

C. It may also occur with potassium depletion and can be corrected by replacement of potassium chloride.

D. Deficiencies and excesses of elemental hydrogen generally do not represent nutritional problems as the element is so ubiquitous in all organic compounds.

SUGGESTED READINGS

Burch, R.E., Hahn, H.K.J., and Sullivan, J.F.: Newer aspects of the roles of zinc, manganese, and copper in human nutrition. Clin. Chem., *21:*501, 1975.

Burch, R.E., and Sullivan, J.F.: Symposium on trace elements. Med. Clin. North Am., *60:*652, 1976.

Comar, C.L., and Bronner, F.: Mineral Metabolism: An Advanced Treatise. vol. 2. New York, Academic Press, 1964.

Halsted, J.A., Smith, J.C., Jr., and Irwin, M.I.: A conspectus of research on zinc requirements of man. J. Nutr., *104:*305, 1974.

Hantman, D., *et al.:* Rapid correction of hyponatremia in the syndrome of inappropriate secretion of antidiuretic hormone: an alternative treatment of hypertonic saline. Ann. Intern. Med., *78:*870, 1973.

Lindeman, R.D.: Hypokalemia, causes, consequences, and correction. Amer. J. Med. Sci., *272:*5, 1976.

Lindeman, R.D., and Papper, S.: Therapy of fluid and electrolyte disorders. Ann. Intern. Med., *82:*64, 1975.

Mertz, W., and Cornatzer, E.: Newer Elements in Nutrition. New York, Marcel Dekker, 1971.

Nielsen, F.H., and Sandstead, H.H.: Are nickel, vanadium, silicon, fluorine, and tin essential for man? Amer. J. Clin. Nutr., *27:*515, 1974.

Prasad, A.S.: Trace Elements in Health and Disease. (I. Zinc and Copper; II. Essential and Toxic Elements.) New York, Academic Press, 1976.

Reinhold, J.G.: Trace elements—a selective survey. Clin. Chem., *21:*476, 1975.

Schrier, R.W.: Renal and Electrolyte Disorders. Boston, Little, Brown & Co., 1976.

Schroeder, H.A.: The Trace Elements and Man. Old Greenwich, Conn., The Devin-Adair Company, 1973.

U.S. recommended daily allowances for dietary supplements of vitamins and minerals. Federal Register, *41:*46172, 1976.

Underwood, E.J.: Trace Elements in Human and Animal Nutrition. ed. 3. New York, Academic Press, 1971.

Wacker, W.E.C., and Parisi, A.F.: Magnesium metabolism. N. Engl. J. Med. *278:*658, 1968.

20. TOTAL PARENTERAL NUTRITION AND ELEMENTAL DIETS

Philip D. Schneider, M.D.

Henry Buchwald, M.D., Ph.D.

TOTAL PARENTERAL NUTRITION (HYPERALIMENTATION)

I. Definition

A. Total parenteral nutrition (TPN) is the long-term maintenance or improvement of a patient's nutritional status solely by the intravenous infusion of basic nutrients.

II. Basic Principles

A. Total parenteral nutrition is never an emergency and is not without risk.

B. The decision to begin TPN must be based on a thorough understanding of the individual patient's nutritional status and of basic nutritional principles.

C. If TPN is deemed appropriate, rigorous adherence to certain tenets of long-term intravenous technique, coupled with continuous clinical and laboratory assessment, will avoid potentially dangerous complications and will maximize the benefit.

III. Nutritional Assessment

A. Assessment of the nutritional status of the patient is a prerequisite for initiating TPN.

B. A thorough history is mandatory.

1. The physician must investigate specifically for abnormalities of the cardiovascular system, liver, kidneys, and endocrine system.

2. It should be determined whether the patient has experienced a weight change and, if so, over what period of time this change has occurred.

C. Physical examination must be thorough and must include assessment of any abnormality of the heart, liver, kidneys, or endocrine system.

1. The physician should look specifically for evidence of jaundice, edema, wasting, and for possible abnormal fluid or nutrient losses (e.g., as a result of gastrointestinal-cutaneous fistulas).

D. Laboratory studies should include, as a minimum, a complete blood count and determination of serum electrolytes, glucose, BUN, creatinine, albumin, and liver function studies such as SGOT, alkaline phosphatase, and bilirubin.

E. Radiological studies, aside from the routine chest radiograph, should include intestinal barium studies, scanning studies, sonograms, and other special procedures.

F. Techniques for the investigation of specific tissue losses secondary to undernutrition have been developed.

1. These include determination of the triceps skin fold, the circumference of the upper arm, and the 24-hour urine creatinine-height ratio as indices of the lean body mass and the status of the body fat stores.

2. The application of such tests requires standard charts against which the patient's measurements can be compared.

G. A rough assessment of the patient's baseline nutritional status can be made utilizing the body weight to define three broad classifications: normal, moderately impaired, and severely impaired.

1. Normal nutritional status refers to the patient without recent weight loss.

2. Moderately impaired nutritional status includes those patients who have lost up to 5% of body weight within 4 weeks or 10% of body weight within 4 months.

H. A general loss of 50% of body weight in the non-obese represents an approximate weight loss of one-fourth to one-third of the lean body mass and is incompatible with life.

I. Loss of 10% of body weight represents moderate nutritional depletion.

1. At this level of undernutrition, immune function is hampered, healing is impaired, and synthesis of important body proteins is curtailed.

2. Improving nutrition will play a beneficial role in the patient's clinical course.

J. A typical hospitalized patient who is nutritionally normal at the beginning of hypocaloric infusion will approach 10% loss of body weight after 4 weeks of such hypocaloric infusions.

IV. Basic Nutritional Requirements

A. Energy Requirements

1. Basic requirements to meet routine energy expenditures are 25 to 30 cal./kg./day. A 70-kg. man, for example, would have a basic caloric requirement of 1,750 to 2,100 cal./day to maintain his weight.

a. This calories-kilogram ratio applies to the majority of hospital patients.

b. With enteral therapy, as opposed to intravenous therapy, caloric intake minimally greater than the caloric expenditures will provide for weight gain.

c. With intravenous nutrition, on the other hand, calorie increases in the range of 20 to 50% above baseline are required to provide comparable increments of weight gain.

2. Increased calories will be required for additional activity, hypermetabolic states, and for anabolism.

a. An increase in total calories of approximately 10% for each Fahrenheit degree temperature elevation above normal will be required to maintain weight in the presence of fever.

b. A normal postoperative patient will require 50% more calories to pro-

vide adequate healing and to prevent catabolism.

c. Septic patients will require 75 to 100% increases in their calories compared with baseline estimates.

d. Major burns place the greatest caloric demands on patients with requirements of 150 to 175% over the estimated basal caloric requirements.

3. With prolonged fasting or hypocaloric infusion, loss of fat stores and loss of lean body mass, particularly muscle, contribute to the total weight loss seen.

a. Fat stores provide fatty acids, which in turn supply two carbon compounds to serve as general fuel to fill body energy requirements.

b. Muscle is lost supplying amino acids which are metabolized to maintain blood glucose levels, liver glycogen, and carbohydrate intermediates for biochemical pathways.

4. If parenteral therapy is begun, and body weight falls, or if body weight remains stable, but additional weight gain is desired, caloric intake can be increased appropriately.

a. If, for example, a 70-kg. man whose basal caloric requirement is 2,000 calories is losing weight on intravenous nutritional support, caloric requirements should be increased 25 to 50%.

b. The effect of a calorie increase is evaluated at the end of 1 or 2 weeks. Further increases in calories can be made if appropriate.

5. Energy requirements are met with TPN solutions comprised of carbohydrates, amino acids, and lipids.

B. Volume Requirements

1. Fluid volumes in TPN generally will markedly exceed those calculated for maintenance fluid balance for an individual patient.

a. This greater volume is essential in order to deliver a large number of calories with the solutions currently available.

2. Abnormal fluid losses, however, may not be adequately replaced by the base-

line TPN infusion, and additional fluid replacement may be necessary.

3. Infusions of 5% dextrose solutions and/or electrolyte solutions can be given by a separate intravenous line in order to meet the fluid requirements.

4. Additional fluid volume also may be required during the introduction of TPN when the hypercaloric solution volumes may not supply the necessary fluid to meet volume requirements.

C. Specific Basic Nutrient Requirements

1. Carbohydrate

a. This is supplied in the form of glucose and generally can be considered to provide the majority of calories in TPN solutions.

b. Glucose, which occurs as a monohydrate, supplies approximately 3.4 cal./g. (usually rounded off to 4 cal. for purposes of calculation).

c. The glucose concentration of the usual TPN solutions is 20 to 30 g./100 ml.

2. Amino Acids

a. Amino acids are supplied in the form of protein hydrolysates or solutions of synthetically derived individual amino acids.

b. Protein supplies 4 cal./g., but the protein contribution to the calories of a TPN solution is small.

c. Nitrogen requirement is approximately 0.12 to 0.15 g. of nitrogen per kg. of body weight per day.

(1) With 5% protein hydrolysate solutions, this would place the requirement of nitrogen at 1 g. of hydrolysate per kg. of body weight per day.

(2) Slightly less amino acid solution (0.5 to 1.0 g./kg.) is required if used instead of hydrolysate because amino acids are more efficiently used for protein synthesis.

d. Blood products, such as plasma and albumin, are inefficient and expensive nitrogen sources compared with the available amino acid solutions, and they have no place in long-term parenteral hyperalimentation, except in the initial stages when preexistent hypoproteinemia or anemia are being corrected.

e. In situations in which weight gain is desirable, 0.2 g. of nitrogen per kg. or 1.5 g. of 5% hydrolysate solution per kg. of body weight will provide enough amino acids for anabolism.

f. The optimal ratio of non-protein calories to grams of nitrogen is approximately 120 to 180:1 for anabolism or maintenance of lean body mass.

3. Fat Requirements

a. The precise minimal requirement for fat in the diet is not known.

b. It is believed that essential fatty acids should comprise 1 to 2% of the total daily diet calories.

c. Lipid emulsions infused at 1.5 to 2 g. of lipid per kg. per day will supply 30 to 40% of the calorie intake, as is the case in an average North American oral diet.

d. In these quantities, the requirements for the essential fatty acids should be met.

e. During the course of parenteral nutrition, fat requirements probably can be met adequately with 2 to 3 L. of fat emulsion administered intravenously per week.

f. If desired, a larger portion of the patient's caloric need can be derived solely from the fat emulsion.

(1) Since fat supplies approximately 9 cal./g., a greater number of calories can be supplied with a 10 or 20% solution of fat emulsion than can be supplied with the corresponding volume of amino acids in hypertonic glucose.

g. Potential toxicity limits the amount of lipid that can be given to an adult patient to approximately 2 g./kg./day.

4. Electrolyte Requirements

a. Electrolyte requirements in TPN are no different, on the whole, from those in normal parenteral therapy.

b. Particular attention must be paid to maintaining adequate levels of potassium, calcium, magnesium, and phosphorous in patients receiving TPN.

5. *Vitamin Requirements*

a. Minimum daily requirements for most vitamins are well established (see Chap. 8).

b. Vitamin requirements in TPN will be increased in instances in which the patient began therapy moderately to severely malnourished.

c. A 10-ml. ampule of any of the currently available intravenous water-soluble vitamin preparations for every 2L. of parenteral nutrient solution is adequate.

d. There is no need to supply more than one 10-ml. ampule per week of a fat-soluble vitamin preparation because this can lead to hypervitaminosis A and D.

e. It should be noted that available parenteral preparations do not contain Vitamin K, and this vitamin should be given intramuscularly weekly or biweekly.

f. Vitamin B_{12} and folate are present in insufficient amounts in TPN solutions. Consideration of their replacement on an appropriate schedule should be made.

D. Basic TPN Solutions. A typical solution, which would fulfill the above nutrient requirements and supply approximately 1,000 cal./L. of solution in the appropriate calorie-nitrogen ratio, is illustrated below.

1. Individual caloric needs can be adjusted by increasing or decreasing the volume of fluid a patient receives each day.

2. In addition to this solution, for long-term parenteral nutrition, 1 L. of lipid emulsion should be administered approximately every other day to supply essential fatty acids.

Basic TPN Solution

		Calories
Glucose	250 g.	1,000
Protein equivalent	36 g. (6 g. N)	120
K^+	15 mEq.	
Na^+	30 mEq.	
Mg^{++}	4 mEq.	
Ca^{++}	5 mEq.	
Cl^-	22 mEq.	
$PO_4^=$	30 mEq.	
Multivitamin solution	10 ml.	

Therefore, 1010 ml. solution = 1,120 calories

1. Increased calories are provided by increasing the volume infused over 24 hours.

2. Electrolyte concentrations may be varied from bottle to bottle to allow for possible incompatibilities and to meet daily requirements.

3. Electrolytes may be varied on a daily basis.

4. Fat-soluble vitamin solutions are given only once weekly.

5. One L. of 10% or 500 ml. of 20% Intralipid (Vitrum) is administered 2 to 3 times weekly.

6. $PO_4^=$ concentrations in currently available protein hydrolysates or synthetic amino acid solutions are sufficient for the needs of most patients. $PO_4^=$ need only be added in severe hypophosphatemia.

V. Managing TPN

A. Basic Principles

1. The decision to begin TPN should not be made lightly as there is significant morbidity and mortality associated with its use.

2. The patient's nutritional status should be such that the patient's requirements cannot be supplied adequately by enteric means.

3. Physicians who undertake the responsibility and the task of administering TPN or elemental diets to their patients must make a commitment not only of themselves but also of their hospital staff and pharmacy to provide for the safe and effective preparation and utilization of these products.

4. Total parenteral nutrition is never an emergency procedure. Hospitals that cannot undertake the continuous expense of the technique or that cannot guarantee the requisite quality in solutions preparation and in TPN administration should not undertake this particular mode of therapy.

B. Procedure

1. The following procedures are recommended, once the decision to place the patient on TPN is made.

2. Baseline chemistry determinations are made, and a laboratory monitoring schedule is established (see Table 20-1).

3. Anemia and hypoproteinemia are corrected.

4. The nursing staff receives protocols of instructions, including those for catheter care, routine laboratory tests, and cautions to be observed for patients receiving TPN.

Table 20-1. **Laboratory and Clinical Monitoring of TPN**

Determination	Frequency	
	Initial Period	Stable Period
Laboratory Determinations		
Blood		
Serum electrolytes	Daily	3 times weekly
(Na^+, K^+, Cl^-, HCO_3^-)		
Blood urea nitrogen	3 times weekly	2 times weekly
Blood glucose	Daily	2 times weekly
Serum osmolarity	Daily	2 times weekly
Serum inorganic phosphate	Daily	2 times weekly
Serum calcium	3 times weekly	2 times weekly
Serum magnesium	3 times weekly	2 times weekly
Liver function	3 times weekly	Weekly
SGOT		
Alkaline phosphatase		
Bilirubin		
Serum proteins with A/G fraction	2 times weekly	Weekly
Complete blood count	2 times weekly	Weekly
Serum iron and iron-binding capacity	Once	Monthly
Arterial blood gases	As indicated	As indicated
Blood ammonia	As indicated	As indicated
Urine		
Glucose	4–6 times daily	2 times daily
Specific gravity	2–4 times daily	Daily
Clinical Determinations		
Body weight	Daily	Daily
Complete intake and output	Daily	Daily
Physical examination	Daily	Daily
Cultures	As indicated	As indicated

5. Provisions are made for daily weight determinations and appropriate fluid balance (intake and output) measurements.

6. A parenteral catheter is inserted. As a rule, a central venous catheter is necessitated by the high osmolarity of the infused solutions. An exception to this is made possible by the recent utilization of peripheral lipid emulsions (see p. 301, Section E.)

7. A radiograph is obtained whenever a central venous line is used, to insure proper positioning of the catheter in the superior vena cava and to rule out possible complications of catheter placement.

    a. Aside from the obvious need to place the catheter somewhere other than the subclavicular or jugular position in patients with neck surgery or tracheostomy, the subclavian position of the delivery catheter offers several advantages, including patient comfort and ease and effectiveness of catheter care.

    b. There is no substitute for experience in placing such catheters. For those lacking experience, there is no substitute for proper understanding of the anatomy involved and skilled instruction in placing subclavian catheters.

C. Formulation of the Hyperalimentation Solution

1. Protein requirements are calculated.

2. Basal energy requirements are estimated, and additional calories are allowed for hypermetabolism or sepsis.

3. Electrolyte requirements are calculated, and particular attention is paid to calcium and magnesium requirements, as well as to insuring adequate phosphate content in the parenteral nutritional solution.

D. Administration of Hyperalimentation Solutions

1. Solutions administration is initiated by continuous infusion at one-half to two-thirds of the calculated caloric requirements per day to allow for adaptation to the large glucose load.

2. The number of calories infused per day is gradually increased to the previously calculated level.

    a. For patients who begin TPN in severe metabolic deficiency, a gradual increase is definitely required.

    b. Primarily, this allows the pancreatic islets to augment insulin output and prevent glucose spillage in the urine and the resulting complication of an osmotic diuresis.

    c. During the course of this build-up particular attention must be paid to potassium, magnesium, and phosphate levels in the blood.

3. Healthy individuals can be raised to the calculated maximum calorie requirement over a 2- to 3-day period.

4. Nutritional repletion is a slow process. Once the desired caloric level is achieved, a period of 10 days to 2 weeks should be allowed to pass before a decision to further increase caloric requirements is made.

5. If the infusion falls behind schedule, no attempt to catch up should be made. The infusion should be continued at the calculated desirable rate.

6. Blood sugars and fractional urines must be observed carefully.

    a. Fractional insulin coverage with regular insulin may be instituted if persistent urine sugar spills of 3+ to 4+ are encountered in association with concurrent blood sugars above 200 mg./100 ml.

    b. In patients who are not diabetic, an appropriate scale of regular insulin therapy, if necessary, would begin with four units of regular insulin for a 3+ urine sugar spill and eight units for a 4+ spill, with increases as appropriate.

    c. Spills of 1+ and 2+ are not routinely covered.

7. In the course of therapy, should laboratory tests disclose any abnormalities, appropriate changes in the composition of the nutrient solutions must be made.

8. In the absence of abnormal endogenous insulin secretion or exogenously administered insulin, TPN may be tapered

over a few hours to one day when discontinued. Longer tapering is indicated when levels of endogenous insulin are high or exogenously administered insulin is present. It should be stressed that abrupt cessation of TPN is contraindicated.

E. Total Parenteral Nutrition via Peripheral Vein

1. The availability of Intralipid (Vitrum), a soybean fat emulsion, has made TPN via peripheral vein possible by obviating the need to use hypertonic glucose solutions to supply necessary calories.

 a. Adequate peripheral veins are required because it is recommended that the peripheral intravenous sites be rotated at least every 72 hours.

2. Marked hypermetabolic states are best treated by a central catheter because the amount of calories that can be delivered peripherally is limited.

3. The caloric limit is based on the recommended limit of fat administration of 2 g./kg./day in order to prevent toxicity reactions (e.g., fat embolization syndrome, acutely, or severe fatty infiltration of the liver, chronically).

4. Individual patient tolerance or intolerance of infiltration lipid emulsions must also be taken into account.

5. The basic regimen for total peripheral parenteral nutrition would involve infusion of protein hydrolysate or amino acid solutions, 10 or 15% glucose solutions and 10 or 20% lipid solutions.

 a. Approximately 3,000 cal./day can be supplied by a total intravenous volume of approximately 3,500 ml.

 b. A typical regimen would include 1 L. of 10 or 15% carbohydrate solution with vitamins, 1 L. of amino acid solution with electrolytes, 500 ml. of a 20% fat emulsion, and, again, 1 L. of a 10 to 15% carbohydrate solution. These solutions are administered via peripheral vein sequentially over a 24-hour period.

6. Peripheral parenteral nutrition must be approached with the same rigorous

patient assessment and laboratory analyses as TPN via central vein.

VI. Complications of TPN

A. Basic Types

1. Mechanical complications secondary to the central venous catheter
2. Septic complications
3. Metabolic complications

B. Mechanical Complications

1. Complications of catheter insertion
 a. Pneumothorax
 b. Hemothorax
 c. Major artery lacerations
 d. Brachial plexus injury
2. Complications related to indwelling central venous catheters
 a. Subclavian venous thrombosis
 b. Air embolism
3. Prevention of mechanical complications
 a. Careful technique and caution in insertion of the central venous catheter
  (1) Much has been written on the subject of subclavian catheter insertion technique (see Suggested Readings, p. 304).
  (2) This is a procedure that must be well taught and well learned.
 b. Careful taping and sealing of all catheter connections
 c. Use of an alarm and a sensing device which will detect cessation of flow if a continuous infusion pump is utilized to provide a constant rate of solution infusion

C. Septic Complications

1. Septic complications constitute the most frequent and the most potentially dangerous complications in patients receiving TPN.
2. Sepsis constitutes the major concern when considering placing patients on TPN.
3. Sources of sepsis include both bacterial and fungal infections.
 a. Etiology is generally invasion of the venous system through the skin at the catheter entrance site.
 b. Additional sources of sepsis in-

clude ongoing septic foci in the patient, such as intra-abdominal abscesses, urinary tract infections, and contaminated nutrient solutions.

4. Prevention of septic complications

a. Proper mechanical and antibiotic ointment care of the catheterization site, daily changes of the intravenous tubing, and the use of in-line antimicrobial filters

b. Absolute adherence to the principle that the central line should not be utilized for drawing blood or infusing solutions other than the nutrient solutions

c. Additional precautions, including taking the patient's temperature four times daily, taking routine cultures of blood and urine for temperature elevations, and removing and culturing the central catheter when evidence suggests it may be a source of sepsis

5. If septic complications ensue, it is likely that the complication will be solved by removing the central catheter and waiting 24 to 48 hours before reinserting it at another site.

a. Peripheral parenteral nutrition may have to be started, to prevent abrupt cessation of the caloric load to a system geared for hypermetabolism.

b. Antibiotic therapy is instituted if sepsis persists.

D. Metabolic Complications

1. The major and most frequent metabolic complications include

a. Hyperglycemia, with glycosuria and osmotic diuresis. These are caused by too rapid an infusion of calories in the initial period of TPN, the presence of diabetes mellitus with inadequate insulin coverage, sepsis.

b. Hyperosmolar, non-ketoacidotic coma. This occurs secondary to large or rapid glucose infusions in patients with or without diabetes who may be septic or dehydrated.

(1) The etiology appears to be pancreatic exhaustion and resultant hypoinsulinemia.

c. Electrolyte abnormalities. A broad range of electrolyte abnormalities can occur, as might be expected in ill patients who are receiving all their nutritional support intravenously. Of particular importance are the following:

(1) Hypokalemia, which can be exacerbated by protein anabolism

(2) Hypophosphatemia, which can induce a variety of metabolic complications (e.g., parcsthesias, dysarthria, stupor, coma, and death)

(3) Hyperchloremic metabolic acidosis, a complication known to occur with certain synthetic amino acid preparations

(a) This is believed to be related to the cation gap which results from mixing the hydrochloric acid salts of synthetic amino acids in solution.

2. Recognition of metabolic complications is dependent upon

a. Clinical observations

b. Recognition of sepsis

c. Close observation of laboratory results, which are obtained on a routine basis (see Table 20-1).

d. In the absence of the laboratory capacity to determine osmolarity, this may be estimated by using the following formula:

$$\text{osmolarity (mOsm.)} = 2(\text{Na}^+ + \text{K}^+) + \frac{\text{Glucose}}{18} + \frac{\text{BUN}}{2.8}$$

e. Osmolarity of 285 to 300 mOsm./L. is normal. Values of 350+ are seen in hyperosmolar coma associated with blood sugars of 1000+ mg./100 ml.

3. Management of metabolic complications

a. Hyperglycemia or hyperosmolar, non-ketoacidotic coma are managed by appropriate additions of insulin, as well as hypotonic fluids.

b. Electrolyte and acid-base abnormalities are managed by appropriate adjustments in basic nutrition solutions.

    c. Treatment of ongoing septic processes, if present, is primary.

ELEMENTAL DIETS

I. Definition

    A. Elemental diets are powdered food sources that are reconstituted with water and supply a patient's nutritional requirements in the form of glucose and short oligosaccharides, amino acids, or protein hydrolysates, and a minimum of fat with sufficient essential fatty acids to supply 100% of estimated normal requirements.

    1. The various available elemental diets include varying quantities of electrolytes.

II. Indications

    A. The use of elemental diets is relatively new, and broad indications and guidelines have yet to be established.

    B. The nutrients, in the form they are provided, are absorbed in the proximal small bowel and require little, or no, enzymatic preparative digestion.

    C. The use of these diets is appropriate for those patients who have a normally functioning gastrointestinal tract and for those who have digestive or absorptive malfunctions (e.g., pancreatic insufficiency, short-bowel syndrome, inflammatory bowel disease, or enteric fistulas).

III. Composition of an Elemental Diet

    A. Several diets are available (see Table 20-2). Of the several listed, Precision LR is probably the most palatable. It has the disadvantage, however, of having a protein source which is not elemental.

    B. When reconstituted as directed, all solutions are hyperosmolar.

    C. Minimum daily vitamin requirements are met by the fully reconstituted solutions.

    D. These diets may be administered orally or by nasogastric tube, gastrostomy, or jejunostomy.

Table 20-2. **Composition of Three Elemental Diets (Per 1000 Calories)**

	Vivonex (Eaton)	Flexical (Mead-Johnson)	Precision LR (Doyle)
Nitrogen (g.)	3.4	3.5	3.7
Protein (g.)	21	22	23
source	Synthetic amino acids	Protein hydrolysate	Egg albumin
Carbohydrate (g.)	213	155	226
source	Glucose oligo-saccharides	Starch, sucrose oligosaccharides	Sucrose maltodextrin
Fat (g.)	1.5	34	0.7
source	Linoleic acid	Soy oil, medium-chain triglycerides	Vegetable oil
Na^+ (mEq.)	37	15	27
K^+ (mEq.)	30	38	20
Mg^{+2} (mEq.)	16	14	15
Ca^{+2} (mEq.)	22	25	22
Cl^- (mEq.)	51	36	83
$(PO_4)^{-3}$ (mEq.)	43	44	41

IV. Administration

A. All diets are best infused slowly and continuously.

    1. Bolus volumes of these solutions delay gastric emptying and cause diarrhea.

B. Slow infusion is best accomplished during the day and should be discontinued at night, to avoid the possibility of aspiration, particularly in debilitated patients.

C. Because of their hypertonicity, the solutions should not be administered initially at full strength.

    1. At the beginning of therapy, a concentration of 15 to 25% is infused slowly.

    2. Volume and concentration can be increased as tolerated.

    3. Tolerance is judged by the presence or absence of nausea, vomiting, cramps, or diarrhea and by attention to laboratory values which indicate hyperosmolarity and dehydration.

        a. Hyperosmolarity of these solutions precludes their use in infants.

D. It is well to follow a program of monitoring laboratory studies in a manner similar to that described for monitoring TPN.

E. The calculated amount of calories infused is based on the calculation of basal minimal requirements, plus the calories required for hypermetabolism and fever (see Energy Requirements, p. 296).

V. Complications

A. These are largely related to gastrointestinal physiological effects related to the hyperosmolarity of the solutions.

B. Adverse metabolic effects such as hyperglycemia or hyperosmolar coma can occur.

C. Hypervitaminosis K is occasionally noted.

SUGGESTED READINGS

Dudrick, S.J., Wilmore, D.W., Vars, H.M., and Rhoads, J.E.: Long-term parenteral nutrition with growth, development, and positive nitrogen balance. Surgery, *64:*134, 1968.

_____: Can intravenous feeding as the sole means of nutrition support growth in the child and restore weight loss in an adult? Ann. Surg., *169:*974, 1969.

Fischer, J.E. (ed.): Total Parenteral Nutrition. Boston, Little, Brown & Co., 1976.

Lee, H.A. (ed.): Patenteral Nutrition in Acute Metabolic Illness. New York, Academic Press, 1974.

21. NUTRITION AND LIVER DISEASE

Dennis Philip Quinlan, M.D.

Carroll M. Leevy, M.D.

The practitioner caring for a patient with liver disease must be concerned with nutritional abnormalities, the nature of which depends on the etiology and severity of the hepatic disorder.

Hepatic functional and/or morphologic changes secondary to a deficit, excess, or imbalance of nutrient intake can be corrected by proper nutritional therapy. Such treatment may also be beneficial in patients with liver necrosis, cholestasis, fibrosis, or neoplasia accompanied by secondary alteration of nutrient balance.

BASIC PRINCIPLES

I. Pathology

A. Hepatic steatosis (fatty infiltration) results from both undernutrition and overnutrition. Obese patients with fatty liver who are treated by intestinal bypass may develop cirrhosis.

B. Deficiencies of nicotinic acid, folic acid, vitamin B_6, vitamin B_{12}, and zinc cause subclinical liver injury with a decrease in hepatic enzymes or interference with DNA synthetic capacity.

1. Such changes may represent the earliest abnormalities in liver injury due to infective agents, drugs, or alcoholism.

C. At the other end of the spectrum, large doses of niacinamide or chronic vitamin A intoxication produce morphologic changes in the liver, which, if not interrupted, become clinically overt.

D. Liver cell necrosis evokes a loss of hepatic stores of protein, carbohydrate, fat, minerals, and vitamins, with a transitory rise in serum levels of these constituents. Persisting necrosis leads to depletion of liver and body nutrients and often produces overt clinical and laboratory abnormalities.

E. Cholestasis, by interfering with the excretion of bile salts required for emulsification and absorption of dietary fat, leads to a deficit of fat-soluble vitamins.

1. Biliary obstruction also leads to hyperlipidemia and accumulation of copper.

F. Cirrhosis with fibrosis and vascular shunts reduces hepatic uptake, assimilation, and storage of nutrients.

G. Catabolic effects of hepatic neoplasms are responsible for nutrient depletion.

H. Inborn errors of metabolism leading to liver disease are also regularly accompanied by nutrient imbalance.

II. Recognition of Malnutrition in Liver Disease

A. Signs and Symptoms

1. Conventional evidence of malnutrition regularly is present in patients with severe liver disease.

2. Of particular importance is the frequent coexistence of liver, pancreas, and intestinal disease, each of which contributes to nutrient depletion.

3. Clinical features may permit recognition of both nutrient imbalance and liver disease.

4. The most common signs and symptoms are:

a. Glossitis, due to a deficiency of nicotinic acid, riboflavin, folic acid, vitamin B_6, protein, or iron

b. Hemorrhagic tendency, due to vitamin C or K depletion

c. Testicular atrophy or loss of taste, due to zinc depletion

d. Delirium or hallucinations, resulting from nicotinic acid or thiamine deficiency

e. Anemia, due to iron, folic acid, or vitamin B_6 deficiency

5. Patients with hepatitis, cirrhosis, or other hepatic disorders associated with liver failure may exhibit somnolence, euphoria, asterixis, constructional apraxia, or coma. These findings are due to abnormalities in protein and fat metabolism.

6. Muscle weakness and wasting secondary to protein and mineral depletion are common.

7. Fluid accumulation due to salt and water retention occurs in later stages of liver disease.

8. Occasionally, overt evidence of beriberi, pellagra, or scurvy is present with all of the classic features of these conditions in addition to evidence of liver failure.

B. Laboratory Studies. These should be obtained to confirm the presence of nutritional abnormalities and to monitor response to treatment in the patient with malnutrition and liver disease. The following specific tests are recommended:

1. Vitamin Deficiency

a. Patients with fatty liver, cirrhosis, and chronic hepatitis often exhibit a decrease in circulating levels of folic acid, thiamine, and vitamin B_6.

b. Less commonly, riboflavin and nicotinic acid deficiencies are present in such patients.

c. Low serum levels of vitamins A, D, E, and K are characteristic of patients with chronic biliary obstruction.

d. Diagnostic and therapeutic perspective is increased by obtaining the following tests, which are available in the clinical laboratory:

(1) Serum folic acid, blood smear for macrocytosis and hypersegmented polymorphonuclear leukocytes, and bone marrow for myeloblastosis

(2) Serum pyridoxine, serum pyridoxal 5–phosphate, urinary pyridoxic acid, and serum glutamic pyruvic transaminase activity

(3) Red blood cells transketolase,

blood thiamine, or urinary excretion of thiamine

(4) Prothrombin time and its change in response to vitamin K

(5) Circulating or urinary levels of riboflavin and serum glutamic reductase activity

2. Protein Intolerance

a. Although patients with liver disease and mental changes have alterations in protein, fat, carbohydrate, and mineral balance, most attention has been focused on protein intolerance because of therapeutic implications.

b. Protein tolerance may be assessed by evaluating response to a protein test meal or ammonium chloride and by measuring serum amino acids with a calculation of the ratio of aliphatic to aromatic amino acids.

(1) Protein tolerance test: Obtain fasting blood for blood ammonia and urea, and give 60 g. protein orally. Obtain blood for ammonia and urea at hourly intervals for 4 hours. In normal subjects, there is a transitory rise in blood ammonia without a change in blood urea during the first 2 hours, followed by a decrease in blood ammonia and an increase in urea.

(2) Evaluation of amino acid patterns, aliphatic-aromatic amino acids ratio. Plasma levels of phenylalanine, methionine, tyrosine, valine, leucine, and isoleucine should be measured. The ratio of aliphatic to aromatic amino acid is normally 2.5:3.5; it may decrease to 1.0:1.5 in hepatic insufficiency.

3. Hematologic Abnormalities

a. Anemia, coagulation disturbances, and abnormal lymphocyte reactivity are common in liver disease.

b. A complete blood count with peripheral blood smear and morphologic indices are desirable to evaluate the type and cause of anemia in liver disease.

c. For hypochromic microcytic anemia, serum iron, vitamin B_6, and hemoglobin patterns should be obtained.

d. Folic acid and vitamin B_{12} should

be measured in patients with macrocytic anemia.

e. A battery of clotting factors is needed to assess the cause of a bleeding tendency. In addition, it is desirable to measure vitamin C and to evaluate response of blood clotting abnormalities to specific replacement therapy.

f. Patients with liver disease and increased susceptibility to infections should have studies of serum immunoglobulins, skin tests, or lymphocyte reactivity to specific antigens.

TREATMENT REGIMENS FOR DISEASES OF THE LIVER

I. General Considerations

A. A balanced diet with specific supplements is needed to repair damaged cells and to produce new hepatocytes in patients with active liver disease.

B. Although nutritional therapy is of utmost importance in proper management of patients with liver disease and its complications, other aspects must also be considered to provide them with proper care and treatment.

C. Symptomatic and supportive therapy is needed while awaiting repair or regeneration of liver cells.

D. Ideally, a high-carbohydrate, high-protein diet with medium-chain triglycerides should be provided. It may be necessary, however, to modify intake to avoid the adverse consequences of high protein intake.

E. Response to treatment may be best evaluated by serial measurement of serum aminotransferases (SGPT and SGOT), serum albumin, clearance of exogenous dyes (indocyanine green 0.5 to 2.5 mg./kg.), serum bilirubin, and serum bile acids.

II. Ascites

A. Ascites in liver disease results from an increase in hydrostatic pressure and lymphatic blockade. There is usually a lowered colloid osmotic pressure with secondary hyperaldosteronism, reflected in decreased urinary sodium.

B. Treatment consists of eliminating retained salt and water while attempting to improve hepatic reserve.

C. A pretherapy diagnostic paracentesis

Table 21-1. **Fruit and Vegetable Diet Sample Menu***

Morning	*Mid-Morning*
Orange juice	Grapefruit juice
Apple	Applesauce
Canned peaches	
Noon	*Mid-Afternoon*
Baked potato	Apple juice
Cooked brussel sprouts	$\frac{1}{2}$ cantaloupe
Cooked peas	
Lettuce with sliced tomato	
Evening	
Baked potato	
Cooked squash	
Cooked string beans	
Green pepper/avocado/asparagus	
Lettuce wedge	
Apple juice	

Cook all vegetables by boiling without salt or sodium additives.
Do not use canned vegetables.
Do not use frozen peas or lima beans.

*All foods are to be eaten.

is essential to be certain that the peritoneal fluid is not infected and to differentiate ascites of liver disease from that due to tuberculous peritonitis, constrictive pericarditis, or metastatic cancer, all of which require specific therapy.

D. Treatment of noninfected ascites consists of sodium restriction and judicious use of diuretics.

E. Response should be monitored by daily measurement of body weight, abdominal girth, sodium and potassium intake, and urinary excretion.

F. Few patients are refractory to specific and symptomatic therapy.

1. Restriction of sodium

a. Initially, even in the hospital, the patient should be given a low sodium intake, such as is achieved on a fruit and vegetable diet (35 mg.). A sample diet is shown in Table 21–1.

b. Rice, matzoth, and other readily available low-sodium foods should be added little by little until a 200 to 500 mg. sodium diet is obtained.

c. The cooperative patient should be taught to monitor sodium intake, using a daily diary.

2. Diuretics should be given to accelerate sodium loss.

a. One must be constantly aware of the potassium depletion which occurs with some diuretics.

b. In these instances, oral potassium supplements, in the form of potassium chloride, potassium citrate, or potassium phosphate, should be provided.

c. Patient and physician should monitor urinary sodium losses.

(1) Non-response should lead to an increase in the diuretic dosage, change in diuretics, or both.

Table 21-2. **Restricted Sodium, 40 Grams Protein Diet**

Total Daily Intake	Sodium (mg.)	Protein (g.)	Fat (g.)	Carbohydrate (g.)
Milk–8 oz.	125	8	10	12
Meats–2 oz.	60	14	10	—
Bread, Cereal (salt-free) –6 servings	30	12	—	90
Fruits–6 servings	—	—	—	60
Vegetables–4 half-cup portions	20	6	—	28
Fats (salt-free)–9 tsp.	—	—	45	—
Sugar–6 tsp.	—	—	—	30

Table 21-3. **Sample Menu—40 Grams Protein Diet**

Morning	Noon	Evening
Orange juice–8 oz. Cereal (salt-free) with $\frac{1}{2}$ cup milk Tea/coffee with 2 tsp. sugar	1 oz. meat 2 slices of bread with salt-free margarine Vegetable (1 serving) Fruit (1 serving) Tea/coffee with 2 tsp. sugar	1 oz. meat Rice Vegetable Salad Fruit
Mid-Morning Fruit	*Mid-Afternoon* Fruit	*Snack* $\frac{1}{2}$ cup milk 1 slice toast with salt-free margarine

(2) In selected patients with general anasarca, renal failure, or pulmonary edema, hemodialysis may be indicated to restore normal fluid balance.

(3) Replacement of water-soluble vitamins is of critical importance in these instances.

3. Patients with ascites refractory to salt restriction, diuretics, and a nutritious diet should be considered for repeated paracentesis with infusion of salt-poor albumin to prevent hypovolemia and hypotension.

a. A surgical procedure, such as construction of a peritoneal-jugular shunt (La Veen), is desirable to facilitate control of the ascites.

III. Hepatic Encephalopathy

A. Basic Principles

1. Hepatic encephalopathy should be suspected in all patients with chronic liver disease or severe acute liver disease.

2. Patients exhibiting mental changes should be suspected of having hepatic encephalopathy if there is overt evidence of liver disease and absence of other causes of mental aberration.

3. Electroencephalograms, brain scans, computerized tomograms, and spinal fluid examinations are desirable for objective evaluation of the nature and severity of encephalopathy.

4. Therapy should be monitored by daily evaluation of mentation. This may be judged at the bedside by ascertaining the presence or absence of asterixis and constructional apraxia (handwriting, trail test, or reproduction of the five star match test).

B. Treatment of Hepatic Encephalopathy

1. Correction of deficits of nutrients known to produce mental changes (niacinamide, thiamine, and phosphate)

2. Reduction in protein intake in an effort to decrease blood ammonia

3. Provision of adequate glucose and oxygen for brain metabolism

4. Simultaneously, an effort should be made to eliminate etiologic factors and provide general supportive measures.

C. Recommended Dietary Program

1. Give carbohydrates, intravenously or orally, in amounts to supply basal caloric needs, without protein, for 48 hours.

2. Add protein hydrolysates which yield a maximum of 20 g. of protein for 48 to 96 hours. Aminosol or Freamine may be used for this purpose.

3. Provide a balanced dietary intake with protein up to 40 g. daily if mentation improves. Table 21–2 lists the 24-hour dietary allowances on such a diet. Table 21-3 shows a sample menu for such a diet.

4. Give parenteral supplements of B-complex vitamins, vitamin C, and zinc. These vitamins and minerals should be given in the amounts shown in Table 21-4. Correct deficits of other minerals if they exist.

Table 21-4. **Recommended Vitamin and Mineral Supplements for Liver Disease Patients**

Supplement	Dosage
Vitamin C	100–500 mg./day
Folic acid	1.0 mg.
Thiamine	5–25 mg.
Riboflavin	3–15 mg.
Niacinamide	20–50 mg.
Pantothenic acid	10–20 mg.
Pyridoxine	7.5–25 mg.
Vitamin D (consider use of 25-hydroxycalciferol)	400 I.U.
Zinc sulfate	10–25 mg.
Calcium phosphate (with deficiency)	1–2 g.
Magnesium sulfate (with deficiency)	0.5–1.0 g.
Ferrous sulfate	10–30 mg.

5. In patients, refractory to the above regimen, who exhibit a marked increase in serum aromatic amino acids, infuse amino acid mixture containing large amounts of branched-chain amino acids and 20% glu-

cose. At the present time, these solutions must be individually constituted by the hospital pharmacy because no commercially available preparations are on the market. The composition of one solution that has been used in clinical trials is shown in Table 21-5.

Table 21-5. **F080 (Fischer J.E.)**

	g./L.
Isoleucine	4.50
Leucine	5.50
Valine	4.20
Threonine	2.25
Methionine	0.50
Phenylalanine	0.50
Tryptophan	0.38
Lysine HCl	3.80
Alanine	3.75
Arginine	3.00
Histidine	1.20
Proline	4.00
Serine	2.50
Glycine	4.50
Cysteine HCl	< 0.20

Suggested amino acid solution to be used in 20% glucose solution for patients with advanced liver disease refractory to treatment.

6. Give blood-ammonia-lowering drugs, which decrease ammonia production from protein degradation in the colon and its entry into the blood.

　　a. Lactulose—4 g., three times daily, 30 minutes before meals, as tolerated

　　b. Broad spectrum antibiotics—tetracycline (250 mg., four times daily) or neomycin (6 g. daily)

7. Provide glucose and oxygen, and correct deficits of 2,3-DPG and other nutrients to restore normal cerebral oxidative capacity.

IV. Malabsorption Syndrome

A. Steatorrhea (fatty stools) and intestinal malabsorption are common in patients with chronic liver disease with biliary obstruction.

　　1. The steatorrhea of liver disease

should be differentiated from that due to pancreatic or primary intestinal disease.

2. Bile salts and medium-chain triglycerides are helpful in some patients with steatorrhea attendant to obstructive jaundice. Medium-chain triglycerides in oil are readily available for oral use. Bile salts are available as Ox Bile Extract, also for oral administration.

3. Cholestyramine resin, which is utilized to decrease bile acids in patients with obstructive jaundice, chelates vitamin D and other nutrients, and this should be noted.

B. In addition, it is necessary to provide fat-soluble vitamins.

1. A,D,E, and K. These vitamins may be given orally, and the preparation chosen should supply 2500 I.U. of vitamin A, 200 I.U. of vitamin D, and 15 to 400 I.U. of vitamin E. Vitamin K may be given intramuscularly in a dose of 2 to 5 mg. Because conversion of vitamin D_3 (the form commonly supplied in most preparations) may be impaired with severe liver injury, 25-dehydroxycholecalciferol may be helpful in these instances.

2. Effectiveness of therapy should be monitored by pre- and posttherapy vitamin levels and by an evaluation of the metabolic effects of administered treatment on plasma prothrombin, serum calcium, and other abnormal laboratory tests.

V. Reduced Hepatic Synthetic Capacity

A. Severe liver injury is characterized by decreased ability to synthesize key proteins, including albumin, coagulation proteins, and a variety of enzymes.

B. Restoration of this capacity requires repair of liver damage. Until this occurs, it is essential to provide replacement therapy.

C. Daily infusion of salt-poor albumin is necessary to correct acute deficits and to restore normal blood volume.

　　1. This is essential either with massive liver cell necrosis or after partial hepatec-

tomy because the liver is unable to make albumin.

    2. A dose of 25 to 50 g. of albumin is usually needed daily. Such therapy should be monitored by serum albumin measurements.

    D. Serum gamma globulin (5 to 10 ml.) should be administered to patients with acute liver injury, recurrent infection, or gram negative sepsis and hypogammaglobulinemia.

    E. Deficits of fibrinogen and other proteins needed for coagulation should be corrected.

    F. It is necessary to provide the vitamins and minerals listed under general therapy (see Table 21-4). In the patient with acute liver injury, correction of deficits of nucleogenic vitamins and minerals (folic acid, vitamin B_6, vitamin B_{12}, and zinc) is of critical importance and may be a key factor responsible for recovery.

VI. Anemia

    A. Anemia of liver disease is most commonly due to iron deficiency resulting from blood loss.

    B. A large number of patients with chronic liver disease have anemia due to folic acid, vitamin B_6, and vitamin B_{12} deficiencies.

    C. Documentation of the cause of anemia is essential so that iron is not given in absence of a deficiency state.

    D. Peripheral and bone marrow blood morphology, serum iron, serum folic acid, vitamin B_6, and vitamin B_{12} are desirable to assess the type and cause of an anemia.

    E. Therapy should consist of iron, folic acid, vitamin B_{12}, or vitamin B_6, when there is a demonstrated deficiency of any of these nutrients.

    1. With B_{12} deficiency, a single intramuscular dose of 1000 μg. of B_{12} is usually curative.

    2. Folic acid deficiency should be treated with a daily oral dose of 5 mg.

    3. If iron deficiency exists, treatment with iron must be prolonged beyond the time required to attain a hematologic response to ensure that the iron stores of the body are repleted. A dose of 300 mg. daily of ferrous sulfate by mouth for a period of 9 months is usually required.

    4. Pyridoxine (vitamin B_6) should be given in an oral dose of 25 mg./day.

    F. In patients who have general malnutrition, absorption is impaired. In these instances, it is important to correct body deficits by parenteral preparations. If iron dextron is to be given parenterally, the usual precautions attendant to its administration must be followed.

VII. Neuropathy

    A. Liver disease with secondary malnutrition is commonly accompanied by peripheral neuropathy due to decreased intake, absorption, or assimilation of the vitamins and minerals needed to maintain normal nerve function.

    B. Deficiencies of thiamine, nicotinic acid, vitamin B_6, and pantothenic acid have been found in such patients.

    C. In 80% of instances, thiamine depletion is responsible. There is often an associated deficiency of other vitamins and minerals, and general replacement is required for restoration of normal nerve function.

    D. Parenteral thiamine (5 mg.), nicotinic acid (20 mg.), vitamin B_6 (25 mg.), and pantothenic acid (20 mg.) are indicated, followed by oral supplements when general nutrition has been improved.

VIII. General Therapy for Liver Disease Without Complications

    A. Liver disease produces an increased demand for nutrients, an increased loss of nutrients, and less efficient utilization of nutrients.

    1. For these reasons, it is desirable to specifically focus on nutritional aspects of patients with liver disease and to provide

a well balanced diet and supplemental nutrients.

B. Patients with deficits may initially profit from large doses of vitamins and minerals.

1. There is no evidence, however, that megavitamin therapy will be beneficial after correction of a deficiency state.

2. Extra amounts of vitamin A, vitamin D, and nicotinic acid may produce liver injury.

3. Age and socio-economic conditions may change requirements.

4. Table 21-4 shows the specific supplements that are desirable until the liver is stabilized.

5. Patients with biliary cirrhosis should be considered for supplemental vitamins E, A, and K.

IX. Provision of Nutrient Supplements—Maintenance Dietary Program

A. Once deficits are corrected, the patient with liver disease should have a nutritious diet which will supply vitamin and mineral needs.

1. An example of a recommended balanced diet is shown in Table 21-6.

B. It is preferable to provide frequent, small feedings, calculated to provide the required calories, carbohydrates, protein, vitamins, and minerals, over a 24-hour period.

1. Food provided in this manner is assimilated, and it decreases the risk of transiently increasing portal pressure and precipitation of variceal hemorrhage.

C. Deficits may persist or reoccur in patients with chronic liver disease due to malabsorption or malutilization.

1. In these circumstances, continuous parenteral replacement therapy may be desirable.

2. Patients with hepatic disease and persisting malnutrition have decreased intestinal transport of thiamine hydrochloride and are unable to break down folylpolyglutamates. These vitamins are

Table 21-6. **Suggested Balanced Diet**

Eat Each Day	Amount
Milk Whole, skim, buttermilk, yogurt One oz. hard cheese equals 1 glass whole milk.	2 eight oz. glasses
Protein Group Chicken, turkey, fish, and lean meats, dry peas and beans, cheese or peanut butter (liver once/week), eggs (2–4/week)	5 oz. (2 average servings)
Fruits Vitamin C fruits or juice (orange, grapefruit, tomato) Other fruits (peaches, pears, berries, melons) To include 1 serving of fresh fruit	3 or more servings 2 servings 1 serving
Vegetables Dark green leafy or yellow vegetables Any other, include 1 raw Starch vegetables—potatoes, lima beans, corn	3–4 servings 1/day 1–2 1
Breads and Cereals Whole grain or enriched (bread, cooked or dry cereal, rice, spaghetti, noodles)	4 or more servings
Margarine, butter, oil, or fat	3 or more teaspoons

Approximate calories 1600, protein 65 g., sodium 2000 mg. To increase the caloric intake, the following foods may be added as tolerated: fresh cakes, cookies, other desserts, jams, and jellies.

absorbable in other forms (allithiamines and crystalline folic acid), and with chronic disease, such oral preparations should be used.

X. Nutrition in Prevention of Hepatic Disease

A. Prophylaxis of liver disease and prevention of its progression to an irreversible stage depend upon elimination of etiological factors and improvement of host resistance.

B. A common pathway is probably responsible for liver damage due to infective agents, drugs, alcoholic beverages, and toxins.

1. The noxious agent usually stimulates B- and T-lymphocytes, which in turn evoke humoral and cell-mediated immunologic reactivity.

2. Stimulated T-lymphocytes release lymphokines that are cytotoxic and fibrogenic.

C. In the case of drug- and alcohol-induced liver injury, active metabolites, produced in the endoplasmic reticulum of the liver, are covalently bound to macromolecules. This combination may cause direct toxicity or a hypersensitivity reaction.

D. The incidence and severity of the liver injury depend on the quantity of the noxious agent and host resistance.

E. Nutrition therapy can improve nutritional status and host resistance.

1. Nutrients known to have a specific antagonistic effect on the noxious agent should be provided. For example, large doses of pyridoxine hydrochloride, or pyridoxal 5-phosphate, if available, should be given because this decreases hepatic cytotoxicity of acetaldehyde, a metabolite of alcohol and a common industrial chemical.

2. General host resistance is improved by maintaining total good nutrition, especially adequate tissue levels of vitamin B_6 and folic acid required for lymphocyte reactivity and replication. In patients with hypogammaglobulinemia, it may be necessary also to give gamma globulin and specific immune globulins.

3. Maximum regenerative capacity of hepatocytes should be maintained by providing sufficient protein and by correcting deficits of nucleogenic vitamins and minerals (folic acid, vitamin B_6, vitamin B_{12}, and zinc).

22. NUTRITION IN DENTAL HEALTH

James H. Shaw, Ph.D.

I. The Ten-State Nutrition Survey* of a cross-sectional sample of 38,000 people found a high prevalence of dental caries among Americans of all ages and almost universal prevalence of periodontal disease among older Americans.

II. A tremendous need for dental care was found in many areas of the U.S.

III. Recent research has demonstrated the intimate relationship of the composition and characteristics of the diet to dental caries and possibly to periodontal disease. There is a need for sound nutrition to improve oral health and to decrease the very high incidence of dental caries and periodontal disease.

SOFT TISSUE PATHOLOGY

I. General Principles

A. The various stresses to which oral tissues are subjected, due to food texture, temperature ranges from cold to hot, and variations in physical, chemical, and microbial stimuli, make them more susceptible to breakdown as a result of certain nutritional deficiencies than more protected tissues of comparable nature elsewhere in the body.

B. Pathology of the soft tissues of the mouth has received special attention because its presence in the mouth as an early indication of deficiency states is readily available for observation and evaluation during a physical examination.

C. As a result of the greater public awareness of the need for good nutrition

through balanced diets and particularly through the enrichment of milk with vitamin D, of various products with ascorbic acid, and of cereal grains and their products with various members of the vitamin B-complex, frank nutritional deficiencies have largely disappeared from the American scene.

D. Physicians and dentists are much less likely to look closely for oral deficiency signs today than they were 30 years ago.

II. Clinical Manifestations

A. Vitamin C Deficiency (Scurvy)

1. In a severe deficiency of vitamin C, the gingivitis, swelling, and hemorrhage of the gums are early and definitive signs.

2. The lesions begin on the interdental papillae with hyperemia and a tendency for the dilated thin-walled vessels to hemorrhage. Infection with ulceration, granulations, and necrosis may result.

3. In cases of prolonged deficiency, the diseased gums may become sufficiently large to interfere with mastication and the periodontal membrane and the alveolar bone surrounding the tooth roots disintegrate, causing increased mobility of the teeth and tooth loss.

4. Poor oral hygiene appears to increase the likelihood of gingival abnormalities in scurvy.

5. In the absence of teeth, scorbutic signs are not evident on the dental ridges.

6. If scurvy occurs while teeth are developing, the odontoblasts decrease in height and metabolic activity, so that little or no dentin is formed. The pulp also becomes atrophic and hyperemic.

7. No evidence of increased caries sus-

*Ten-State Nutrition Survey, 1968–1970. III Clinical, Anthropometry, Dental Health Services and Mental Health Administration Center for Disease Control, U.S. Department of Health, Education, and Welfare. Atlanta, Georgia. DHEW Publication (HSM) 72–8131.

ceptibility has been reported to be associated with scurvy.

B. Niacin Deficiency (Pellagra)

1. In acute deficiency, changes in mucous membranes, chiefly in the mouth, are quite characteristic with scarlet glossitis and stomatitis.

2. At first, the tip and margins of the tongue and the buccal mucosa around Stensen's duct become scarlet.

3. If the deficiency is prolonged, the entire tongue and oral mucous membranes develop a bright scarlet hue with tenderness of the mouth, increased salivation, and edema and swelling of the tongue.

4. Ulcers may develop under the tongue, on the lower lip, and opposite the molars.

C. Riboflavin Deficiency

1. The oral evidences of ariboflavinosis are most frequent on the lips and tongue.

2. Cheilosis and angular stomatitis are common in adults and are manifest by chapping, edema, and by vertical markings of the lips, which may become quite atrophic in chronic deficiency states.

3. In atrophic cheilosis, the exposed mucosa becomes like parchment and vertical fissures disappear.

   a. The angles of the mouth are especially affected, becoming erythematous and macerated with dermatitis of the adjacent skin and superimposed infection.

4. Cheilosis also occurs in pyridoxine and iron deficiency states as well as in edentulous persons in whom the vertical dimension has decreased.

5. Riboflavin deficiency probably also causes a magenta coloration of the tongue, which is superimposed upon a chronic glossitis.

D. Vitamin D Deficiency (Rickets)

1. In the rachitic child, the areas of enamel and dentin which are being formed during the deficiency are poorly mineralized.

2. Because remodeling cannot occur in enamel and dentin due to their acellular

nature, the hypomineralized areas cannot be repaired.

3. In mild cases, the hypomineralized areas are only discernible by preparation of ground sections.

4. In more severe or prolonged cases, the inadequately mineralized areas may result in hypoplastic pits or lines on the enamel surface.

5. Some investigators believe that proneness to caries may be increased as a result of enamel hypoplasia.

III. Management

A. Vitamin B-Complex Deficiencies

1. Because the likelihood is high that a B-complex deficiency is present at a subclinical level in any person who exhibits oral evidence of pellagra or ariboflavinosis, treatment should be with a multivitamin preparation containing five to ten times the recommended daily allowance until a remission of the oral signs has occurred.

B. Vitamin C Deficiency

1. The usual therapeutic dose should be in the range of 250 to 1000 mg./day.

C. Vitamin D Deficiency

1. Slow repair of rickets will occur with the provision of 400 I.U. of vitamin D daily.

2. More rapid recovery will occur when four to five times this dosage is provided daily.

3. In cases of refractory rickets, a much higher intake must be provided.

   a. When these high levels are required, the patient must be under the close supervision of a physician, with frequent serum calcium and phosphorus determinations.

   b. Any evidence of an elevation of serum calcium above normal must result in an immediate reduction to maintenance levels in order to prevent vitamin D toxicity.

D. The above therapeutic levels are for the period of repletion and should not be continued indefinitely unless clear evidence of increased need is found.

1. The ultimate objectives for any person with sufficiently frank nutritional deficiencies to have oral manifestations in this area must be to determine whether the deficiency was primary or whether it was conditioned by secondary problems of malabsorption or poor utilization of nutrients and to correct the underlying cause(s) of the deficiency.

2. Accomplishment of these objectives must involve evaluation of why such a gross deficiency has occurred and then design of an appropriate diet composed of foods from the basic four food groups (see Chap. 2), supplemented as necessary by a proprietary product to prevent its recurrence.

DENTAL CARIES

I. General Considerations

A. Dental caries (tooth decay) is a chronic infectious disease in which progressive destruction of tooth substance results from interactions between the metabolic products of microorganisms colonizing the tooth surfaces and the inorganic and organic components of enamel, dentin, or cementum.

B. The carious lesion invariably originates on the external enamel surface of an erupted tooth or on the cementum of a root surface that has been exposed to the oral milieu by recession of the periodontium.

C. Progression of a carious lesion varies from acute and rapid to slow and chronic, depending upon the balance of etiologic factors.

1. The area involved may vary from minute, discrete lesions in pits and fissures on the occlusal surfaces to widespread coverage of the smooth buccal and lingual surfaces.

2. The carious lesion progresses centripetally and is not usually self-limiting.

3. Its rate of development varies from relatively slow to surprisingly rapid in car-

ies-prone children. (The lesion continues to increase in area and depth until the pulp becomes infected, the crown is destroyed, periapical granulomas and abscesses may develop, and the remnants of crown and roots have to be extracted.)

D. Progress of a carious lesion can be slowed or terminated by three methods.

1. The carious lesion develops in such a way that the diseased area becomes self-cleansing and does not retain food debris to serve as nutrients for the flora.

2. The dietary habits and oral hygiene practices of the person are altered sufficiently to deprive the microorganisms of sufficient nutrients for rapid metabolism.

3. Professional mechanical intervention occurs with the removal of decayed tooth substance and its replacement by an inert substance.

E. Even in persons with rampant caries with numerous rapidly progressing lesions on several teeth, no evidence of the development of natural immunity of sufficient capability to cause any clinically discernible reduction in the future occurrence of new carious lesions has been demonstrated.

II. Etiology

The etiology of dental caries is complex and is best described in terms of the epidemiologists's triad: agent, host, and environment, with the recognition of the many interrelationships among these major facets.

A. Agent(s)

1. The mouth harbors many microorganisms due to its warmth, humidity, and the passage of food through it several times a day.

2. The microorganisms that are responsible for dental caries are able to colonize the tooth surface or a carious lesion so that their metabolic products will be held in close proximity to tooth substances.

3. These microorganisms elaborate acid and are able to metabolize rapidly,

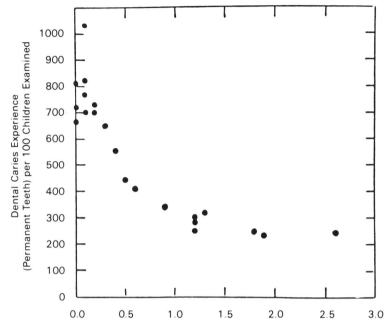

Fig. 22-1. The accumulated lifetime dental caries experience for the permanent teeth of 7257 selected 12- to 14-year-old white children from 21 cities
in four states is plotted against the fluoride content of the public water supply
in those cities. Note the low plateau in dental caries experience which is
attained between 1.0 and 1.5 ppm. of fluoride in public water supplies. (Dean,
H.T., Arnold, F.A., Jr., and Elvove, E.: Domestic water and dental caries.
U.S. Public Health Reports, *57:*1155, 1942)

even when the hydrogen ion concentration
in their surroundings is sufficiently high to
dissolve the minerals in enamel, dentin, and
cementum.

4. These microorganisms have a high
requirement for carbohydrate to enable
them to metabolize rapidly.

5. While numerous oral microorganisms have these general characteristics,
Streptococcus mutans has received special
attention in recent years due to its ability to
produce dextran (polyglucose) from sucrose, the most common sugar in the
human diet.

6. Dextran formed from sucrose enables the appropriate oral microorganisms to
colonize tooth surfaces and serves as a

nidus for the development of plaque on the
surface of the tooth on which the carious
lesion develops.

B. Host

1. The level of caries activity is dependent upon various host factors.

2. Truly genetic relationships do not
appear to be strong. Some evidence of relationships exists insofar as the inheritance of
tooth morphology, structure, and position
in the jaw are concerned.

3. Caries activity and the amount of
tooth destruction of the host are clearly influenced by such familial and cultural relationships as

a. Frequency of eating
b. Snacking habits

c. Use of sugar and sugar-containing foods and confections

d. Oral hygiene

e. Desire or ability to obtain professional dental care

4. The strongest host relationship to dental caries concerns the nutrients available during tooth development.

a. While the presence of all nutrients is necessary for the development of well-formed teeth, the nutrient of greatest importance is fluoride insofar as dental caries resistance is concerned.

b. Fluoride is not present in food supplies in adequate amounts to permit the development of teeth that are relatively resistant to dental caries.

c. The presence of 1.0 ppm. (1 mg./L.) of fluoride in the drinking water in communities in the northern temperate zone throughout the long period of tooth development has been shown to result in about one-third of the dental caries experience in comparable children in areas where the water supply contains 0.1 ppm. of fluoride (see Fig. 22-1).

d. The fluoride ion is equally effective, whether its presence in the water is due to fluoride-bearing soils or to controlled additions in water treatment plants.

e. Fluoride is also effective when provided by the parent in suitable amounts daily in a pharmaceutical preparation. The problem with this method of administration is that few parents have the discipline and concern to provide the fluoride supplement from birth up through the teenage years.

f. Fluoride exerts its beneficial influence by incorporating into the hydroxyapatite crystal lattice to replace some hydroxyl ions.

C. Environment

1. The surroundings in which a person is born and raised have pronounced influences on the extent to which dental caries will occur.

a. The best demonstration of this relationship concerns the presence or absence of appropriate amounts of fluoride in the communal drinking water.

b. As described above, fluoride operates through the host to increase the caries resistance of the teeth.

c. However, the presence or absence of an adequate amount in the communal water supply is an environmental variable that determines the dental caries experience of the children and adults who grow up in the community.

d. There appears to be an indirect relationship of dental caries experience to the annual hours of sunshine, presumably by increasing the amount of vitamin D available and thereby improving mineral metabolism.

e. Hardness of the water and dental caries experience may be directly related.

2. Children in countries where the sugar intake is low tend to have less caries than in countries where sugar intake is high.

a. Likewise in countries where food supplies are inadequate and food consumption presumably is less frequent, caries has a lower prevalence than in countries where food is abundant and food is available to consume more frequently each day.

3. The environment in the mouth around and on the teeth is of special importance.

a. Dental caries is a disease. It does not develop when food is not present in the oral cavity due to tube feeding or when the food does not contain any carbohydrates.

b. The cereal grains, as sources of carbohydrate in the form of starch, have practically no ability to initiate or support the progression of carious lesions.

c. Starch as the only carbohydrate in the diet has a limited ability to support the carious process.

d. Dietary mono- and disaccharides support the very active initiation and progression of carious lesions with generally little differentiation among the various sugars.

e. Sucrose may have a greater ability to support carious lesions in experimental animals, especially on the smooth surfaces of the molars, when *Streptococcus mutans* predominates.

f. Relatively low levels of sugars (5 to 10%) may be adequate to cause rapid progression of lesions when the total carbohydrate content of the diet, primarily as starch, is high.

g. Higher levels of sugars are needed to produce comparable levels of caries progression when the total carbohydrate content is low, and protein and fat are higher.

h. The severity of the carious process increases in proportion to the length of time that food is available for consumption in any 24-hour period.

4. A direct association between caries activity and the frequency of eating sugar-containing foods and confections has been shown in many surveys, including the Ten-State Nutrition survey. These sugar-containing items are most deleterious when their physical nature permits them to adhere to tooth surfaces or other structures in the mouth. The best example of this fact was obtained in the study conducted in Vipeholm, Sweden (see Fig. 22-2).

5. Because the six-carbon sugar alcohols, sorbitol and mannitol, are not metabolized by oral microorganisms as are sucrose or glucose, it was believed generally that these polyalchohols would not be cariogenic as sweetening agents in sugar-free foods as confections.

a. Both sorbitol and mannitol are only about one-half as sweet as sucrose and are commonly used in combination with saccharin to obtain a desirable level of sweetness.

b. Xylitol, a five-carbon sugar alcohol, is as sweet as sucrose and, like the six-carbon alcohols, is not metabolized as readily by oral microorganisms as sucrose and glucose.

c. The suggestion has been made on the basis of clinical impression that sorbitol and mannitol may be cariogenic, especially for carious lesions on root surfaces, when chewing gum or lozenges sweetened with them are used excessively. As yet no adequate clinical study has been conducted to evaluate whether these sugar alcohols are indeed cariogenic.

d. In Finland, xylitol was used as the sweetening agent in place of sucrose in many foods in a total dietary regimen in a two-year study with dental students. A striking reduction in dental caries was observed among the students on the xylitol regimen. In a one-year study in which chewing gum was sweetened with xylitol and sorbitol and other polyols in a ratio of five parts of xylitol to two of sorbitol and other polyols, caries reduction also was observed.

e. Xylitol is used as a sweetening agent in a great many confectionery products in several European countries. In the U.S., xylitol is only available as a sweetener in chewing gum. Use of xylitol in the U.S. is currently limited because its safety upon ingestion has not been established sufficiently to pass the specifications of the Food and Drug Administration.

III. Diagnosis

A. Gross open carious lesions can be observed by the layman even during a casual examination.

1. Diagnosis before one can observe gross lesions is of great importance, not only to minimize tooth loss but, more importantly, to remove diseased tissue early enough that small restorations are adequate and can be retained well and that remaining tooth structure is not weakened excessively.

2. Radiographs are an important adjunct to careful oral examinations as areas demineralized by progressing lesions, especially on the proximal surfaces, often are otherwise concealed to visual or physical exploration.

B. The most careful oral examination accompanied by radiographs is not capable

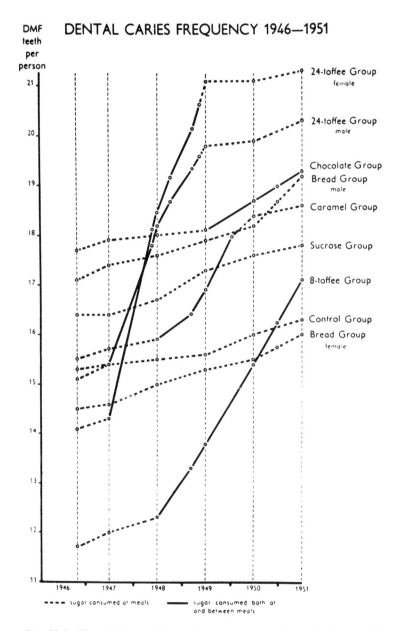

Fig. 22-2. The relation of time of sugar consumption and of type of sugar-containing items to dental caries incidence. Note striking influence of consumption of candy between meals on the dental caries experience. (Gustafson, B.E., *et al.:* The Vipeholm dental caries study: the effect of different levels of carbohydrate intake on caries activity in 436 individuals observed for five years. Acta Ondotol. Scand., *11*:232, 1954)

of revealing the earliest or preclinical lesions.

1. Sizeable progress of the lesion generally has occurred before detection is possible at the current clinical level.

IV. Management

A. Carious enamel and dentin must be removed mechanically to prevent further loss of structure.

B. The filling material must be in very close proximity to tooth substance at all points to prevent gross leakage of oral fluids between the tooth and the restoration in order to reduce the likelihood of secondary decay around the margins of the restoration.

C. The filling material must be shaped in such a way as to prevent any impingement on adjacent soft tissues.

V. Prevention

A. Dental caries affects almost every American at about three times the rate at which adequate treatment is sought or provided. Thus prevention of new lesions is of utmost importance.

B. Preventive procedures need to be directed against each of the three major etiologic factors—agent, host, and environment.

C. The preventive procedure with the best demonstrated effectiveness on a community-wide basis is the provision of adequate fluoride throughout tooth development.

1. Water fluoridation is a relatively inexpensive process.

2. In the northern U.S., 1.0 ppm. fluoride in the drinking water is appropriate.

3. In southern areas, where temperature and water consumption are higher, proportionately lower water fluoride levels are appropriate.

4. In this way, host resistance to the microbial agent and the oral environment is greatly increased.

D. A well-balanced diet of varied foods representative of the four basic food categories throughout tooth development is also important for the formation of teeth of ideal histologic and chemical structure.

1. Like all other tissues, the teeth require adequate amounts of all nutrients throughout their formation.

2. During the development of a tooth, a protein matrix is laid down which subsequently becomes mineralized.

a. As is the case with any mineralization process, the nutrients vitamin D, calcium, phosphorus, and fluoride must be present to insure sound, proper mineralization.

b. Protein-calorie malnutrition in the pre-eruptive phase may contribute to enamel hypoplasia and dental caries in the primary teeth.

c. It is possible that prolonged periods of vitamin A deficiency may result in inadequate bone growth patterns, which result in malalignment and malocclusion of the teeth.

3. Unlike all other tissues in the body, the tooth has no potential for remodeling or replacement to correct developmental deficiencies or to repair injury.

4. Proper nutrition, including adequate fluoride, throughout tooth development is even more important because of this lack of reparative ability.

5. Fluoride may also be provided by pharmaceutical preparations during tooth development to children in communities or rural areas where the water supply does not contain sufficient fluoride or cannot be fluoridated. Appropriate levels for various age groups are shown in Table 22-1.

E. Fluoridated toothpastes, or topical application of fluoride by the dentist or hygienist are important preventive procedures after tooth development.

1. They are less effective than systemic fluoride during tooth development because only the very superficial surface layers of the teeth are available for fluoride incorporation by these topical procedures.

2. Their effectiveness is also limited because each of these procedures demands patient participation and cooperation in contrast to the community-wide benefit of water fluoridation.

F. Modification of the oral environment is also an important preventive measure.

1. Its effectiveness, however, is dependent upon individual concern and cooperation. (In contrast, the benefit of water fluoridation to modify host susceptibility is community-wide.)

2. Oral environmental changes include restricting the use of sugar-containing foods and confectionery items.

3. Foods that are retained on tooth surfaces and elsewhere in the mouth, to serve as metabolites for caries-producing microorganisms, should be restricted or eliminated from the diet.

4. Elimination of undesirable between-meal snacks or replacement with items of low or negligible caries-producing potential, such as fresh fruits and vegetables, nuts, cheese, and popcorn, are essential to modify the caries potential of the oral environment.

5. Such modifications in food habits must be accompanied by systematic and frequent oral hygiene procedures to remove the microbial plaque and food debris which accumulate, even with careful food habits.

G. The oral environmental procedures recommended above operate by reducing the food available to the oral microorganisms and by removing microbial masses that serve to continually replenish the oral microbial flora. Unfortunately, as yet no direct attack upon the microbial flora with an antibiotic or germicidal agent or immunization procedure is feasible.

H. The regular oral examination is an important component of a complete preventive program.

1. The physician should routinely look for open carious lesions and refer the patient to a dentist when appropriate.

2. Regular oral examinations with nutritional advice and treatment should be scheduled at the dental office as frequently as the caries activity of a patient requires.

3. Frequency should be much greater for the caries-prone child than for the adult. Attention to total nutrition is important for most effective management of the child's medical and dental status.

I. With current knowledge of the benefits of fluoride and of modifications of the oral environment, coupled with good oral hygiene, this disease could be largely prevented.

PERIODONTAL DISEASES

I. General Considerations

A. The tissues that support the teeth in the jaws are collectively known as the periodontium or the supporting apparatus.

Table 22-1. **Supplemental Fluoride Dosage Schedule***

	Water Fluoride Content		
Age	0–0.3 ppm.	0.3–0.7 ppm.	0.7–ppm.
6 mos.–2 yr.	0.25 mg.	0	0
2–4 yr.	0.50 mg.	0.25 mg.	0
4–6 yr.	0.75 mg.	0.50 mg.	0.25 mg.
6–8 yr.	1.0 mg.	0.75 mg.	0.50 mg.
8 yr. and over	1.0 mg.	1.0 mg.	1.0 mg.†

*The amount of fluoride prescribed varies accordingly to the patient's age and the level of fluoride in the water supply. For example, a dosage of 0.25 mg./day is recommended for a 1-year-old child who lives in an area which has 0 to 0.3 ppm. fluoride in its water supply.
†Dosage increased because tooth crown formation usually complete (except for third molars).
(Parkins, F.M.: Prescribing fluoride supplements for home use. Table of supplemental dosage schedule. J. Prev. Dent., *4* [6]: 33,1977)

They include:

1. The gum tissue or gingiva, which is normally firm, pale red, and in close apposition as a cuff at the neck of the crown of each tooth

2. The periodontal membrane, which absorbs the shock of mastication and is a fibrous elastic structure surrounding the roots, largely composed of collagen fibers embedded at one end in the cementum on the root surfaces and at the other end in bone

3. The alveolar bone, which is the specialized bone surrounding and supporting the roots of each tooth

B. Any abnormality that leads to a visual change or loss of integrity of any component of the supporting tissues is listed among the category of periodontal diseases. These include:

1. Gingivitis. The most common abnormality of the supporting apparatus of the teeth is a minor inflammatory change of the gingiva, which may be localized or generalized, acute or chronic.

2. Acute Necrotizing Ulcerative Gingivitis (Vincent's Disease, Trench Mouth). This syndrome is an acute pseudomembranous ulceration affecting the marginal gingiva with inflammation and necrosis of the interdental papillae. Its onset is abrupt, painful, and is commonly accompanied by a slight fever, malaise, excess salivation, and fetid breath.

3. Periodontitis and Periodontosis. Pyorrhea and gum disease are used to refer to the gross breakdown of the supporting structures, with progressive loosening and loss of a tooth or teeth.

   a. Whereas dental caries is primarily a problem in the childhood and teenage years, pyorrhea is the major oral problem in the adult population and the major cause of tooth mortality among adults.

   b. Diagnosis of periodontitis and periodontosis is dependent largely upon an oral examination for plaque and calculus accumulations, pocket formation, and tooth mobility. Radiographic examination contributes by providing a means to estimate the extent to which the alveolar bone margin has receded due to resorption.

II. Etiology

A. The causes of some of the periodontal diseases are much less well understood than the causes of dental caries.

1. As in dental caries, the likelihood is high that agent, host, and environmental factors are interrelated in disease causation.

B. The systemic effects of nutritional status on periodontal health are probably quite important.

1. The dependence of the periodontium on an adequate supply of nutrients may be due to the rapid, continuous turnover that occurs in certain periodontal tissues.

2. Severe malnutrition can alter the resistance of periodontal tissues. The severity and progression of periodontal disease are likely to be increased when bacterial irritants are present.

C. Gingivitis

1. There is a strong direct correlation between the indices for evaluating the quality of oral hygiene and the occurrence of gingivitis.

2. The consensus is that the causative relationship of plaque to gingivitis is the irritant action of plaque on the adjacent soft tissues of the gingiva coupled with an immune response to components or metabolic products of the microorganisms in plaque.

3. Experimental vitamin C deficiency in its chronic form leads to gingivitis and bleeding of the gums. No substantial body of evidence indicates that gingivitis as routinely seen in Americans should be considered to be an evidence of scurvy. However, because ascorbic acid deficiency increases the permeability of the mucosal tissues to bacterial toxins, inadequate vitamin C in the diet may contribute to periodontal disease.

4. During pregnancy, mild inflammation of the gingiva may occur with hypertrophy of the interdental papillae. The con-

dition usually arises in the first or second month, may persist throughout pregnancy, and usually disappears after parturition.

5. Gingivitis may also be associated with diabetes and leukemia. In these conditions, systemic alterations may have made the person more prone to a gingival response to unfavorable local circumstances.

6. Hyperplasia of the gingiva with consequent gingivitis may occur with continued use of diphenylhydantoin (Dilantin). It regresses when the drug is discontinued.

D. Acute Necrotizing Ulcerative Gingivitis

1. This problem is invariably associated with a mixed infection of spirochetes and fusiform bacilli in and around the affected tissues.

2. Some clinicians believe in a strong psychosomatic component because the syndrome tends to occur with increased frequency at times of personal stress, such as during examination periods among students, and in persons who have been recently bereaved or who have marital conflicts.

3. Because the organisms found in the necrotic areas are common oral inhabitants, some local or systemic change seems to occur to allow their striking pathologic ascendancy. Substandard nutrition may play a role in these untoward changes.

E. Periodontitis

1. Local irritant factors of plaque and calculus accumulations are involved in the etiology of periodontitis. As pockets of disease appear, sites for more extensive food and microbial accumulation increase with the probability of periodontal abscess formation.

2. Because local conditions that favor periodontal breakdown often are present in persons with little or no evidence of any problem beyond simple gingivitis, host resistance to local irritants or bacterial infection is often invoked to explain lack of more advanced disease.

3. Optimal levels of fluoride in the drinking water do not appear to have any striking beneficial influence on the prevalence of periodontitis, although total nutrition status may.

III. Management and Prevention

A. Depending on the severity and rate of progression of the existing disease entity, treatment may vary from a thorough prophylaxis with a comprehensive home care program in early disease states to extensive periodontal surgery to remove pockets and recontour the gingiva in order to reduce areas where plaque and food debris can be trapped in more advanced disease states.

B. Clinicians do not agree on the dietary recommendations that should be made to the patient during periodontal treatment.

1. Some clinicians stress well-balanced diets with low amounts of fermentable carbohydrates.

2. Others routinely supplement the patient's diet with a vitamin-mineral preparation containing one or two times the recommended daily allowances.

3. Because the concern is for the total needs of the patient, the most prudent approach is to recommend the use of a well-balanced diet comprised of varied food choices from the four major food groups.

4. There should be a minimum of between-meal, high-carbohydrate snack foods and confectionery items.

5. A maintenance level vitamin-mineral supplement should also be provided if dietary evaluation or the physical condition of the patient suggests the need for additional nutrients beyond those provided by the usual diet.

SUGGESTED READINGS

Dunning, J.M.: Principles of Dental Public Health. ed. 2. Cambridge, Harvard University Press, 1970.

Jolliffe, N.: Clinical Nutrition. ed. 2. New York, Harper and Brothers, 1962.

McClure, F. J.: Water Fluoridation: The Search and the Victory. Washington, D.C., National Institutes of Health, 1970.

Nizel, A. E.: Nutrition in Preventive Dentistry: Science and Practice. Philadelphia, Saunders, 1972.

Shaw, J. H., and Sweeney, E. A.: Nutrition in relation to dental medicine. *In* Goodhart, R. S., and Shils, M. E. (eds.): Nutrition in Health and Disease. ed. 6. Philadelphia, Lea and Febiger, 1978.

Sognnaes, R. F., and Shaw, J. H.: Natural history and prevention of oral disease. *In* Leavell, H. R., and Clark, E. G. (eds.): Preventive Medicine for the Doctor in His Community: An Epidemiologic Approach. ed. 2. New York, McGraw-Hill, 1965.

23. NUTRITIONAL DISTURBANCES IN NEUROLOGY AND PSYCHIATRY

Jerry G. Chutkow, M.D.

Most nutritional neuropsychiatric disorders are associated with simultaneous alterations in the metabolism of several nutrients. Often, however, one or another substance has assumed major pathogenic significance based on the results of experimental data, chemical analysis of biologic fluids, and responsiveness to therapy.

I. Secondary Metabolic (Nutritional) Encephalopathy

A. This indicates a generalized or multifocal disturbance in neuronal or glial metabolism (or both) in the brain which results from malnutrition involving an essential nutrient.

B. Such secondary encephalopathies are potentially reversible if the systemic malnutrition is corrected.

C. The clinical picture is usually nonspecific and fluctuates in severity.

1. Included are variable combinations of depression in the level of consciousness, ranging from mild apathetic, lethargic inattention to coma and disorientation to time, distance, place, and person.

2. A generally commensurate impairment of cognition and memory occurs, as well as an unlimited variety of derangements in affect, perception, and thought, which span the entire gamut of psychiatric disorders.

3. Nonlocalizing motor signs such as symmetric hyperreflexia, stato-action tremors, instability of gait, bilateral grasp, and snouting responses may be present.

D. With few exceptions, the electroencephalogram is diffusely slowed, and the cerebrospinal fluid is normal.

II. Secondary Metabolic (Nutritional) Polyneuropathy

A. This is due to the effects of malnutrition on the peripheral nervous system.

B. It is potentially reversible if the systemic malnutrition is corrected.

C. The clinical picture is characterized by the insidious onset of a slowly progressive, predominantly symmetric impairment of appendicular strength or sensation (or both).

1. Mild to very severe hypotonic, hyporeflexic to areflexic paresis; paresthesias; dysesthesias; and diminution of one or more modalities of general somatic sensation may be seen.

2. The legs are usually involved earlier and to a greater extent than the arms; the acral portions of the extremities are affected sooner and more severely than the proximal.

VITAMIN MALNUTRITION

I. Thiamine (Vitamin B$_1$)

A. General Considerations

1. The recommended daily dietary allowance for thiamine is 0.5 to 1.5 mg., depending on the age of the individual. These requirements are best related to total caloric intake.

2. Thiamine pyrophosphate is a cofactor for numerous decarboxylases and transketolases. Of these, pyruvate decarboxylase has received considerable attention.

3. Following severe and prolonged experimental thiamine deprivation, lesions involving the glial cells and myelin sheaths of the central nervous system have been found in man and animals. Peripheral nerves may undergo axonal degeneration in man.

B. Thiamine Deficiency

1. Common Causes

a. Primary hypovitaminosis occurs as a consequence of chronic alcoholism combined with inadequate intake of food, eating polished rice as the main dietary staple, and dietary faddism.

b. Secondary thiamine hypovitaminosis may be found in patients with prolonged, recurrent vomiting; long-standing hyperthyroidism; and chronic debilitating illnesses.

(1) The illnesses frequently are compounded by intestinal malabsorption or excessive urinary loss of thiamine as a result of diuretics, renal disease, or recurrent renal dialysis.

2. Clinical Neurologic Features

a. POLYNEUROPATHY

(1) The sensorimotor polyneuropathy of beriberi, with or without generalized edema due to hypoproteinemia and congestive heart failure, may also involve the torso, facial sensation (trigeminal nerve), and the vocal cords (recurrent laryngeal nerve).

(2) Thiamine deficiency probably plays a major role in the polyneuropathy seen in long-standing alcoholism.

b. WERNICKE-KORSAKOFF SYNDROME

(1) Wernicke's disease may begin insidiously as a mild metabolic encephalopathy that subsequently is complicated, often rather abruptly, by a combination of sixth cranial nerve and supranuclear gaze palsies, vertical and horizontal nystagmus, apathetic global confusion with drowsy inactivity, and prominent cerebellar ataxia of gait.

(2) That form of Korsakoff's psychosis attributable to thiamine deficiency often becomes apparent as the confusional state of Wernicke's disease subsides, although it may develop in the absence of Wernicke's disease.

(a) The patient exhibits retrograde amnesia of varying degree and extent, extending back for months to years, antero-grade amnesia (the inability to retain most new memory traces for more than a few minutes), preservation of islands of memory which are recalled without regard to their proper temporal sequence (pseudo-confabulation), true confabulation in response to challenging questions, and no appreciation of the memory deficit (lack of insight).

(b) Sensorium is normal, and other perceptual-cognitive functions are largely intact.

(3) About 3% of hospitalized chronic alcoholics develop Wernicke-Korsakoff syndrome.

c. INFANTILE BERIBERI

(1) Infants who, during the first year of life, are fed milk that is low in thiamine may exhibit congestive heart failure, polyneuropathy with prominent involvement of the recurrent laryngeal nerve, and a syndrome resembling Wernicke's disease on which is superimposed fever, nuchal rigidity, and convulsions.

(2) The spinal fluid is said to be microscopically, bacteriologically, and chemically normal.

(3) It is seen most commonly in Southeast Asia.

d. STRACHAN'S SYNDROME

(1) The combination of a predominantly sensory polyneuropathy and loss of vision (retrobulbar neuropathy), occasionally associated with deafness and vertigo (stato-acoustic neuropathy), has been observed in the Orient and the West Indies.

(2) Its relationship to thiamine deficiency has not been proven conclusively.

3. Laboratory Tests

a. An erythrocyte transketolase activity of less than 800 μg. hexose/ml./hour (normal = 900 to 1,200 μg. hexose/ml./hour) suggests deficiency.

b. An erythrocyte transketolase activity increase of more than 25% in the presence of thiamine pyrophosphate (normal < 16% increase) is indicative of thiamine deficiency.

4. Nutritional Therapy

a. The recommended therapeutic dose of thiamine is 50 to 100 mg. administered parenterally, followed by 25 mg./day in divided doses by mouth or parenterally for 10 to 14 days, then by 5 to 10 mg./day in divided doses until the patient's nutritional status has stabilized.

b. Patients with alcoholism and illnesses which are expected to produce impaired intake or excessive loss of vitamins would probably benefit from prophylactic vitamin supplementation, including 5 to 10 mg. of thiamine per day in divided doses.

c. Probably all chronic alcoholics, and in particular those who are believed to be suffering from generalized primary hyponutrition, should be given 50 to 100 mg. of thiamine parenterally as part of their initial therapeutic program, as a prophylaxis against the Wernicke-Korsakoff syndrome.

d. All patients suffering from generalized hyponutrition and neurologic symptoms believed to be caused by hypovitaminosis should receive a high-protein, high-carbohydrate diet in increasing amounts as tolerated, aiming for an intake of about 3,000 cal./day.

(1) Because such patients have multiple vitamin deficiencies, general vitamin supplementation should be given, by the appropriate route, in doses ranging from five to ten times the recommended daily allowances.

5. Prognosis

a. Slow improvement of the polyneuropathy can be expected over a period of months, particularly if adequate physical therapy is maintained. The degree of recovery depends on the duration, extent, and severity of the neuropathy.

b. The acute ocular abnormalities of Wernicke-Korsakoff syndrome respond to thiamine within hours and usually subside completely in 2 to 4 weeks.

(1) More than half of the patients, however, have some residual gait ataxia.

c. In most patients with Wernicke's disease, the condition progresses into Korsakoff's psychosis. Of these patients, about 50% recover partially or completely.

C. Thiamine Excess

1. No neurologic disturbances secondary to thiamine excess have been described.

II. Niacin

A. General Considerations

1. The recommended daily dietary allowance for niacin ranges from 5 to 20 mg.-equivalents, depending on age (60 mg. of dietary tryptophan, the precursor of niacin, is equivalent to 1 mg. of niacin).

2. Nicotinamide, the physiologically active form of niacin, is a component of nicotinamide adenine dinucleotide and nicotinamide adenine dinucleotide phosphatase, coenzymes for a large number of enzymes involved in cellular respiration.

B. Niacin Deficiency

1. Common Causes

a. Pellagra due to primary dietary deficiencies may be seen in chronic alcoholics and diet faddists.

b. Although now unusual in the U.S., primary niacin deficiency is seen in areas of the world where corn and maize are the main dietary staples.

c. Secondary hypovitaminosis may develop in patients with gastrointestinal malabsorption and in the malignant carcinoid syndrome.

d. Niacin deficiency is commonly associated with inadequate intake of other vitamins.

2. Clinical Neurologic Features

a. Metabolic (nutritional) encephalopathy is common and characteristic.

(1) Mental symptoms are usually mild (insomnia, moodiness, fatigue, apathy, and depression) and thus nonspecific until the dermatologic and gastrointestinal manifestations of pellagra have appeared, at

which time the mental derangement may become severe.

(2) The nervous system is generally less severely affected in children than in adults.

(3) Seizures and parkinsonian features have been described.

b. Leukoencephalomyelopathy:Hyperreflexic, spastic paresis with extensor plantar responses, ataxia, diplopia, and optic neuropathy have been attributed to niacin deficiency, but the cause-effect relationship is tenuous.

c. Polyneuropathy: Some patients have objective findings of mild peripheral neuropathy. This, however, is due very likely to concomitant thiamine deficiency.

d. Hartnup disease: The relationship between the episodic cerebellar ataxia and metabolic encephalopathy and the impaired formation of nicotinamide from tryptophan is not clear.

3. Laboratory Tests

a. If the analysis is available, urinary N^1-methylnicotinamide of less than 0.5 mg./g. creatinine or 2 mg./24 hours (normal = 1.6 to 4.29 mg./g. creatinine or 12 to 18 mg./24 hours) points to niacin deficiency.

4. Nutritional Therapy

a. Institution of a well-balanced diet is indicated along with general vitamin supplementation as described in the section on thiamine.

b. The recommended therapeutic dose of nicotinamide is 200 to 400 mg./day in divided doses, orally or parenterally, until the clinical manifestations of pellagra subside.

5. Prognosis

a. The dermatologic, enteric, and encephalopathic symptoms begin to clear within hours to days after initiation of therapy.

b. Response to nicotinamide is considered diagnostic of the condition.

c. The course of the peripheral neuropathy should be similar to that described for thiamine deficiency.

C. Niacin Excess

1. No significant neurologic complications have been recorded.

III. Vitamin B_6 Complex (Pyridoxine, Pyridoxal, Pyridoxamine)

A. General Considerations

1. The recommended daily dietary allowance for Vitamin B_6 depends on the age of the individual and ranges from 0.5 to 2.5 mg./day.

2. The phosphorylated forms of the B_6 complex are essential cofactors for a number of enzymes involved in transamination and decarboxylation.

3. Pyridoxal phosphatase is the coenzyme for decarboxylation of glutamic acid to γ-aminobutyric acid, a suspected inhibitory neurotransmitter in the central nervous system.

4. Vitamin B_6 is also important in the conversion of linoleic acid to arachidonic acid.

5. In humans fed 4-deoxypyridoxine, a pyridoxine antagonist, peripheral neuropathy may develop.

B. Vitamin B_6 Deficiency

1. Common Causes

a. Primary hypovitaminosis has been described in infants who are bottle-fed artificial diets that are low in vitamin B_6.

b. Primary deficiencies presumably can occur in any hyponutritional state associated with multiple vitamin deficiencies, including chronic alcoholism.

c. Secondary hypovitaminosis should be anticipated in those conditions that produce malabsorption or increased excretory loss of water-soluble vitamins.

d. Requirements for vitamin B_6 are increased by various drugs including isoniazid (INH), hydralazine, penicillamine, cycloserine, and, probably, also by oral contraceptives.

e. Infants rarely have pyridoxine dependency.

2. Clinical Neurologic Features

a. POLYNEUROPATHY

(1) This syndrome is the one most commonly seen in patients receiving isoniazid.

(2) The relationship between vitamin B₆ deficiency and the nutritional polyneuropathies of primary and secondary hypovitaminosis has not been established.

b. METABOLIC ENCEPHALOPATHY

(1) Nervousness, irritability, and generalized or partial motor convulsions develop in infants who are fed diets that are low in B₆ for 3 days to 10 months or, rarely, in neonates who have an increased metabolic requirement for the B₆ vitamin complex.

(2) The electroencephalogram is markedly abnormal.

3. Laboratory Tests

a. Excretion of urinary xanthurenic acid in excess of 50 μmol./24 hours (normal <50 μmol./24 hours) after a 2.0-g. load with L-tryptophan has been used as evidence of vitamin B₆ deficiency.

4. Nutritional Therapy

a. INFANTS

(1) Five to 10 mg. of pyridoxine per day should be given as a therapeutic trial to infants with convulsive disorders of unknown etiology.

(2) By the end of 6 to 12 months, an infant's diet usually contains adequate amounts of vitamin B₆.

b. ADULTS

(1) The recommended therapeutic dose of pyridoxine is 10 to 50 mg./day combined with general vitamin B-complex supplementation.

(2) Patients taking large doses of isoniazid (20 mg./kg. body weight per day) should receive 50 mg. of pyridoxine a day.

5. Prognosis

a. Pyridoxine promptly stops seizures and causes the electroencephalogram to revert to normal in infants and young children suffering from a lack of or an increased dependency on pyridoxine.

b. The peripheral neuropathies may improve over a period of months, the ulti-

mate degree of recovery depending on the duration, extent, and severity of peripheral nerve involvement.

C. Vitamin B₆ Excess

No neurologic side effects have been described.

IV. Vitamin B₁₂ (Cobalamin)

A. General Considerations

1. The recommended daily dietary allowance for vitamin B₁₂ is 2 μg. in adults, 0.3 μg. in infants, and 2.5 to 3.0 μg. in pregnant and lactating women.

2. Vitamin B₁₂ is required for the conversion of methylmalonate to succinate and of homocysteine to methionine. The former reaction ties cobalamin in with carbohydrate and lipid metabolism; the latter, with the formation of tetrahydrofolate and indirectly with the synthesis of thymidylic acid, a DNA precursor.

3. Vitamin B₁₂ is particularly important in the maintenance of myelin, especially that derived from oligodendroglia.

B. Vitamin B₁₂ Deficiency

1. Common Causes

a. With rare exceptions, the deficiency state results from intestinal malabsorption of vitamin B₁₂, either due to absence of gastric intrinsic factor or secondary to one of a large number of intestinal disorders.

2. Clinical Neurologic Features

a. METABOLIC ENCEPHALOPATHY

(1) Irritability, confusion, and a variety of affective-thought disorders may evolve into dementia of varying severity, even before the hematologic picture of vitamin B₁₂ deficiency is evident—a qualification that is true of all neurologic complications of hypovitaminosis B₁₂.

b. DEMYELINATING MYELO-POLYRADICULONEUROPATHY

(1) Initially, the patient complains of sensory disturbances in the acral portions of the limbs, which slowly progress proximally, suggesting a peripheral neuropathy. The arms may be involved before the legs.

(2) In time, however, evidence of upper motor neuron involvement, and, ultimately, autonomic nervous system involvement appears.

(3) In the more advanced stages, the characteristic neurologic picture is that of subacute combined degeneration of the spinal cord: mixed spastic-ataxic appendicular motor dysfunction; hyporeflexic to areflexic weakness with extensor plantar responses; and multimodality sensory deficits, the proprioceptive and epicritic senses being most severely impaired. Precipitous urinary frequency may be present.

c. BILATERAL OPTIC NEURO-PATHY

(1) Although uncommon, impaired visual acuity with scotomatous visual field defects and optic atrophy has been observed, mainly in males who smoke a great deal and who have a vitamin B_{12} deficiency.

(2) Whether so-called alcohol-tobacco amblyopia is due to vitamin B_{12} deficiency has not been settled.

3. *Laboratory Tests*

a. Serum levels of vitamin B_{12} are less than 170 pg./ml. (normal values = 170 to 760 pg./ml. by radioimmunoassay)

b. Radioactive vitamin B_{12} absorption studies without and with intrinsic factor and the presence or absence of histamine-fast achlorhydria, chemical and roentgenologic indicators of intestinal malabsorption, and the radioactive B_{12} absorption test results will help determine the cause of the deficiency.

4. *Nutritional Therapy*

a. The recommended therapeutic dose of vitamin B_{12} is 100 μg. daily, intramuscularly or deep subcutaneously, for 1 to 3 weeks, followed by 100 μg. three times a week until the blood picture is completely normal.

b. Maintenance doses of 50 to 100 μg. per month appear to be adequate thereafter.

c. The duration of treatment de-pends on the cause of the vitamin B_{12} malabsorption.

d. Patients with pernicious anemia must receive parenteral therapy indefinitely.

5. *Prognosis*

a. Early diagnosis of vitamin B_{12} deficiency, in patients with compatible neurologic symptoms, is essential to prevent serious and permanently incapacitating neurologic deficits.

b. Treatment usually produces improvement except in advanced cases.

c. Progression is always arrested by adequate therapy.

d. The degree of neurologic recovery appears to depend more on the duration of the symptoms than on their severity or extent.

e. Patients with a picture of subacute combined degeneration of the spinal cord should never be given folic acid alone unless one is absolutely sure that the body stores of vitamin B_{12} are normal. Whereas the megaloblastic anemia of pernicious anemia responds to folic acid, the neurologic lesions do not.

C. *Vitamin B_{12} Excess*

1. No neurologic disturbances have been reported with prolonged administration or ingestion of large quantities of vitamin B_{12}.

V. Vitamin A

A. *General Considerations*

1. The recommended daily dietary allowance for vitamin A ranges from 1,500 I.U. in the infant to 5,000 I.U. in the adult.

2. As with all other vitamins, pregnancy and lactation increase the need for vitamin A.

3. Carotenes are the precursors of the various forms of vitamin A.

4. Vitamin A is essential for the integrity of epithelial cells and the formation of the visual pigments, rhodopsin and the iodopsins.

B. Vitamin A Deficiency

1. Common Causes

a. Primary dietary deficiency of vitamin A is found most often in children and is particularly prevalent in tropical regions throughout the world.

b. Secondary hypovitaminosis A occurs as a consequence of intestinal malabsorption, defective conversion of carotene to vitamin A (hypothyroidism and diabetes), rapid destruction (prolonged, sustained fevers), and renal disease (excessive excretory loss).

2. Clinical Neurologic Features

a. Night blindness (nyctalopia)

b. In infants, several neurologic symptoms or lesions have been reported, including mental retardation, facial nerve palsies, hydrocephalus, and increased intracranial pressure.

3. Laboratory Tests

a. A concentration of vitamin A in plasma of less than 10 μg./dl. (normal = 20 to 50 μg./dl.) is evidence of deficiency.

b. A concentration of carotene of less than 20 μg./dl. (normal = 20 to 50 μg./dl.) is also an indication for therapy.

4. Nutritional Therapy

a. The recommended therapeutic dose of vitamin A is 25,000 to 30,000 I.U. orally per day for 1 to 2 weeks.

b. If evidence of keratomalacia, dryness with ulceration, and perforation of the cornea occurring in severe vitamin A deficiency, is present, 100,000 I.U. intramuscularly in a water-dispersible form should be given immediately and continued for several days, followed by 25,000 I.U. orally, as above.

5. Prognosis

Night blindness and early corneal lesions clear completely in a few days.

C. Vitamin A Excess

1. Common Causes

a. Ingestion of 50,000 to 500,000 I.U. of vitamin A per day, depending on the age of the patient, usually for months

b. Infants and adults may become acutely intoxicated after ingestion of 300,000 I.U. or more in a single dose.

2. Clinical Neurologic Features

a. Acute overdosage causes an acute metabolic encephalopathy.

b. Chronic intoxication is often heralded by headache and mild personality changes.

c. Increased intracranial pressure is common to both forms.

d. The clinical picture of longstanding hypervitaminosis A in adults is that of pseudotumor cerebri: headache, palsies of the abducens nerves, and papilledema. In infants and young children, full fontanelles and separation of the cranial sutures are seen.

e. The cerebrospinal fluid is usually normal.

f. The ventricular system is smaller than normal, and no mass lesions can be identified by computerized tomographic scans of the head or by pneumoencephalography.

g. Hypervitaminosis A is the likely diagnosis if the above features are coupled with a compatible history, coarse hair, hepatomegaly, and painful hyperostosis of the extremities and of the occipital regions of the skull.

3. Laboratory Tests

a. Plasma vitamin A may or may not be elevated.

4. Nutritional Therapy

a. Discontinue vitamin A.

5. Prognosis

a. The pseudotumor cerebri should resolve completely.

VI. Other Vitamins

A. Riboflavin

1. Ariboflavinosis is rarely encountered without symptomatic evidence of deficiencies of other B vitamins.

2. Therefore, one cannot convincingly attribute isolated reports of polyneuropathy or electroencephalographic changes to lack of this vitamin.

3. A urinary level of riboflavin of less than 27 μg./g. creatinine (normal = 80 to 270 μg./g. creatinine) suggests a deficiency state.

4. Riboflavin should be given to all patients who have thiamine and niacin deficiencies.

5. The recommended therapeutic dose is 10 to 40 mg./day until the neurologic and dermatologic disturbances subside. Alternatively, dry yeast tablets, 30 g. three times a day, may be used.

B. Pantothenic Acid

1. Symptoms suggesting spinal cord disease or polyneuropathy have been attributed to pantothenic acid deficiency.

2. The relationship is tenuous, at best, in humans, although lesions have been described in the central and peripheral nervous systems in animals that have been fed diets low in pantothenic acid.

C. Vitamin C

1. Scurvy, vitamin C deficiency, usually is found in improperly fed infants and in persons who live alone and cook for themselves (bachelor scurvy).

2. If severe, the generalized bleeding tendency may produce a broad spectrum of transient or permanent neurologic deficits, depending on the site, size, and rate of the intracranial hemorrhage.

3. The recommended therapeutic dose of ascorbic acid is 300 to 500 mg./day, either as the vitamin alone or in one of the citrus juices.

4. Citrus juices generally contain 40 to 50 mg. of vitamin C per 100 ml.

D. Folic Acid

1. Isolated instances of metabolic encephalopathies, neurologic syndromes compatible with subacute combined degeneration of the spinal cord, hereditary ataxia, and neuropathy have been reported in patients with malabsorptive disorders or congenital defects in folate metabolism.

2. In some of these patients, deficiency of vitamin B$_{12}$ has been excluded, and the acute syndromes have improved coincident with administration of folic acid.

3. The relationship between neurologic dysfunction and lack of folic acid is still in doubt. Serum folate of less than 3 ng./ml. (normal = 3 to 12 ng./ml. by radioimmunoassay) suggest folic acid deficiency.

4. The recommended therapeutic dose of folic acid is 5 to 10 mg./day.

5. Vitamin B$_{12}$ deficiency must be rigorously excluded before folic acid is given because folic acid has an adverse effect on the neurologic complications of B$_{12}$ deficiency.

E. Generalized Vitamin B-Complex Deficiency and the "Burning Feet Syndrome"

1. The central feature of this syndrome ("hot feet," "happy feet") is the complaint of severe burning paresthesias and aching of the feet, worse at night, with dysesthesias (distortion of sensation).

2. Patients commonly seek relief by soaking their feet in cold water.

3. Hyperhidrosis (excessive sweating) and vasomotor disturbances may be present.

4. Other clinical and electromyographic findings of peripheral neuropathy are usually lacking.

5. Although this syndrome has been attributed to generalized B-vitamin deficiency, a definitive relationship has not been established.

6. A therapeutic trial of B-vitamin supplementation has been recommended.

MINERAL MALNUTRITION

I. Sodium

A. General Considerations

1. The role of sodium in the regulation of the exchange of water across cellular membranes, both systemically and in the central nervous system, is well known.

2. While the movement of sodium from plasma to the cerebrospinal fluid appears to be regulated in part by active transport, the blood-C.S.F. barrier has little

homeostatic function in the presence of hyponatremia or hypernatremia.

3. Sodium is also essential for the generation of the action potential in excitable tissues.

B. Sodium Deficiency (Hyponatremia)

1. Common Causes

a. A net depletion of the sodium content of soft tissues usually is due to an uncompensated loss of sodium through the kidney or in perspiration. This may be the result of the excessive use of diuretics, regulatory hormonal failure, renal disease, prolonged fever, or poor acclimatization.

b. Dilutional hyponatremia secondary to excessive ingestion of water or to its retention produces the same neurologic picture.

2. Clinical Neurologic Features

a. Altered peripheral neuromuscular excitability. The symptoms are nonspecific and include coarse fasciculations or cramps and hyporeflexic weakness of appendicular muscles.

b. Metabolic encephalopathy: Apathy and disorientation may progress rapidly to convulsions, coma, and death, depending on the acuteness of onset and severity of the hyponatremia.

3. Laboratory Tests

a. Symptoms usually occur when the concentration of serum sodium has decreased to the range of 115 to 127 mEq./L., depending on the rate of sodium loss or dilution.

b. At serum levels of 90 to 105 mEq./L., most individuals exhibit severe central neurologic abnormalities.

4. Nutritional Therapy

a. Identifying and treating the cause for the depletion of sodium is of utmost importance.

b. The route, preparation, and rate used for replacement of sodium losses must be adjusted to any underlying cardiac, renal, or endocrine dysfunction.

c. If water overload is present, the intake of water may have to be restricted.

5. Prognosis

a. The clinical features of uncomplicated hyponatremia resolve rapidly after the electrolyte imbalance has been corrected.

C. Sodium Excess (Hypernatremia)

1. Common Causes

a. Primary sodium hypernutrition is rare and usually results from inadvertent administration of excessive salt to infants and repeated ingestion of sea water.

b. Hypernatremia almost always reflects uncompensated loss of water in excess of sodium and may be a complication of severe diarrhea, prolonged sweating, extensive dermatologic disease, posterior pituitary failure, osmotic diuresis, prolonged coma with inadequate water intake, or renal disease.

2. Clinical Neurologic Features

a. DIFFUSE METABOLIC ENCEPHALOPATHY

(1) The clinical picture of hyperosmolar encephalopathy is dominated by progressive obtundation, meningeal signs (due to blood in the cerebrospinal fluid), rigidity, and focal or generalized convulsions.

(2) Patients who are not in coma often complain of thirst.

(3) The classic features of dehydration (loss of skin turgor and dry mucous membrane) usually complete the clinical picture.

3. Laboratory Tests

a. Hypernatremia is defined as a concentration of serum sodium greater than 150 mEq./L. However, symptoms are usually not seen until sodium is in excess of 155 mEq./L.

4. Nutritional Therapy

a. Emergency treatment should begin with plasma-expanding solutions in volumes large enough to correct hypovolemia, followed by a more gradual replenishment of calculated total body water deficits.

b. Careful monitoring of serum electrolytes, hematocrit, and urinary output is important in order to avoid overhydration and the precipitation of hyponatremic, hypo-osmolar encephalopathy.

5. *Prognosis*

a. The outlook for functional recovery depends on the presence and extent of parenchymal or extraparenchymal intracranial hemorrhages and vascular occlusions.

b. Infants and children are much more susceptible to such vascular complications than are adults.

II. Potassium

A. *General Considerations*

1. The ratio of extracellular to intracellular concentration of potassium determines the resting membrane potential of nerve and muscle cells.

2. Changes in potassium metabolism do not usually affect the central nervous system, because of the protective blood-brain-cerebrospinal fluid barriers.

B. *Potassium Deficiency (Hypokalemia)*

1. *Common Causes*

a. With rare exception, net deficits of total body potassium are due to uncompensated loss through the kidneys or gastrointestinal tract.

b. Such losses may occur in renal failure or tubular dysfunction, or they may result from an increase in secretion of endogenous mineralocorticoids or an excess administration of exogenous mineralocorticoids.

c. Use of diuretics, diabetic ketoacidosis, repeated vomiting, diarrhea, and gastrointestinal fistulas can contribute to potassium deficiency.

2. *Clinical Neurologic Features*

a. Severe potassium depletion may produce variable degrees of hypo-excitability of the peripheral somatic motor and autonomic nervous system, as evidenced by mild- to severe hypotonic, hyporeflexic paresis.

b. Appendicular muscles are involved to a greater degree than truncal, and

muscles innervated by the cranial nerves are often spared.

c. Abdominal distention, reflecting gastrointestinal atony, is common.

d. A metabolic myopathy may occur with subacute and chronic potassium depletion.

3. *Laboratory Tests*

a. The serum concentration of potassium is almost always reduced.

b. The severity of the hypokalemia does not correlate well with the degree of depletion of cellular potassium.

c. Hypochloremic alkalosis may be present.

d. The electrocardiogram shows progressive depression of the S-T segment, an inversion of a rounded T wave, and a prominent U wave.

4. *Nutritional Therapy*

a. The cause of the hypokalemia must be determined and corrected whenever possible.

b. Potassium chloride may be admindministered orally or parenterally, depending on the urgency for treatment and the cause of the electrolyte disturbance.

5. *Prognosis*

a. The paresis is reversible with therapy.

C. *Potassium Excess (Hyperkalemia)*

1. *Common Causes*

a. Potassium intoxication is usually seen in renal failure or as the consequence of the inadvertent administration of excessive amounts of potassium parenterally.

2. *Clinical Neurologic Features*

a. Hypotonic, hyporeflexic appendicular paresis rapidly progressing to flaccid, areflexic quadriplegia with less severe involvement of truncal muscles, and relative sparing of muscles supplied by cranial nerves, may accompany rising extracellular levels of potassium.

b. Patients often complain of paresthesias and may have impairment of vibratory and position sense.

c. The picture simulates that of a

rapidly evolving, predominantly motor, metabolic peripheral neuropathy.

d. Abrupt cardiac arrest is an ever-present threat.

3. Laboratory Tests

a. Changes in the electrocardiogram characterized by the development of tall, "tented" T waves, decreasing amplitude of the P wave culminating in atrial asystole, and progressive widening of the QRS that may terminate in ventricular standstill appear in mild form at serum potassium levels of 6 to 8 mEq./L.

b. Cardiac standstill is probable at a concentration of 9 to 10 mEq./L.

c. The neuromuscular manifestations become evident when hyperkalemia is severe.

4. Nutritional Therapy

a. In acute situations, the infusion of 1 L. of 10% glucose in water containing 50 units of crystalline insulin is recommended.

b. If the patient is acidotic, and there are no cardiovascular contraindications, 100 to 300 mEq. of sodium bicarbonate may be given.

c. One to 2 g. of calcium lactate may decrease the toxic effects of potassium on the heart.

d. Long-term treatment includes low-potassium diets, 20 to 30 g. of sodium polystyrene sulfonate (Kayexalate) orally every 6 hours, cathartics, and renal dialysis when indicated.

5. Prognosis

a. Hyperkalemia is potentially life-threatening.

b. All neurological symptoms are reversible when the hyperkalemia is corrected.

III. Calcium

A. General Considerations

1. Calcium is essential for the stability of excitable cellular membranes, the release of peripheral (and perhaps central) neuro-transmitters, and excitation-contraction coupling in muscle.

2. The concentration of calcium in the cerebrospinal fluid is relatively independent of acute fluctuations of calcium levels in plasma, by virtue of carrier-mediated transport across the choroid plexuses.

3. The transport of calcium into the brain has not been well studied.

B. Calcium Deficiency

1. Common Causes

a. Nutritional depletion of total body calcium can result from hypovitaminosis D secondary to inadequate exposure to sunlight coupled with primary dietary deficiency of the vitamin.

b. Intestinal malabsorption of calcium due to disease of the small bowel, pancreas, or liver also leads to hypocalcemia.

c. Neonatal hypocalcemia usually begins between the fifth and tenth days of life; childhood tetany due to vitamin D deficiency is seen most often between the ages of 4 months and 3 years.

d. Hypoparathyroidism is another etiological mechanism.

e. The concentration of calcium in blood serum rarely is beyond the normal limits of 9 to 11 mg./100 ml. of serum.

2. Clinical Neurologic Features

a. PATHOGENESIS

(1) The neurologic syndrome of calcium deficiency is caused by a decrease in the concentration of ionized calcium in the systemic extracellular fluid when symptoms are referable to the peripheral nervous system.

(2) A decrease in the levels of calcium in the cerebrospinal and parenchymal interstitial fluid of the central nervous system is presumably present when the manifestations indicate a central disturbance.

b. PERIPHERAL NEUROMUSCULAR HYPERIRRITABILITY

(1) The syndrome of overt tetany includes paresthesias, spontaneous muscle twitching progressing to cramps, and epi-

sodic carpal, pedal, or laryngeal spasms, occurring alone or in combination.

(2) Whether massive tonic contractions of muscle resembling the tonic phase of a grand mal fit can occur with tetany has not been resolved.

(3) Latent tetany is present when carpal spasm *(main d'accoucheur)* can be induced by ischemia of the arm with or without superimposed respiratory alkalosis (Trousseau's sign) and, of less diagnostic reliability, when facial twitching can be precipitated by percussion of the facial nerve (Chvostek's sign).

c. SECONDARY METABOLIC ENCEPHALOPATHY

(1) Seizures are most often seen in children and may occur in the absence of tetany.

(2) Usually the convulsions are grand mal, but they may be partial (focal) motor, sensory, or complex (psychomotor seizures) and may be followed by evanescent postictal neurologic deficits (Todd's phenomenon).

3. *Laboratory Tests*

a. Hypocalcemic tetany usually appears when the total calcium concentration is less than 7.0 mg./dl. (assuming a normal albumin concentration) or when the level of ionized calcium is less than 4.3 mg./dl. (normal = 5.9 to 6.5 mg./dl.).

b. In hypovitaminosis D, plasma 25-hydroxycholecalciferol is less than 10 ng./dl. (normal = 20 to 48 ng./dl.).

c. In tetany, the electromyogram shows fibrillations and fasciculations, plus doublet, triplet, and multiple muscle-action potentials that progress to a full interference pattern.

d. When metabolic encephalopathy is present, the electroencephalogram may show generalized or focal paroxysmal dysrhythmias superimposed on a slow background activity.

4. *Nutritional Therapy*

a. The cause of the hypocalcemia must be determined before rational treatment can be instituted.

b. If the problem is hypovitaminosis D, supplementation of the diet with sufficient vitamin D to provide 400 I.U./ day, coupled with adequate dietary calcium and exposure to sunlight, is adequate.

c. In an emergency, 1 to 2 g. of calcium as a 10% solution of calcium chloride can be administered slowly intravenously.

5. *Prognosis*

a. The acute neurologic symptoms usually clear promptly after correction of the hypocalcemia.

b. Long-standing, untreated hypocalcemia may be associated with permanent mental defects.

C. *Calcium Excess*

1. *Common Causes*

a. There are two major nutritional causes of hypercalcemia.

(1) Vitamin D intoxication—ingestion of vitamin D considerably in excess of 400 I.U./day by infants and children, and often as much as 50,000 to 100,000 I.U./day for prolonged periods of time by adults.

(2) The milk-alkali syndrome

b. Numerous medical conditions may produce hypercalcemia. These include hyperparathyroidism, metastatic and nonmetastatic neoplasms, and disease of bone complicated by immobilization.

2. *Clinical Neurologic Features*

a. Secondary metabolic encephalopathy

(1) Although a variety of psychiatric symptoms have been attributed to mild hypercalcemia, unequivocal evidence of a diffuse encephalopathy is uncommon before the concentration of calcium in serum reaches 14 mg./100 ml.

(2) Above this level, the degree of depression of the central nervous system corresponds reasonably well to the severity of the hypercalcemia.

(3) A marked confusional state progressing to coma develops with calcium concentrations in excess of 16 mg./dl.

(4) Rapidly deteriorating renal

function usually contributes to the clinical situation.

(5) Seizures of any type and focal neurologic signs are said to be rare.

b. Depressed function of the peripheral neuromuscular and autonomic nervous systems

(1) The appearance and severity of myopathic-like proximal limb girdle weakness, of more generalized hypotonic, hyporeflexic appendicular paresis, and of intestinal hypomotility, tend to parallel the rising concentration of serum calcium.

(2) The threat of cardiac asystole is great at calcium levels in the range of 16 mg./dl.

3. *Laboratory Tests*

a. Serum calcium levels are readily available.

b. Changes in serum and urinary electrolytes, parathormone levels, and various infusion procedures have been used to unravel the cause of hypercalcemia (see Chap. 20).

4. *Nutritional Therapy*

a. Vitamin D and calcium intake must be stopped or markedly decreased.

b. Severe hypercalcemia is a potentially lethal condition if not corrected promptly.

c. Mithramycin, glucocorticoids, oral and intravenous phosphates and furosemide have been used to treat hypercalcemia.

5. *Prognosis*

a. Ultimately, the outcome depends on the cause of the hypercalcemia.

b. The encephalopathic symptoms usually subside over a period of several days after the serum calcium has been successfully lowered.

c. The peripheral manifestations also respond well.

d. Severe, irreversible mental retardation has been described in infantile hypercalcemia secondary to excessive intake of vitamin D.

IV. Magnesium

A. General Considerations

1. Magnesium is an activator of numerous enzymatic reactions.

2. It also antagonizes the effect of calcium on the release of peripheral neurotransmitters and appears to regulate the sensitivity of post-synaptic membranes in the central nervous system.

3. Magnesium appears to play an important role in the contraction of skeletal muscle.

4. The central nervous system is protected from the harmful consequences of acute fluctuations in the concentration of magnesium in the systemic fluids by means of a tight blood-brain barrier, as well as a carrier system in the choroid plexuses which transports magnesium into the cerebrospinal fluid.

B. Magnesium Deficiency

1. *Common Causes*

a. A prolonged negative magnesium balance is most often due to the combination of long-standing intestinal malabsorption and inadequate intake, as in prolonged parenteral fluid therapy and in chronic alcoholism with or without alcoholic hepatopathy.

b. Excessive use of diuretics by patients with congestive heart failure can lead to low serum magnesium levels.

c. Hypomagnesemia may accompany a variety of other conditions, including acute tubular necrosis, hyperparathyroidism, and diabetic ketoacidosis.

d. The prevalence of primary magnesium hyponutrition is currently a subject of debate.

e. Neonatal hypomagnesemia is an uncommon but well established disorder that has many causes.

2. *Clinical Neurologic Features*

a. Metabolic encephalopathy: A confusional state with myoclonus, tremors, and convulsions may develop acutely or subacutely in patients with prolonged uncorrected magnesium losses. A syndrome characterized by multiple neurotic complaints, hypochondriasis, and anxiety has been attributed to magnesium deficiency. The connection between this particular psychopathy and mild degrees of magnesium deficiency is still in doubt.

b. Latent or overt tetany: Tetany which does not respond to or is made worse by administration of calcium and which improves after treatment with magnesium has been reported in some, but not all, patients with hypomagnesemia.

3. *Laboratory Tests*

a. Hypomagnesemia is frequently mild and asymptomatic.

b. A decrease in serum concentration of magnesium should be viewed as significant and should be treated promptly if a patient has signs of central or peripheral neurologic hyperirritability that is unresponsive to calcium therapy. Usually, in such cases, the concentration of magnesium is definitely and, often, markedly low.

c. Isolated hypomagnesemia is rare. Commonly, other electrolyte imbalances are present, particularly hypokalemia.

d. According to recent experimental studies and a few clinical reports, if the concentration of magnesium is low in the cerebrospinal fluid (less than 2.0 mEq./L. when measured by atomic absorption spectrophotometry) in a patient with a metabolic encephalopathy, it is likely that magnesium deficiency is either the sole cause of or is contributing to the neurologic problem.

4. *Nutritional Therapy*

a. Patients on prolonged parenteral fluid therapy should receive from 100 to 200 mg. of magnesium per day.

b. In adults with a metabolic encephalopathy believed to be due to magnesium deficiency, $MgSO_4$ or an equivalent amount of magnesium chloride or magnesium acetate can be given intramuscularly or by slow intravenous drip. The suggested amount of magnesium administered per day in divided doses may range from 1,200 to 1,500 mg. in the first 24 hours, 600 to 700 mg. on the second day, and 350 to 400 mg. thereafter until the patient's condition stabilizes and the predisposing factors are treated (2 ml. of a 50% solution of $MgSO_4$ contains 49 mg. of magnesium per milliliter).

c. In neonates and young children, the suggested dose of magnesium in an emergency is 0.5 ml. (0.25 to 1.0 ml.) of 50% $MgSO_4$ given intramuscularly. This may be repeated two or three times per day, depending on the clinical response of the infant. Therapeutic maintenance doses for infants should be approximately 0.25 ml./kg. of 50% $MgSO_4$ per day initially. This should be diluted to about a 10% concentration.

d. The dose of magnesium must be adjusted for changes in renal function, and serum levels of magnesium should be monitored closely.

5. *Prognosis*

a. The neurologic symptoms clear rapidly with correction of the hypomagnesemia.

C. *Magnesium Excess*

1. *Common Causes*

Hypermagnesemia may appear in the course of renal failure; after parenteral or oral administration of magnesium salts, particularly to patients with depressed renal function; and after $MgSO_4$ enemas in rare instances.

2. *Clinical Neurologic Features*

a. Serum magnesium levels two to three times normal are usually asymptomatic.

b. Beyond this point, increasingly severe hypermagnesemia is accompanied by a progressive blockade of peripheral neuromuscular, neuroeffector, and autonomic ganglionic chemical transmission, thereby producing a hyporeflexic, hypotonic weakness of the somatic muscles and hypotension.

c. Acute hypermagnesemia probably has no direct effect on the function of the central nervous system.

3. Laboratory Tests

a. The serum magnesium is always elevated in symptomatic magnesium intoxication.

4. Nutritional Therapy

a. One to 2 g. of a 10% solution of calcium chloride administered slowly and intravenously will usually ameliorate or completely reverse the symptoms of acute magnesium intoxication.

b. Acute hypermagnesemia usually resolves if the patient's renal function is good.

c. Clinically symptomatic chronic hypermagnesemia is probably rare and occurs only in patients who have renal failure, particularly after the administration of magnesium-containing antacids or cathartics.

5. Prognosis

a. The neurologic symptoms of hypermagnesemia are completely reversible.

b. The ultimate outlook, therefore, depends on the cause of the condition.

V. Iodine

A. General Considerations

1. The recommended daily requirement for iodine necessary to maintain optimal synthesis of thyroid hormones is about 200 μg./day for children and 70 to 100 μg./day for adults.

2. These figures will vary from one region to another, depending on the quantity of goitrogenic substances in the diet.

B. Iodine Deficiency

1. Common Causes

a. Inadequate dietary intake of iodine is most commonly seen (if iodized salt is not used) in remote geographic areas which have no access to the sea (high plateau regions) where iodine has been leached from the soil.

2. Clinical Neurologic Features

a. The neurologic manifestations of severe iodine deficiency are those of hypothyroidism.

b. Endemic cretinism produces a secondary metabolic encephalopathy manifested by delayed or arrested psychomotor development. This usually becomes apparent between the sixth and twelfth months of life. Deaf mutism is prominent, and a variety of upper motor neuron findings may be present.

(1) When these features are coupled with the classic facial, cutaneous, and skeletal findings of cretinism, the diagnosis is evident.

c. If severe hypothyroidism is present in endemic goiter of adulthood, the patient may present with a metabolic encephalopathy characterized by pronounced psychomotor slowing, various psychiatric symptoms with paranoid overtones, and cerebellar ataxia.

(1) Peripheral neuropathic symptoms including sensorineural hearing loss, appendicular paresthesias, and compressive bilateral carpal tunnel syndromes are common.

(2) Some patients have evidence of a metabolic myopathy with generalized myotonic weakness. Children may also have muscular hypertrophy.

(3) Myxedema coma of the elderly is a rare complication of hypothyroidism, regardless of the cause.

3. Laboratory Tests

a. The combination of low serum thyroxine and triiodothyronine levels, high thyroidal uptake of radioactive iodine, and decreased urinary excretion of iodine is characteristic of iodine deficiency.

4. Nutritional Therapy

a. Iodine replacement using iodized salt is the recommended form of treatment.

5. Prognosis

a. Endemic cretinism must be treated early if permanent residua are to be avoided.

b. The neurologic complications of hypothyroidism accompanying endemic goiter in the adult are reversible.

VI. Trace Metals

A. Copper

1. There are no recorded nutritional disorders of copper in human beings clearly associated with reproducible neurologic symptoms.

2. Copper deficiency arising from defective transport of copper across the intestinal mucosa in trichopoliodystrophy (Menkes' kinky hair syndrome) and chronic copper retention in hepatolenticular degeneration (Wilson's disease) are due to heritable defects in the metabolism of copper.

B. Zinc

1. Zinc deficiency in humans has been associated with habitual dietary avoidance of meat and other animal products, excessive demands during pregnancy, chronic alcoholism, liver disease, intestinal malabsorption, chronic renal disease, and recurrent febrile illnesses.

2. Impairment or perversions of taste and smell are the most commonly described disturbances.

3. Zinc-responsive, acute alterations in mentation and pancerebellar dysfunction have been reported following oral administration of histidine, an amino acid that causes excessive urinary excretion of zinc, with and without azauridine.

4. Serum and urinary concenttrations of zinc are low in zinc deficiency, (normal serum concentration of zinc averages about 90 ± 10 µg./dl. and urinary zinc, 530 ± 80 µg./24 hours when measured by atomic absorption spectrophotometry).

5. The recommended therapeutic dose of zinc is 20 mg. as $ZnSo_4$ twice daily.

C. Manganese

1. Chronic inhalation of manganese-containing dust, an occupational hazard of manganese mining and ore crushing, produces a chronic progressive encephalopathy manifested by emotional instability, memory impairment, generalized muscular weakness, and an extrapyramidal syndrome resembling parkinsonism upon which is superimposed dystonic posturing of the trunk and limbs.

2. Manganese workers should be removed from contact with the ore dust as soon as the initial symptoms appear.

3. L–dopa has been reported to be effective in the treatment of the extrapyramidal symptoms.

D. For more information on trace metals, see Chapter 19.

PROTEIN-CALORIE MALNUTRITION

I. General Considerations

A. Primary protein and, therefore, essential amino acid hyponutrition may cause defective growth and function of the central nervous system in infants and small children suffering from kwashiorkor.

1. Deficient caloric intake produces marasmus or inanition.

B. In general, the nutritional needs of the central nervous system are maintained whatever the expense to the less essential systems in the body.

C. There are experimental data to indicate that permanent defects may result if starvation occurs during those periods when the cells of the brain are undergoing active differentiation and maturation (e.g., during the first 2 years of life; see Chap. 26).

D. Prolonged total caloric deprivation in the adult, on the other hand, often has no immediate or long-term functional and biochemical effects.

II. Clinical Neurologic Features

A. Kwashiorkor usually appears between the ages of 1 and 3 years, often after a child has been transferred from breast milk to a high-carbohydrate, low-protein diet.

B. If the syndrome is severe (generalized edema; desquamating hyperkeratosis;

sparse, silky, golden-red hair; xerostomia; and multisystem dysfunction), the child becomes apathetic and irritable and may evidence delayed appearance or regression in psychomotor developmental milestones, presumably because of a secondary metabolic encephalopathy.

C. Approximately one-third of these patients have localized or generally slow electroencephalograms.

D. Interestingly, anywhere from 6 days to several weeks after the onset of treatment, a syndrome termed kwaski shakes may develop. It consists of coarse tremors, rigidity, appendicular postural disturbances, hyperreflexia, and myoclonus, all of which may persist for an additional 3 to 6 weeks.

III. Laboratory Tests

A. Levels of plasma proteins and amino acids are decreased.

IV. Nutritional Therapy

A. The patient should be provided with a diet that includes 2 to 3 g. of protein/kg./day, preferably in the form of milk.

B. Dehydration, hypoglycemia, and electrolyte imbalances including magnesium deficits must be corrected.

V. Prognosis

A. Many of the encephalopathic symptoms are reversible.

B. The incidence of persistent defects in higher mental function has not been determined.

SUGGESTED READINGS

Burch, R.E., and Sullivan, J.F. (eds.): Symposium on trace elements. Med. Clin. North. Am., *60:*653, 1976.

Chutkow, J.G.: Metabolism of magnesium in the central nervous system: Relationship between concentrations of magnesium in cerebrospinal fluid and brain in magnesium deficiency. Neurology (Minneap.), *24:*780, 1974.

Dodge, P.R., Prensky, A.L., and Feigin, R.D.: Nutrition and the Developing Nervous System. St. Louis, C. V. Mosby, 1975.

Henkin, R.I., Patten, B.M., Re, P.K., and Bronzert, D.A.: A syndrome of acute zinc loss: Cerebellar dysfunction, mental changes, anorexia, and taste and smell dysfunction. Arch. Neurol., *32:*745, 1975.

Löken, A.C.: Vitamin deficiencies. *In* Minckler, J. (ed.): Pathology of the Nervous System. vol. 2. New York, McGraw-Hill, 1971.

Victor, M., Adams, R.D., and Collins, G.H.: The Wernicke-Korsakoff Syndrome: A Clinical and Pathological Study of 245 Patients, 82 With Post-Mortem Examinations. Philadelphia, F. A. Davis, 1971.

Vimken, P.J., and Bruyn, G.W. (eds.): Handbook of Clinical Neurology, vol. 28. Metabolic and Deficiency Diseases of the Nervous System, Part II. New York, North-Holland Publishing, 1976.

24. CUTANEOUS ASPECTS OF NUTRITIONAL DISORDERS

Albert M. Lefkovits, M.D.

In nutritional diseases, as in other systemic illnesses, the skin reflects internal disorders. In the U.S. and other industrialized countries, cutaneous manifestations of malnutrition tend to occur primarily in association with alcoholism, general inanition, gastrointestinal malabsorption, and lack of knowledge about nutrition.

The steadily rising proportion of elderly people living alone and in restricted economic circumstances who lack incentive to prepare nutritious meals and who select soft foods, often of high carbohydrate content because of poor dentition, will undoubtedly lead to more frequently recognized nutritional problems.

DERMATOLOGICAL MANIFESTATIONS OF NUTRITIONAL DISORDERS

Table 24-1 summarizes the most frequently encountered states of nutritional deficiency and excess with cutaneous manifestations.

The following comments pertain only to the clinical cutaneous manifestions. These deficiency states tend to be seen in combination with each other more frequently than separately, which modifies their appearance.

I. Cutaneous Aspects of General Protein Deficiency

A. Protein deficiency occurs both as part of general caloric starvation, called marasmus, and in the presence of adequate caloric intake, known as kwashiorkor.

B. In underdeveloped countries, marasmus and kwashiorkor constitute important predisposing factors in high infant- and childhood mortality.

C. Marasmus causes an emaciated "skin-and-bone" or "monkey" facies, with loss of subcutaneous fat, giving a listless, vacuous look to the comparatively prominent eyes. The thin, dry skin does not have the edema which is characteristic of kwashiorkor.

D. Kwashiorkor is endemic throughout large areas of India, Asia, and Africa. A few cases may be seen in Europe and the U.S.

1. The edema, giving rise to the apparent "swollen belly," is due to hypoalbuminemia.

2. Gamma globulin may be increased, accompanied by low alpha- and beta globulins.

3. Aside from edema, muscle wasting, diarrhea, and retardation of mental and physical development are generally seen.

4. The many cutaneous signs include cheilosis, circumoral pallor, and generalized edema.

a. The skin develops erosive desquamation and then exfoliation, and the skin becomes a reddish brown color.

b. This gives rise to a dermatosis variously described as "flaky," "enamel paint," "crazy paring," or "

c. The dry, lusterless, brittle hair thins out and may take on a light red-brown color and then turn grey, or develop the "flag sign" or *signe de la bandera* in which bands of light and dark pigmentation alternate, reflecting periods of better and worse nutrition.

d. The typically stiff and curled hair of the African child may soften and straighten.

(Text continues on p. 347.)

Table 24-1. Cutaneous Manifestations of Nutritional Deficiency Disorders

Nutritional Substance and Recommended Daily Allowance	Dietary Source	Signs of Deficiency State	Reported Consequences of Excessive Intake	Comments and Reported Therapeutic Uses
Vitamin A 5,000 I.U.	Milk, butter, eggs, liver (carotene in vegetables, tomatoes, carrots)	Follicular hyperkeratosis (pirynoderma), dryness of skin, (ocular manifestations include Bitot's spots, xeropthalmia, impaired night vis on, blurring, and dryness of the cornea)	Swelling and fragility of bone and cartilage, alopecia, patchy erythema, purpura hepatotoxicity, pseudotumor cerebri	Pityriasis rubra pilaris, ichthyosis, ichthyosiform erythroderma, skin manifestations usually associated with other nutritional deficiencies, alcoholism malnutrition
Vitamin B$_1$—thiamine, aneurin 1 mg.	Unrefined cereal and rice, peas, beans, nuts, liver, pork, kidney, fresh green vegetables	Beriberi, edema, redness and burning of the tongue, peripheral neuropathy, burning feet		Generalized inanition
Vitamin B$_2$—riboflavin 2.5 mg.	Milk, liver, green vegetables, egg white	Sebor-hea-like dermatitis, glossitis, stomatitis, perleche, dermatitis of the scrotum or vulvae, (oro-oculo-genital syndrome)		
Vitamin B$_6$—pyridoxine 2–3 mg.	Yeast, grain, egg yolk, meats, liver, vegetables	Dermatitis, acrodynia, convulsions, anemia (clinical deficiency uncommon)		Deficiency may be induced by isoniazid, hydralazine hydrochloride
Vitamin B$_{12}$ 1–2 µg.	Widely distributed in animal tissue, especially liver, kidney, meat, fish	Infrequent hyperpigmentation, neuritis, macrocytic anemia most common manifestation.		Deficiency seen in absence of intrinsic factor and in post-gastrectomy patients
Niacin equivalent 1–2 mg.	Yeast, liver, meat, poultry, peanuts, legumes	"The three D's,"—dermatitis, dementia, diarrhea, photosensitivity (Casal's necklace)		Deficiency seen in carcinoid syndrome, Hartnup disease, homocystinuria, competitive inhibition by INH
Biotin 150 µg.	Liver, kidney, yeast, milk, egg yolk	Only seen in experimental volunteers Non-pruritic desquamation, lingual pallor and atrophy.		

Nutrient (dose)	Sources	Clinical findings	Comments
Vitamin C 1 mg./kg.	Citrus fruits, leafy vegetables, kidney, liver, roe, milk	Scurvy-delayed wound healing, swelling and bleeding of gums, perifollicular hemorrhages, broken curled hairs (cork-screw hair), hematomas, anemia	Scattered reports of renal stones, gastritis and esophagitis, induction of B_{12} deficiency
Vitamin D 400 U.S.P. Units	Homogenized milk	Rickets	Hypercalcemia reported in patients with sarcoidosis
Vitamin E 0.5 mg./kg. for children 10–30 mg. for adults	Vegetable oil	No documented clinical deficiency in humans, but laboratory evidence of impaired biochemical function has been reported.	Deficiency associated with pancreatic disease and malabsorption.
Vitamin K 1–2 mg.	Dark green leafy vegetables, tubers, seeds, some fruits	Hematuria, ecchymoses, bleeding, purpura	
Calcium 0.8–1.4 g.	Dairy products, dark green vegetables	Patchy alopecia of the scalp, axillary and pubic areas; eyebrows and eyelashes, cutaneous and oral candidiasis	Deficiency associated with malabsorption and hypoparathyroidism
Zinc 10–15 mg.	Meat, seafood (especially oysters and herring), milk, nuts, legumes, whole grains, wide natural distribution	Photophobia, glossitis, stomatitis, onychodystrophy, secondary bacterial and yeast infections, deficient host defense mechanisms, especially macrophage and monocyte function, defective neutrophil chemotaxis, delayed wound healing, hyperkeratosis	Deficiency associated with hyperalimentation syndrome; acrodermatitis enteropathica.

(Continued)

Table 24-1. Cutaneous Manifestations of Nutritional Deficiency Disorders (Continued)

Nutritional Substance and Recommended Daily Allowance	Dietary Source	Signs of Deficiency State	Reported Consequences of Excessive Intake	Comments and Reported Therapeutic Uses
Iron 10–15 mg.	Eggs, meat, especially liver, green vegetables	Atrophic glossitis, alopecia, anemia	Hemosiderosis seen in patients with porphyria cutanea tarda symptomatica, hemochromatosis due to increased Fe absorption from intestines, maybe associated with alcoholism and aminoacidurias Symptoms may be exacerbated.	
Protein 70–85 g.		Kwashiorkor appears in children after weaning: severe protein deprivation with adequate caloric intake, "swollen belly," impaired mental and physical development, "crackled skin" with hyperpigmentation, thin, light hair, prematurely gray or light red brown Marasmus is protein deprivation in generalized starvation: dry, thin, wrinkly, inelastic skin, skin-and-bones appearance, eventual death		

e. Finally, the eyebrows may become affected.

5. Kwashiorkor means the "sickness of the weanling," due to the fact that it typically starts after the child no longer has access to its mother's milk. The most effective therapeutic approach is dietary supplementation with a high quantity of good quality protein.

II. Cutaneous Lesions and Vitamin A

A. Vitamin A deficiency often presents with diminished night vision and can progress in extreme cases to produce keratomalacia and xerosis of the cornea and conjunctiva (xerophthalmia).

B. The skin changes, marked by hyperkeratinization, roughness, and dryness, are called follicular hyperkeratosis, phrynoderma, or toad skin.

1. Microscopically, the hair follicles may be blocked with large horny plugs, the sweat glands can atrophy and sometimes can display keratinizing metaplasia.

2. It should be noted that some physicians feel these changes are due not only to vitamin A deficiency but may be linked to deficiencies of linoleic acid, vitamin B-complex, or vitamin C.

C. American physicians are more likely to encounter an excessive intake of vitamin A than a deficiency state. This is due to ready access to potent oral vitamin A preparations, and excessive intake can lead to alopecia, pseudotumor cerebri, hepatotoxicity, patchy erythema, and purpura.

D. On an empirical basis, vitamin A therapy has been used with varying degrees of success in several disorders of keratinization of the skin. The usual daily dose administered is 25,000 to 50,000 I.U. taken orally.

E. Topical treatment with retinoic acid, a derivative of vitamin A is helpful in some cases of acne vulgaris and Darier's disease.

III. Hypercarotenemia

A. Yellow or orange discoloration of the skin may occur when the total serum carotenoid concentration exceeds 250 µg./100 ml. (normal range 80 to 120 µg./ml.).

B. It is caused by grossly excessive ingestion of carrots, yellow leafy vegetables, citrus fruits, and tomatoes.

C. Hypercarotenemia does not affect the sclera or mucous membranes. There is also an absence of pruritus. These characteristics may be used to differentiate it from jaundice.

D. The pigmentation is caused by excretion of carotenoids in sebum and sweat which are then reabsorbed by the stratum corneum. Consequently, the changes are most marked where sweat and sebaceous glands are abundant and the stratum corneum is thickest.

E. When due to the excessive consumption of tomatoes, in which lycopene constitutes 90% of the carotenoid pigments, the condition is more properly designated lycopenemia and has been reported in association with vacuolization of the liver.

F. Finally, derangement of carotenoid metabolism has been reported with some cases of hypothyroidism and hyperlipemia.

G. Obviously, while these associated metabolic disorders must be treated, hypercarotenosis itself does not affect general health and usually disappears promptly with discontinuance of excessive carotenoid ingestion.

IV. Cutaneous Lesions and the B Vitamins

A. Basic Principles

1. Because the B vitamins are generally distributed as a group in foods, it is more common to see multiple, rather than any single, B-vitamin deficiencies.

B. Thiamine (B₁)

1. The chief cutaneous manifestations

of thiamine deficiency consist of erythema, edema, a burning sensation of the tongue, and edema of the ankles, face, and hands associated with a peripheral neuropathy.

2. Consumption of polished rice and chronic alcoholism are frequent predisposing factors.

3. The many other manifestations of severe thiamine deficiency, wet beriberi and dry beriberi are discussed in Chapter 27 and Chapter 23.

C. Riboflavin (B₂)

1. Oro-oculo-genital syndrome covers the spectrum of manifestations of a riboflavin deficiency, consisting of

   a. Magenta tongue (smooth, purplish-red, tender)

   b. Perlèche, or maceration and fissuring at the angles of the mouth

   c. Cheilosis, or vertical fissuring of the vermilion border of the lips

   d. Conjunctivitis and epithelial keratitis with amblyopia

   e. Dermatitis of the scrotum or vulvae

   f. Rather severe, greasy seborrheic dermatitis-like involvement of the ear lobes, malar area, alae nasi, and nasolabial fold.

2. The prompt response to therapy with 5 mg. of riboflavin daily is striking.

D. Niacin (Nicotinic Acid)

1. Niacin deficiency results in pellagra, known by the "three D's"—dermatitis, diarrhea, and dementia.

2. Pellagra was first described by Casal in 1730, and the events culminating with Golderger's studies constitute one of the most fascinating chapters in medical history.

3. Exacerbation of the dermatological manifestations correlates with sun exposure and local pressure and trauma.

   a. The lesions begin with erythema, itching, and burning.

   b. Vesiculation, cracking, and scaling often ensue, followed by brittleness, hyperkeratosis, and hyperpigmentation of the involved areas, with an underlying pink skin.

   c. The symmetrical distribution of the lesions on the sun-exposed areas and their sharp line of demarcation is noteworthy.

   d. Dermatological signs

      (1) Casal's necklace, a sharply defined band-like eruption around the neck

      (2) a boot-like eruption of the front and back of the legs

      (3) involvement of the feet extending from the toes to the malleoli

      (4) involvement of the dorsa of the hands and forearms to form a "gauntlet" or "glove"

   e. "Goose skin" with fissuring of the palms overlying thickened, scaling, hyperpigmented skin of the fingers, marks the involvement of the hands.

   f. The neck and face are also frequently affected, but there is an area of normal skin below the hair line.

   g. Interestingly, even in the absence of sun exposure, the elbows, knees, forearms, nape of the neck, eyelids, and scrotum or perineum may be involved, closely resembling the oro-oculo-genital syndrome of riboflavin deficiency.

4. Glossitis, present as a raw, beefy, painful, swollen tongue, is frequently accompanied by angular stomatitis and cheilosis.

5. Proctitis is also a frequent accompaniment.

6. Traditionally, pellagra was seen in areas where maize or corn constituted the chief dietary staple, and, for this reason, was a widespread problem among poorer economic groups in the southern U.S., where corn bread constituted an important part of the diet.

7. Pellagra can be seen in alcoholism, Hartnup disease, carcinoid syndrome, and in patients treated with isoniazid.

8. The diagnosis should present no difficulty when the classic features enumerated above are seen, but, at times, pellagra

must be differentiated from various photosensitivity eruptions and even kwashiorkor.

9. Therapy, consisting of 500 mg. of niacinamide a day for 2 to 3 weeks, produces rapid and dramatic improvement.

E. Pyridoxine (B₆)

1. Pyridoxine deficiency in industrialized countries is more likely to result from secondary causes than from inadequate nutritional intake.

2. These secondary factors include

a. Alcoholism

b. Loss of vitamins through excessive oxidation or renal clearance

c. Impaired phosphorylation due to inhibition by deoxypyridoxine

d. Chemical inactivation of the phosphorylated vitamin, as in patients receiving isoniazid and hydralazine hydrochloride

e. Intestinal malabsorption

f. Occasionally, defective intracellular transport

3. Increased metabolic demands encountered in pregnancy or febrile states may create a relative deficiency.

4. Urticaria and asthma have been reported in xanthurenicaluria, an apparently recessive condition in which aprokynureninase has been implicated in causing relative pyridoxine deficiency.

5. The requirements for pyridoxine are increased by anovular drugs.

6. Cutaneous manifestations include seborrhea-like dermatitis, which is most pronounced around the mouth, nose, nasolabial folds, eyes, and eyebrows and which spreads to the neck.

a. The perineum, scalp, buttocks, and shoulders may be involved.

b. Glossitis and cheilosis resembling that seen, respectively, in niacin and riboflavin deficiency have been noted.

F. Cyanocobalamin (B₁₂)

1. B₁₂ deficiency has been held to be responsible for symmetrical hyperpigmentation of the palms, dorsal aspects of the hands, wrists, and forearms, extensor surface of the thighs and legs, and face.

2. This hyperpigmentation, seen together with macrocytic anemia, has been reported among Indian and Nigerian populations but not in Caucasian populations.

3. Finally, B₁₂ deficiency has been noted in patients with vitiligo who lack extrinsic factor.

G. Biotin

1. Biotin deficiency, induced experimentally, produces a transient nonpruritic, scaling dryness and desquamation, along with lingual pallor and atrophy of the lingual papillae.

H. Vitamin C (Ascorbic Acid) Deficiency—Scurvy

1. Adequate ascorbic acid is important for the normal development and maintenance of teeth, bone, collagen, and the connective tissue around the capillaries.

2. Infantile scurvy is most commonly seen between 6 and 12 months of age and results from inadequate formulas.

3. The elderly living alone and not eating fruit and vegetables are most likely to develop adult scurvy.

4. In infants, pseudoparalysis, tenderness of the legs, and nervous irritability are the most common presenting signs.

5. Bleeding around the gums and from the body orifices may be seen.

6. Adults develop perifollicular petechiae and hyperkeratotic papules, associated with broken-off "corkscrew" hairs.

7. Easy bruisability, ecchymoses over the shins, and subungual splinter hemorrhages develop.

a. Both decreased perivascular collagen and vacuolar degeneration of the capillary endothelial cells, resulting in the discontinuity of the endothelial lining, contribute to red cell extravasation.

8. In later stages, especially in patients with preexisting periodontal disease, the gums develop spongy edema, ulceration, apthae, and tend to bleed easily.

9. Addisonian pigmentation has also been described, along with woody edema in chronic adult cases.

10. Therapy should be initiated with

300 mg./day for infants and 100 mg. to 500 mg. for adults, both in divided doses.

V. Cutaneous Lesions and Vitamin K

A. Vitamin K deficiency may result in easy bruisability and ecchymosis.

B. The differential diagnosis from other bleeding disorders is made by appropriate hematological tests, which show prolonged prothrombin time corrected by vitamin K administration.

C. Malabsorption states including sprue can interfere with absorption of this fat-soluble vitamin (as well as of vitamins A and E).

D. Additionally, oral anticoagulants including Coumadin and salicylates antagonize the pharmacological action of vitamin K.

VI. Cutaneous Lesions and Linoleic Acid

A. Linoleic acid and other essential fatty acid deficiencies have been experimentally produced in both rats and, in normal, full term, healthy infants fed a diet deficient in linoleic acids, producing dry scaling skin with perianal irritation and intertrigo.

B. These changes were reversed by restoring linoleic acid to the diet.

C. However, because of the adequate distribution of linoleic acid in milk and cereal grains, this deficiency has not been seen clinically.

VII. Zinc

A. The role of zinc, as of other trace elements, is just beginning to be understood.

B. Apparently functioning as a coenzyme, zinc deficiency produces scaling and parakeratosis.

1. In humans, deficiency appears to be related to impaired wound healing and increased susceptibility to infection.

2. Recently, zinc deficiency has been shown to play an important role in acrodermatitis enteropathica.

a. This is a potentially fatal, genetically transmitted infantile disease characterized by failure to thrive, alopecia, diarrhea with malabsorption, and vesiculobullous lesions around the body orifices and extremities often with secondary candidiasis.

b. A similar syndrome in adults recently seen in patients receiving intravenous hyperalimentation is also responsive to zinc.

3. Reports of the efficacy of oral zinc in acne vulgaris requires corroboration.

VIII. Calcium

A. Calcium deficiency can result in patchy alopecia of the scalp, axillary and pubic area, and of the eyebrows and eyelashes with cutaneous and oral candidiasis.

B. Deficiency of calcium is usually associated with malabsorption and hypoparathyroidism.

IX. Iron

A. Iron deficiency resulting in microcytic anemia produces an atrophic glossitis.

B. Additionally, cases of alopecia, especially in women, are apt to be associated with iron deficiency.

SUGGESTED READINGS

Cairns, R. J.: Metabolic and nutritional disorders. *In* Fitzpatrick, T.: Textbook of Dermatology. pp. 1870–1888. Oxford University Press, 1972.

Ginsburg, R., Robertson, A., and Michel, B.: Acrodermatitis enteropathica. Arch. Dermatol., *112*:653, 1976.

Hansen, A.E., *et al.:* Role of linoleic acid in infant nutrition. Pediatrics, *31*:171, 1963.

Jacobs, E. C: Oculo-oro-genital syndrome: A deficiency disease, Ann. Intern. Med., *35*:1049, 1951.

Kay, R.G., Tasman-Jones, C., Pybus, J., Whiting, R., and Black, H.: A syndrome of acute zinc deficiency during total parenteral alimentation in man. Ann. Surg. *183*:331, 1976.

Lever, W. F., and Schaimberg-Lever, G.: Histopathology of the Skin. ed. 5. p. 157. Philadelphia, J. B. Lippincott, 1975.

Lynch, W., and Roenigk, H.: Acrodermatitis enteropathica. Arch. Dermatol., *112*:1304, 1976.

McLaren, D. S.: The vitamins. *In* Bondy, P. K.: Duncan's Diseases of Metabolism. ed. 6. pp. 1280–1320. Philadelphia, W. B. Saunders, 1969.

Moschella, S.: Diseases of nutrition and metabolism. *In* Moschella, S. L., Pillsbury, D. M., and Hurley, H. J. J.: Dermatology. pp. 1237–1248. Philadelphia, W. B. Saunders, 1975.

Stimson, W. H.: Vitamin A Intoxication in adults. N. Engl. J. Med., *265*:369, 1961.

25. NEW CONCEPTS ON CALCIUM, VITAMIN D, AND SKELETAL DISORDERS

Louis V. Avioli, M.D.

I. Vitamin D Metabolism

A. The functions of vitamin D in the body are

1. Increasing the intestinal absorption of calcium and phosphorus

2. Facilitating the mineralization, modeling, and remodeling of bone

B. Vitamin D must be activated by both the liver and kidneys before exerting its biological activities.

C. Following the ultraviolet conversion of 7-dehydrocholesterol to cholecalciferol (vitamin D_3) in the skin, the cutaneously synthesized vitamin D_3 then mixes in the blood with the vitamin D_3 and vitamin D_2 (ergocalciferol) which have been absorbed from dietary sources.

D. The combined vitamins D_2 and D_3 then are converted by a hepatic microsomal system to 25-hydroxycholecalciferol ($25OHD_3$) and 25-hydroxyergocalciferol ($25OHD_2$) respectively.

E. Both $25OHD_3$ and $25OHD_2$ (hereafter designated 25OHD) are transported in protein-bound forms to the renal cortex.

1. There they are further metabolized to 1,25-dihydroxycholecalciferol ($1,25(OH)_2D$).

F. Both 25OHD and $1,25(OH)_2D$ serve as biological forms of vitamin D which regulate calcium and phosphorous absorption from the intestine and bone mineralization and growth.

G. It is now established that 25OHD normally circulates at concentrations averaging 20 ng./ml., whereas $1,25(OH)_2D$ blood levels approximate 30 pg./ml.

II. Vitamin D Requirements

A. Despite a wide variation in both the mineral requirements and skeletal turnover of growing children, young adults, and pregnant lactating females, it has been estimated that a vitamin D intake of 400 I.U./day produces satisfactory calcium and phosphate retention in each of these groups.

B. Vitamin D_2 (ergocalciferol) or vitamin D_3 (cholecalciferol) are equally potent as dietary supplements.

C. The recommended daily dose of 400 I.U. actually may exceed the amount needed to maintain skeletal integrity and calcium homeostasis in adults.

D. It is recognized that vitamin D metabolites gain access to the fetus and that neonatal circulating levels of 25OHD correlate directly with maternal levels.

E. Whereas prematurity might cause a delay in the hepatic hydroxylation of vitamin D to 25OHD, the 2-day-old neonatal liver appears to be quite capable of performing the enzymatic 25-hydroxylation.

F. The vitamin D requirement of a healthy adult has never been clearly defined but probably does not exceed 200 I.U./day.

1. Under ordinary circumstances, this requirement is readily met by the average diet and casual exposure to sunshine.

G. Major dietary sources of vitamin D are limited to foods of animal origin. Liver oils and body oils of fish constitute the richest natural source.

H. Vitamin D is also present in good quantities in the livers of cattle, pigs, sheep, and chickens.

1. Other meats, human milk, and non-irradiated cow's milk are all poor sources (see Table 25-1).

III. Vitamin D-Deficiency Disorders

A. Following the discovery that antirachitic activity could be produced in animals and food by ultraviolet radiation, dietary or nutritional rickets was virtually eliminated as a major medical problem.

B. Nutritional rickets, or osteomalacia, is relatively rare in adults.

1. The mature skeleton with its relatively slow turnover rate is able to withstand short periods of vitamin D deficiency without deleterious effects.

2. Vitamin D depots are often more than sufficient to maintain normal mineral homeostasis.

C. Nutritional or conditioned deficiencies of vitamin D may develop in adults of any age when the diet contains less than 70 I.U. of vitamin D per day.

D. The usual dietary history obtained when vitamin D deficiency is found is of total avoidance of fatty foods or being a strict vegetarian.

E. Immigrants, premature infants, elderly females, and persons who routinely ingest food with excessive phytic acid content appear to be most susceptible to the nutritional form of osteomalacia.

1. This disorder characteristically responds to small doses of vitamin D.

F. In contrast to the relative rarity of simple vitamin D-deficiency syndromes, a variety of disorders have been described with increasing frequency which can be related either to a malabsorption of vitamin D or to disturbances in its metabolic rate.

G. Clinical disorders of vitamin D may represent either exaggerated or blunted responses to vitamin D.

1. Insufficient knowledge of the metabolism of vitamin D and the relative insensitivity of bioassay techniques have led to the above characterizations.

2. It is commonplace to speak of an abnormal sensitivity to vitamin D in patients with sarcoidosis or idiopathic hypercalciuria.

3. A resistance to vitamin D is present in familial hypophosphatemic rickets, renal osteodystrophy, gluten-sensitive enteropathies, and primary biliary cirrhosis.

Table 25-1. **Vitamin D Content of Unfortified Foods (I.U./100 g. unless otherwise stated)**

Butter	35
Cheese	12–15
Cream	50
Egg yolk	25 I.U./average yolk
Halibut	44
Herring, fresh, raw	315
canned	330
Liver, beef, raw	9–42
calves, raw	0–15
lamb, raw	17–20
pork, raw	44–45
chicken, raw	50–67
Mackerel, fresh, raw	1100
Milk, cow's	0.3–4 I.U./100 ml.
human	0–10 I.U./100 ml.
Oysters	5 I.U./3 to 4 medium-sized
Salmon, fresh, raw	154–550
canned	220–440
Sardines, canned	1150–1570
Shrimp	150

Yendt, E.: Vitamin D. *In* International Encyclopedia of Pharmacology and Therapeutics. vol. 1. pp. 197-235. New York, Pergamon Press, 1970)

4. An antagonism exists between glucocorticoids and vitamin D.

H. The availability of sensitive, quantitative assays for 25OHD and 1,25(OH)$_2$D has not only led to a more sophisticated analysis of the underlying disorders of vitamin D metabolism in some of the above described clinical syndromes, but it has also provided a rational means for therapeutic intervention.

IV. Vitamin D and Gastrointestinal Disorders

A. Osteopenia, which includes both osteomalacia and osteoporosis, is relatively common after gastric surgery.

  1. Estimates of the incidence of bone disease vary between 14 and 26% depending on the diagnostic criteria used.

  2. The pathogenesis of the bone disease following gastrectomy still is virtually unknown.

  3. Inadequate intake of calcium and protein, steatorrhea, and a malabsorption of calcium and vitamin D are considered the most likely etiologic factors.

  B. It has now been established that no quantitative relationship exists between the amount of fecal fat and the proportion of ingested calcium excreted in the feces.

  1. It has also been demonstrated that vitamin D absorption may be normal or only slightly abnormal in gastrectomized patients with osteomalacia.

  2. Steatorrhea alone probably is not the major cause of the impaired vitamin absorption because vitamin D absorption can be normal in patients with steatorrhea.

  3. The intestinal absorption of calcium in gastrectomized patients may, in fact, be increased, and it may not be responsive to vitamin D.

  C. Vitamin D and Liver Disease With Jaundice

  1. There appears to be little doubt that a high incidence of osteopenia exists in patients with chronic obstructive jaundice.

  a. Some of these patients respond poorly to vitamin D therapy.

  2. Although osteomalacia has been well documented in patients with primary biliary cirrhosis, osteoporosis appears to be a more common cause for the progressive bone disease in these patients.

  3. Although parenteral vitamin D therapy may stimulate the defective intestinal absorption of calcium, it apparently does not halt the progression of bone disease in patients with primary biliary cirrhosis.

  4. Vitamin D preparations generally are ineffective in curing experimental rickets in animals with experimentally induced chronic jaundice.

  5. There is a variety of potential reasons for the osteopenia attending hepatobiliary disorders and the observed resistance to vitamin D therapy.

  a. Bile salt deficiency may also promote the formation of insoluble calcium "soaps" of unabsorbed fatty acids in the intestinal lumen and, as such, may compromise the absorption of dietary calcium.

  b. The liver is essential for the first in a series of biologic hydroxylations of vitamin D to biologically active metabolites.

  (1) In the absence of the liver, 25OHD is not produced.

  c. Patients with hepatocellular dysfunction demonstrate an unusually slow plasma disappearance of vitamin D and a decreased formation of vitamin D-glucuronide conjugates.

  d. Despite these preliminary observations, relatively little is known of the metabolism and biologic activity of vitamin D$_3$ and its metabolites in biliary cirrhosis or of the mechanisms responsible for the resistance of patients, thus afflicted, to parenteral doses of vitamin D$_3$.

  6. Recent experience, with patients who have biliary cirrhosis with osteomalacia, reveals a malabsorption of vitamin D and extremely low circulating levels of 25OHD.

  a. Whereas vitamin D therapy in

pharmacological doses of 400 to 800 I.U./ day often proves ineffective, immediate biological responsiveness (i.e. elevation in plasma calcium, inorganic phosphatate, and alkaline phosphatase) has been obtained during 25OHD therapy with doses of 5000 I.U./day.

7. Current studies indicate that the hepatocellular dysfunction in this disorder may condition the metabolic conversion of vitamin D and contribute to the progressive osteomalacia component of the osteopenia attending chronic biliary cirrhosis.

D. Vitamin D and Liver Disease Without Jaundice

1. While there appears to be some general agreement concerning the role of vitamin D in the pathogenesis of the osteopenia of patients with long-standing biliary obstruction, such is not the case concerning its role in the pathogenesis of chronic anicteric hepatic disease.

2. These patients demonstrate a significant decrease in bone mass.

3. The increased incidence of osteopenia in cirrhotic patients is consistent with the observations that

a. An increase in pancreatic fibrosis occurs in patients with alcoholic cirrhosis.

b. Intestinal malabsorption and steatorrhea frequently complicate the course of anicteric patients with liver disease.

c. Pancreatic insufficiency results in the intestinal malabsorption of calcium and vitamin D.

4. Chronic alcoholics may be more predisposed to vitamin D deficiency because the chronic ingestion of ethanol stimulates hepatic cytochrome P-450 microsomal enzyme systems. This can lead to an accelerated biologic degradation of vitamin D and 25OHD.

5. Chronic inanition, malnutrition, and decreased fat stores, so often characteristic of the clinical course of patients with long-standing liver disease, may result in a decrease in the available body stores of vitamin D and 25OHD because adipose and muscle tissues serve as large depots for these substances.

6. Elevated levels of calcium-complexing ligands in the plasma of cirrhotic patients and the associated decrease in ionized calcium, might very well contribute to the progressive decrease in bone mass seen in these patients because this constellation of biochemical abnormalities tends toward progressive parathyroid overactivity and a stimulated resorption of bone.

E. Vitamin D and the Intestine

1. The potpourri of conflicting evidence regarding the relationship between gastrointestinal and hepatic dysfunction and osteopenia may result from an inadequate appraisal of intestinal cell functions.

2. The intestinal response to vitamin D depends on the integrity of the mucosal cell.

3. There is a resistance to vitamin D observed in certain patients with celiac disease when gluten-free diets are discontinued.

a. This resistance is also seen in others with tropical sprue and folic acid deficiency.

b. It exemplifies the permissive requirement of cellular integrity for the maximal expression of vitamin D metabolites on intestinal calcium absorption.

V. Vitamin D and Anticonvulsant Therapy

A. The prolonged use of anticonvulsant medication has been shown to result in rickets and osteomalacia.

B. Significant hypocalcemia, hyperphosphaturia and hyperphosphatasia with increased urinary glucaric acid have been reported in 19 to 30% of epileptic populations.

C. Bone biopsies, when obtained, reveal florid osteomalacia, which responds to dietary vitamin D supplementation.

D. Plasma levels of 25OHD are decreased in patients receiving anticonvulsant medications, although circulating 1,25(OH)$_2$D levels are normal.

    1. The lowest values are seen in blacks and in persons with low dietary intakes and limited sunlight exposure.

    E. The incidence of osteomalacia in patients on anticonvulsants can be reduced considerably by increasing vitamin D intake to levels of approximately 2,000 to 5,000 I.U./day.

    F. Anticonvulsant-induced rickets and osteomalacia appear to stem from drug-stimulated hepatic microsomal P-450 enzymatic activity, with resultant accelerated degradation of vitamin D and 25OHD to inactive substances.

    G. Since a variety of commonly used medications, including muscle relaxants, oral antidiabetic agents, anticonvulsants, tranquilizers, and sedatives, are capable of inducing hepatic microsomal degradative enzymatic activity, the potential for drug-induced vitamin D-deficiency states exists in a number of clinical situations.

VI. Vitamin D, Calcium, and Chronic Renal Insufficiency

    A. Chronic renal insufficiency is characteristically attended by derangements in skeletal metabolism and in the homeostatic control of calcium, inorganic phosphate, magnesium, and a variety of other minerals.

    B. The following abnormalities are found:

    1. An impaired gastrointestinal absorption of calcium

    2. Parathyroid overactivity

    3. An acquired resistance to the biological action of vitamin D

    4. A steadily progressive form of bone disease which presents both histologically and radiographically as a mixture of osteomalacia, osteosclerosis, osteoporosis, and osteitis fibrosa cystica

    C. Although it is difficult to determine exactly when the alterations in skeletal and mineral metabolism associated with chronic renal impairment become resistant to vitamin D therapy, it becomes clinically detectable when glomerular filtration rates are reduced to 15 or 25 ml./minute.

    1. At this level of reduced renal functional mass, uremic patients reveal alterations in vitamin D metabolism, which include a limited ability to synthesize biologically active metabolites.

    2. Because a reduction in renal mass leads by necessity to a reduction in the generation of 1,25(OH)$_2$D from 25OHD, the resultant decrease in the circulating level of this extremely potent biologically active metabolite results in decreased intestinal malabsorption of calcium.

    D. Although the plasma levels of 25OHD increase in uremic patients during vitamin D therapy, patients on chronic hemodialysis can be separated into those with normal circulating 25OHD levels and osteitis fibrosa cystica, and others with low 25OHD levels and osteomalacia.

    E. Vitamin D therapy by itself has been shown to reverse the osteomalacia of bilaterally nephrectomized patients on chronic hemodialysis.

    1. The use of 25OHD, in doses of 6000 to 12,000 I.U./day, has proven to be effective therapy for uremic bone disease in patients refractory to vitamin D in equivalent doses.

    2. Thus, even in the absence of the kidney, 25OHD is effective in reversing the skeletal pathology.

    F. The osteomalacic component of the osteodystrophy of uremic adults is less resistant to 25OHD$_3$, and, therefore, this compound is used in its treatment.

    1. A dose of 30 to 500 μg./day for 3 to 9 months effectively reverses the skeletal abnormalities of uremic adults undergoing intermittent hemodialysis.

    2. Concomitant increments in intestinal calcium absorption occurs together with a decrease in circulating alkaline phosphatase and PTH.

    3. The use of 25OHD$_3$ in doses of 25

to 200 μg./day also effectively reverses the skeletal lesions toward normal in uremic children who are resistant to vitamin D in doses of 345 to 386 μg./day.

4. Although 100 to 200 μg. daily doses of 25OHD$_3$ are still considerably higher than those required to heal dietary rickets or the rickets attending malabsorption syndromes, they are much lower than those of vitamin D$_2$ or D$_3$ used unsuccessfully in azotemic osteodystrophy.

G. The use of 1,25(OH)$_2$D$_3$ has been successful in vitamin D-resistant uremic patients with osteodystrophy. Improvements in bone mass and calcium absorption and a decrease in circulating PTH have been documented on doses of 0.68 to 2.7 μg./day.

1. Limited long-term therapeutic trials with this agent are promising.

2. In one instance, a 14-year-old child, given 0.68 μg. daily for over 3 months, demonstrated progressive healing of the skeletal lesions radiographically (detectable after 4 weeks of therapy) and a fall in alkaline phosphatase.

3. This response was attended by a complete reversal of the secondary hyperparathyroidism and osteomalacic bone lesions noted on iliac crest biopsy specimens prior to the intervention of 1,25(OH)$_2$D$_3$ therapy.

4. Of additional interest is the observation that, during the 1,25(OH)$_2$D$_3$ treatment period, muscular weakness also improved both clinically and by electromyographic testing.

H. The most recent synthetic vitamin D$_3$ analogue used for the treatment of vitamin D-resistant renal osteodystrophy is a 1α=hydroxycholecalciferol (1α=OHD$_3$).

1. This analogue has biological activity comparable on the basis of weight to 1,25(OH)$_2$D$_3$ in the stimulation of intestinal calcium transport and bone calcium mobilization in the normal and anephric state.

2. Unlike 1,25(OH)$_2$D$_3$, which is more effective when administered intravenously than orally, the response to oral 1α=OHD$_3$ is rapid with daily doses of 2.5 μg. effectively reversing the skeletal defects of patients with nutritional osteomalacia in 8 to 10 days.

3. Doses as small as 10 μg./day for 2 to 3 days in uremic patients have been associated with a two- to threefold increase in calcium absorption, an elevation in serum calcium, and a fall in circulating alkaline phosphatase.

4. Prolonged treatment (i.e. 9 to 10 weeks) with daily doses of 1.0 to 2.0 μg. reveals progressive increments in both calcium absorption and skeletal mineral. In the anephric state, 1α–OHD$_3$ is biologically effective, although it appears to be rapidly metabolized in the liver to 1α–25(OH)$_2$D$_3$, which is considered to be the ultimate metabolically active form.

26. NUTRITION AND MENTAL DEVELOPMENT

Pedro Rosso, M.D.

Jorge A. Bassi, M.D.

BASIC PRINCIPLES

I. Undernutrition is the primary cause of the high rates of infant morbidity and mortality in developing countries.

A. In the U. S., a food supply of high quality is readily available for the consumer's selection. It is difficult, therefore, to rationalize the fact that undernutrition also exists in this country.

B. In contrast with the developing nations, in the U.S., the discrepancy between the capacity to meet the nutritional needs of all the people and the existence of undernutrition is not primarily economical in nature, but rather cultural and sociological.

C. Regardless of its ultimate cause, however, in both cases the milieu in which undernutrition appears is a deprived family.

II. The combination of inadequate food intake and deprived family environment has a devastating effect on the growth and development of a child, especially on his intellectual development.

III. Recent evidence indicates a causal relationship between undernutrition and deficient mental function.

A. Early undernutrition has an adverse effect both on the central nervous system and on the intellectual capacity of the affected child.

NORMAL BRAIN GROWTH

I. The total number of cells of an organ can be measured by determining its DNA content.

A. After the number of cells has been determined, the average weight per cell, RNA content per cell, and lipid content per cell can be determined by measuring the total amount of each of these components and dividing by the quantity of DNA.

B. The result is expressed chemically as a weight-DNA, protein-DNA, RNA-DNA, or lipid-DNA ratio.

C. An increase in total organ DNA content during development represents one aspect of growth, namely, an increase in the number of cells.

D. In contrast, increases in the weight-DNA or protein-DNA ratio and, in certain cases, the lipid-DNA ratio represent another aspect of growth, namely, an increase in cell size or cell mass.

II. Growth from conception to maturity can be divided into three phases.

A. In the first phase, there is rapid cell division with cell size remaining constant.

B. In the second phase, both cell number and cell size increase as DNA and protein content rise, but because of a decrease in the rate of DNA synthesis, protein rises out of proportion to DNA.

C. In the third phase, there is an increase in cell size as DNA synthesis stops and protein continues to accumulate.

D. Growth finally ceases when protein synthesis and degradation come into equilibrium.

E. These phases do not change abruptly but merge gradually, one into the other.

III. Studies indicate that the rate of DNA increments in the human brain is linear prenatally, begins to slow down shortly after birth, and reaches a plateau after the first year of life (see Fig. 26-1).

A. It has been shown that there are two peaks of DNA synthesis that occur normally during the development of the human brain.

1. The first peak is reached at about 26 weeks of gestation, and the second peak is reached around birth.

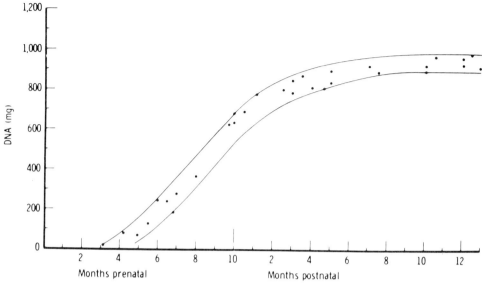

Fig. 26-1. Amount of DNA in the brain of normal human fetuses and children. Each dot represents one brain (Winick, M.: Changes in nucleic acid and protein content of the human brain during growth. Pediatr. Res., 2:352, 1968)

2. These peaks correspond to the maximum rate of neuronal division and the maximum rate of glial division, respectively.

B. Available data indicate that the rate of cell division postnatally is about the same in cerebrum and cerebellum and that cell division stops at about the same time in both areas, that is, between 12 and 15 months of age.

C. In the brain stem, DNA synthesis continues at a slow but steady rate until at least 1 year of age.

D. Thus, in most regions of the brain, the total number of cells present in adults is largely determined by the end of the first year of life. (see Fig. 26-2).

UNDERNUTRITION AND BRAIN GROWTH

I. Experiments have demonstrated that when undernutrition is imposed during the proliferative phase of growth, the rate of cell division is slowed, and the ultimate number of cells of every organ, including the brain, is reduced.

A. This change is permanent and can not be reversed once the normal time for cell division has passed.

B. In contrast, undernutrition imposed during the period of hypertrophic growth will curtail the cellular enlargement, but, on subsequent rehabilitation, the cells will regain their normal size.

C. Total brain cell number can be permanently reduced by 15 to 20% when undernourishment occurs throughout the entire period of lactation.

D. No matter what feeding regimen is attempted thereafter, this reduction in cell number persists.

E. It is possible to retard fetal growth by restricting food intake or the percentage of protein in the maternal diet. After that there is a progressive decrease in cell number in all organs.

F. The reduction in brain cell number is proportional to the reduction in the number of cells in the other organs.

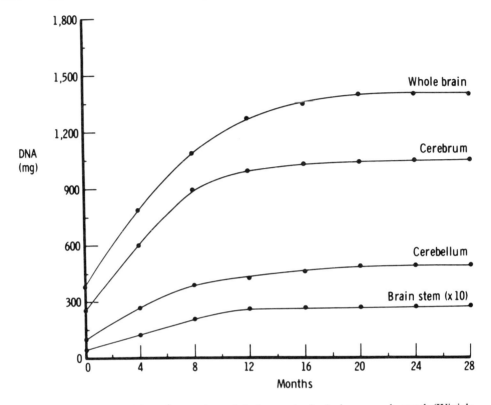

Fig. 26-2. DNA content in various regions of the human brain during normal growth (Winick, M.: Malnutrition and Brain Development. p. 44. New York, Oxford University Press, 1976)

G. By term, brain cell number is only 85% of normal.

H. These findings demonstrate that the magnitude of the effect of undernutrition depends largely on the rate of cell division.

II. The effects on the brain of the exposure to postnatal undernutrition as well as prenatal undernutrition are extreme (see Fig. 26-3).

A. Undernutrition applied constantly throughout the entire period of brain cell proliferation will result in a profound reduction in brain cell number, greater than the sum of effects produced during various parts of the proliferative phase.

B. It appears that the duration of undernutrition as well as the severity during this early critical period is extremely important in determining the ultimate cellular makeup of the brain.

C. Deficiencies in specific nutrients such as vitamin A, vitamin B$_6$, folic acid, zinc, and magnesium may also affect fetal development and involve, among other tissue, those of the nervous system.

III. In the human brain, there is a type of response to undernutrition similar to that which has been described in lower animals. During proliferative growth, cell division is curtailed; during hypertrophic growth, the normal enlargement of cells is prevented.

A. In the brains of infants who died of undernutrition during their first year of life, wet weight, dry weight, total protein, total RNA, total cholesterol, total phospholipid, and total DNA content were proportionally reduced. Thus, the rate of DNA synthesis was slowed, and cell division was curtailed, reducing the number of cells.

B. Because the reduction in the other

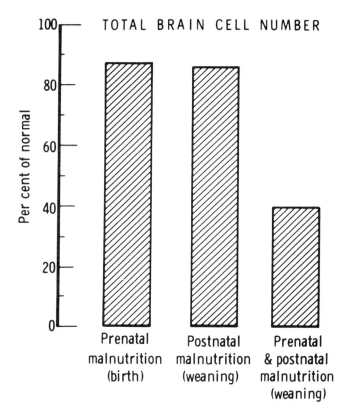

Fig. 26-3. The effects on the brain of prenatal undernutrition, postnatal undernutrition and undernutrition during both periods (Winick, M.: Nutrition and nerve cell growth. Fed. Proc., *29*:1510, 1970)

elements was proportional to the reduction in DNA content, the ratios were unchanged, and the size of cells as well as the lipid or RNA content of the individual cell was not altered.

C. If under nutrition persists beyond about 8 months of age, not only the number of cells but also their size will be reduced.

1. In addition, the lipid per cell is also reduced (see Fig. 26-4).

2. Total cholesterol or phospholipid content is reduced, hence, the number or length of myelin sheaths is reduced.

3. But because both cholesterol and phospholipid concentration are unaffected, the thickness of those myelin sheaths that are present is unaffected (see Fig. 26-5).

D. The major effect of undernutrition is to interfere with cellular growth, while continued undernutrition reduces cell size. In neurons, this would be associated with a reduction in the number or length of processes, and myelination would be proportionally curtailed. This indicates that dendritic branching may be retarded by early undernutrition.

IV. In the developing human brain, early undernutrition affects both cell division and myelination, the vulnerable periods coinciding with the maximum rate of synthesis of DNA and of myelin.

A. All brain regions seem to be vulnerable. This varies depending on the timing at which the maximum rate of

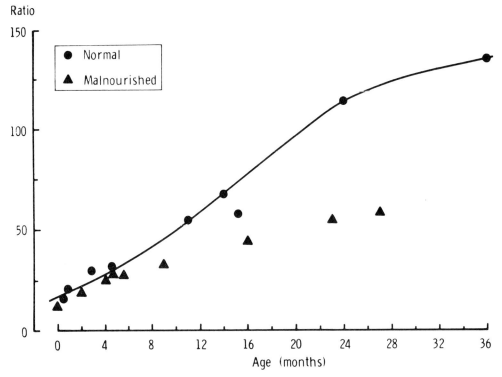

Fig. 26-4. Lipid-DNA ratio in normal and undernourished children at different ages (Russo, P., *et al.*: Changes in brain weight, cholesterol, phospholipid, and DNA content in marasmic children. Am. J. Clin. Nutr., *23*:1275, 1970)

synthesis of DNA in the particular region takes place.

B. All neural cell types so far studied are affected by undernutrition if they are dividing at the time that the insult occurs.

V. Maternal undernutrition inhibits cell division in the human fetus so that fetal growth is retarded, and birth weight is reduced.

VI. Three patterns emerge from available information on infants who died after exposure to severe postnatal undernutrition.

A. Breast-fed infants who are malnourished during the second year of life have a reduced protein-DNA ratio but a normal brain DNA content.

B. Full-term infants who died of severe food deprivation during the first year of life have a 15 to 20% reduction in total brain cell number.

C. Infants who weighed 2000 g. or less at birth and who died of severe undernutrition during the first year of life have a 60% reduction in total brain cell number.

1. It is possible that the children in this category were also deprived in utero and fall into the doubly deprived category.

2. It is also possible that these were true premature infants and that the premature infant is much more susceptible to postnatal undernutrition than the full-term infant.

UNDERNUTRITION AND MENTAL DEVELOPMENT

I. The effects of undernutrition early in life on subsequent mental capacity and behavior has been investigated in several countries.

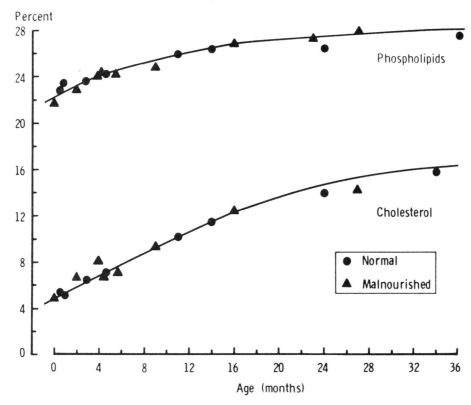

Fig. 26-5. Cholesterol and phospholipid concentration per 100 g. dry tissue in normal and undernourished children at different ages. (Rosso, P., *et al.*: Changes in brain weight cholesterol, phospholipid, and DNA content in marasmic children. Am. J. Clin. Nutr., *23*:1275, 1970)

A. Most of these studies have focused on measuring intelligence because testing procedures are readily available and because the demonstration of persistent intellectual deficits would have immediate social impact.

B. In studies of malnutrition and mental functioning, there is a tendency to overlook the fact that the term undernutrition may cover deficits in one or more nutrients.

C. The age at which a person is deprived of food intake, the severity and the repetition of the food deprivation, and concomitant deprivations of a non-nutritional nature, all affect psychological functioning.

D. Undernutrition occurs within the context of massive deprivation. In most in-

stances, the specific effects of undernutrition on brain development in humans are inseparable from effects of the environment. Adequate nutrition generally is part of a good environment. Undernutrition occurs primarily in poor environments in which many other factors may also limit the person's development.

E. The measurement of psychological deficits cannot be precise because undernutrition affects the several areas of psychological function differently.

II. Several studies done throughout the world suggest that early undernutrition in a deprived environment interferes with subsequent learning ability.

A. Among poor children, the better

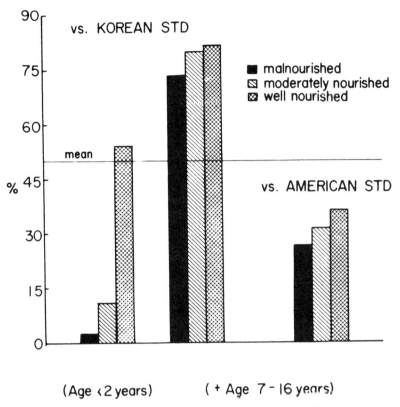

Fig. 26-6. Changes in weight in adopted Korean children.

nourished, taller ones generally score higher in I.Q. tests than the previously undernourished, shorter children.

B. The lowest I.Q.'s are usually associated with the poorest prior nutritional status.

C. It is not clear, however, to what extent the reduced I.Q. is purely the result of the prior episode of malnutrition and to what extent it is due to other factors.

D. In populations of uniform socio-economic backgrounds in Mexico and Guatemala, performance on psychological tests was found to be related to dietary practice and not to differences in personal hygiene, housing, cash income, crop income, proportion of income spent on food, parental education, or other social or economic indicators.

E. Moreover, performance of both preschool and school children on the Terman, and Goodenough draw-a-man tests was positively correlated with body weights and heights.

F. Because the shorter children did not come from families significantly lower in socio-economic status, housing, and parental education than those of the taller children, it was concluded that the most important variable reflected by the short stature was poor nutrition during early life and that this also led to the lag in development of sensory integrative competence.

G. The exact time span when undernutrition has the most serious effect on the brain is not yet known. In a study done in Jamaica, all of the children from a low-income group undernourished at any time

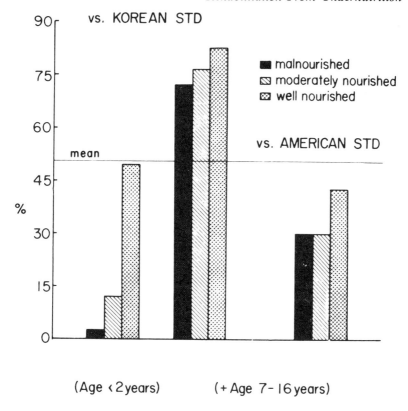

Fig. 26-7. Changes in height in adopted Korean children.

during the first 2 years of life had significant behavioral abnormalities at school age.

REHABILITATION FROM UNDERNUTRITION

I. There are indications that the deleterious effects on development of early undernutrition can be reversed. In order to examine the effects of environmental enrichment on the development of undernourished children, a population of Korean children, some of whom were severely undernourished during the first year of life and were then adopted by families in the U.S., has been studied.

A. All of the infants were adopted before their second birthday by American families. The adoptions were entirely random on a first come, first served basis. The foster parents had no idea of a child's previous nutritional history.

B. The children were classified as malnourished, moderately malnourished, and well nourished.

1. By the time these children reached 7 years of age, there were no differences in average weight among the three groups (see Fig. 26-6). All had reached normal by Korean standards.

2. Changes in height were similar to those in weight except that the undernourished children remained slightly but significantly smaller (see Fig. 26-7).

3. The mean I.Q. of the previously undernourished groups was 102.05. The marginally nourished children achieved a mean I.Q. of 105.95. This is not a statistically significant difference.

4. The previously well-nourished chil-

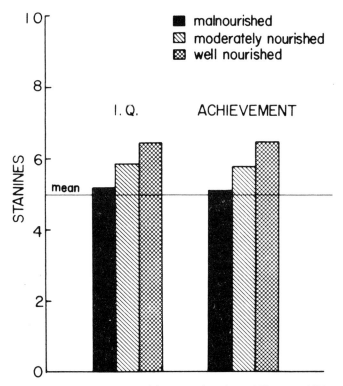

Fig. 26-8. Intelligence and achievement in adopted Korean children.

dren reached a mean I.Q. of 111.68, which does represent a significant difference from the undernourished children.

C. When achievement in these three groups was compared, the results were similar.

1. Both the severely undernourished and the marginally undernourished children were achieving exactly at expected norms for American children of the same age and the same grade (see Fig. 26-8).

2. The previously well-nourished children were achieving slightly, but significantly, better.

II. These findings show that severely undernourished children, when reared in a middle-class environment, before their second birthday can catch up in height and weight and reach an I.Q. and school achievement level which is perfectly normal for well-nourished children raised in an industrialized nation.

A. The data also suggest that when well-nourished children are placed in a more stimulating environment they do even better. Their I.Q. scores and achievement scores are not only higher than those of the undernourished children but also are higher than the norms for American children in general.

B. From a practical standpoint, the importance of this study lies in its pointing out the reversibility of effects of early undernutrition.

C. In all previous studies, when the child was returned to his or her previous environment, the I.Q. was 70 or below at school age.

D. In a study in Colombia, severely undernourished children after recovery have been placed in an enriched environment at about 2 years of age. The children are exposed to all types of stimulating learning and play experiences. Their nutrition has been kept adequate.

1. Preliminary results show that the test levels of the stimulated undernourished children are higher than those of the children from the higher socio-economic group who were not stimulated.

2. Results show that the well-nourished, stimulated children have the highest learning capacity.

III. Nutritional State of Pregnant Women and Young Infants and Mental Development in Nutritionally Deprived Populations

A. A study was being done in three rural Guatemalan villages. One village received a food supplement in the form of a high-protein supplement drink that was consumed by the young children and the pregnant mothers. A second village was supplied with a supplement of some caloric value but no protein content. Both villages were given medical care. The third village received medical care only.

1. Growth rates were increased in the children receiving the high-protein supplement.

2. Moreover, the women who get a protein supplement during pregnancy have babies whose birth weight is significantly higher than that of babies born in the non-supplemented village.

3. Finally, it would appear that the development of the children is better in the protein supplemented village than in the other villages.

B. In rural Mexico, food supplements have been given to children of families carefully selected to represent the norms of their community.

1. When the growth rate of the supplemented children was compared with that of their previously studied, unsupplemented, poorly nourished siblings, a marked increase was observed.

2. The supplemented children also demonstrated marked superiority in physical strength, independence, attentiveness, and ability to perform certain behavior tests.

3. They tended to explore their environment more thoroughly, play with toys more frequently, and interact with adults better than nonsupplemented children.

IV. These nutrition intervention studies indicate that improvement in the diet during either pregnancy or early life will significantly and favorably affect birth weight, subsequent growth rate, and subsequent behavior.

A. Although all aspects of diet are implicated, significant amounts of high quality protein are of especial importance.

B. Because the diet during pregnancy and early life is an important determinant of future mental development, intellectual capacity, and learning capability, the diet at this time of life should be carefully directed and not left to chance.

27. THE NUTRITIONAL MANAGEMENT OF ALCOHOLISM, DRUG ADDICTION, AND ACUTE TOXICITY SYNDROMES

Carlo H. Tamburro, M.D.

America's two largest addiction problems, alcoholism and excessive use of drugs, both medical and non-medical, are major causes of malnutrition in adults, despite the adequate availability of food. Nutritional deficiency frequently is instituted by suppression of the appetite by chronic or excessive use of alcohol, barbiturates, narcotics, and like drugs. These drugs add to the nutritional abnormalities by interfering with the absorption and utilization of foods. Secondary acute and chronic illnesses such as liver disease, gastrointestinal disorders, and chronic infection add to the nutritional abnormalities by increasing the nutrients required for body defense and tissue repair. They can also lead to excessive loss of nutrients.

DEFINITIONS

I. Normal Nutritional State

A. The clinical nutritional status of an individual can be assessed in a semiquantitative fashion by a number of indicators.

    1. Weight-height ratio

    2. Dietary history including quantitative and qualitative composition

    3. Medical history of congenital or acquired diseases associated with malnutrition

    4. Arm circumference

    5. Muscle circumference (see Table 27–1)

    6. Triceps skin fold (see Table 27–1)

B. The clinical appearance of a patient under careful medical examination will often reveal subtle early signs of malnutrition.

    1. In the early stage of alcoholism and drug abuse there usually is an absence of such physical findings, and often a negative medical and normal dietary history is given.

    2. These negative findings are, at best, gross clinical assumptions of a normal nutritional state in the alcoholic or drug user.

II. Abnormal Nutrition or Malnutrition

A. Overnutrition

    1. This clinical condition is most often associated with affluent areas of the world.

    2. Clinically, it is manifested by an excess total body weight in comparison to bone size and height. This is due to an excessive caloric intake and is associated with increased total body fat.

    3. This abnormal nutritional state is epidemiologically and biostatistically associated with increased incidence of cardiovascular disease, cerebrovascular disease, cancer, and with a shortened life span.

    4. Overnutrition or obesity is not uncommon among the alcohol and drug abusers of an affluent society.

        a. The excessive alcohol consumed interferes with the dietary composition by adding empty or functionless calories to the person's total food intake.

        b. Overnutrition is more commonly seen in the early stages of alcohol excess. Drug abuse or addiction, however, is more often associated with undernutrition.

        c. The presence of either nutritional state is greatly dependent upon the financial status of the individual, cost of drug or alcohol, and the presence of protective family structure.

B. Undernutrition

    1. This clinical state is most often manifested by a decreased body weight in comparison to bone size and height.

    2. The early stages of undernutrition

should be looked for as an almost required accompaniment to alcohol- and drug-related medical disease and disorder.

ETIOLOGY

Clinical causes of malnutrition in alcoholism, drug addiction, and toxicity syndromes can be divided into five categories. Any one of these may lead to malnutrition. Clinically, however, more than one of these factors are almost always operative in these disorders.

I. Decreased Intake

A. The loss of appetite due to illness, and foods selected because of economic status, geographic location, and religious and ethnic backgrounds are the major causes of inadequate dietary intake.

B. In alcoholics and addicts, ethanol and drugs interfere with the normal appetite mechanism as well as with customary work and social habits.

C. Grossly inadequate histories are noted more frequently among hospitalized alcoholics and addicts than among patients with other medical disorders.

II. Malabsorption

A. Alcoholics and drug addicts both have a high incidence of liver injury, gastrointestinal lesions, and pancreatic disease, all of which contribute to abnormalities in gastrointestinal absorption.

B. Gastrointestinal mucosal damage and dysfunction result from direct alcohol or drug toxicity.

1. This leads to impaired gastrointestinal transport of dietary fats, proteins, vitamins, and minerals.

C. Absorptive defects are accentuated further by altered bile and pancreatic secretion in those patients with liver disease and pancreatic disorders.

III. Malutilization

A. In addition to abnormalities in absorption, both the alcoholic and the drug addict have difficulty in the proper utilization of the nutrients they do absorb, usually due to the presence of both liver disease and pancreatitis.

B. In the acute phases of hepatic injury, whether induced by ethanol, drugs, or the hepatic virus, there is a decreased ability to

Table 27-1. **Standard Values for Arm and Muscle Circumference and Triceps Skin Fold**

	Men*	Women*	Depletion Status
Mid-upper Arm	> 26	> 26	none
Circumference	18–26	18–26	moderate
(cm.)	< 18	< 18	severe
Muscle	> 23	> 20	none
Circumference†	16–23	14–20	moderate
(cm.)	< 16	< 14	severe
Triceps Skin	> 11	> 15	none
Fold	7.5–11	10–15	moderate
(mm.)	< 7.5	< 10	severe

*Adults only
†Calculation of muscle circumference
$C = \pi D$ C = Circumference
               π = 3.14
               D = Diameter
Mid-upper arm circumference ÷ 3.14 = Arm diameter
Arm diameter − Tricep skin fold thickness = Muscle diameter
Muscle diameter × 3.14 = Muscle circumference

convert the available nutrients into their metabolically active forms.

1. This leads to impaired nucleic acid synthesis, interferes with nutrient utilization for cellular energy production, and prevents the adequate cellular repair needed in these patients.

IV. Increased Utilization

A. The frequent presence of hepatic infections, cirrhosis, hepatitis, gastrointestinal and pancreatic disease, as well as toxic injury directly to other body systems, leads to increased nutritional demands in both the alcoholic and drug addict.

B. Reparative processes for these diseases increase the requirements for protein, lipids, carbohydrates, vitamins, and minerals.

C. This increased utilization further depletes body stores and worsens the malnutrition already present in these conditions.

V. Increased Loss

A. Clinical injury to the gastrointestinal tract, liver, pancreas, and kidney by alcohol and drug excess can also lead to an increased loss of essential nutrients due to recurrent nausea and vomiting, diarrhea, fever, and excess renal excretion.

B. These conditions add to the already inadequate nutritional state.

MANAGEMENT

I. Definitions

A. Alcoholism

1. Alcoholism may be defined in practical clinical terms as excess alcohol consumption which produces physical, mental, or biochemical derangements in the body.

2. This may be induced in some persons with as little as 3 to 5 oz. of whiskey or its equivalent per day.

3. It is the alcohol content of the beverage that constitutes the major danger.

4. The fact that 1 oz. of whiskey has approximately the same alcohol content as one 12-oz. can of beer or one 4-oz. glass of wine is often missed by most medical personnel, as well as by the general public.

B. Drug Addiction

1. Clinically definable as the intermittent or chronic excessive use of drugs or chemicals so as to develop a continuing physical or psychological dependency.

C. Acute Toxicity Syndrome

1. This is the acute excessive use of drugs or chemicals which produce immediate or rapid, generalized or organ specific injury.

II. Management of Protein Abnormalities

A. Indications

1. The management of protein deficiency is the key element in the treatment of severe alcoholism- and chronic drug abuse-associated nutritional disorders.

B. Definition

1. Protein deficiency is defined as an impairment in either the availability or the utilization of essential amino acids at the subcellular, cellular, physiological, or clinical levels.

C. Basic Principles

1. Alcohol and dietary deficiency both have effects on the intestinal absorption of protein.

2. Alcohol produces histological abnormalities in the intestinal mucosa, decreases the intestine absorptive capacity, and alters intestinal motility, especially when large doses are ingested.

3. Ingestion of small doses for prolonged periods, even with an adequate diet, produces a consistent decrease in vitamin B_{12} absorption and ultrastructural changes

in the intestinal mucosa. On occasion, it can result in malabsorption of other vitamins or substances.

4. The development of protein malnutrition in the alcoholic is a process which begins when the alcohol consumed exceeds the body's ability to detoxify it, thus causing cellular injury.

5. Gastrointestinal mucosal cells have a rapid turnover. Clinical studies have shown increased regeneration of these cells and increased secretion of gastric acid and other enzymes at low (< 1 oz. alcohol) short-term alcohol consumption.

6. At higher doses (2 ozs. or more), mucosal cell turnover is impaired, thus impairing normal absorption.

7. The hepatocellular toxicity of alcohol also causes injury to the rough endoplasmic reticulum, mitochrondria, and cell membranes, interfering with adequate syn-

thesis of building proteins, enzymes, carrier proteins, lipoproteins, and reparative proteins.

8. With chronic alcohol ingestion, intercellular proteins can be degraded or changed so that they are no longer recognized as normal body constituents, thus causing the immunological system to destroy its own tissue cells.

9. Alcohol injury to the protein synthesizing capability of body cells plays a vital role in the development of complications such as increased infection, particularly gram-negative sepsis, decreased response to antibiotics and drugs, increased difficulty with fluid, electrolyte, and acid-base balance, prolonged use of critical care facilities, delayed discharge, and the inability to return to work.

D. Criteria for Diagnosis. The major methods for diagnosing abnormalities in

Table 27-2. **Useful Laboratory Tests for Assessing Nutritional States**

Proteins, Serum	Normal Range
Total	6.0–8.0 g./dl.
Albumin	3.5–5.5 g./dl.
Prothrombin time	2 sec. above control
Iron-binding capacity	250–410 mg./dl. (20–55% saturation)
Transferrin	100 mg./dl.
Red Blood Cell Studies	
Hematocrit, males	40–54 ml./dl.
Hematocrit, females	37–47 ml./dl.
Reticulocyte count	25,000–75,000/cu. mm. 0.5–1.5% of R.B.C.
Mean corpuscular volume (MCV)	80–105 μ^3
Carbohydrate, Blood	
Glucose, fasting true	60–100 mg./dl.
Glucose, serum/plasma	70–115 mg./dl.
Pyruvate (plasma)	1.0–2.0 mg./dl.
Lipids, Serum	
Total, lipids	450–850 mg./dl.
Cholesterol	150–250 mg./dl.
Fatty acids	190–420 mg./dl.
Phospholipids	6–12 mg./dl.
Triglycerides	0–250 mg./dl. (age dependent)

the protein status of the alcoholic are: (see also Table 27–2)

1. Serum Albumin Levels

a. This is probably the most practical and most easily available routine parameter for assessing protein status.

b. Even in the early stages of alcoholism, the mean albumin level is lower than normal—usually between 3.5 and 4 mg./dl.

c. In contrast, the age equivalent non-alcoholic serum albumin levels range between 3.8 and 5.2 mg./dl.

d. As the alcoholism and subsequent protein malnutrition progress, the albumins fall further and may be as low as 1.2 mg./dl.

e. Decreasing albumin level is clinically accompanied by peripheral edema, ascites, muscle wasting, weakness, apathy, and anorexia, which in turn contributes further to the decreased protein intake, disordered protein distribution in the body, ineffective protein utilization, and excess protein loss due to malabsorption and diarrhea.

2. Prothrombin Time and Protein Clotting Factors

a. The protein-synthesizing capacity of the liver is reflected by the prothrombin time and the concentration of the protein clotting factors.

b. Prothrombin time abnormalities most often accompany acute hepatocellular injury or chronic destruction, such as cirrhosis.

c. In the acute phase of severe liver injury, such as in the acute toxicity syndrome, the albumin is normal in the presence of an abnormal prothrombin time. The fall in albumin occurs later.

d. In contrast, in chronic disease the albumin level is the first to decrease and is later followed by an abnormality in the prothrombin time.

e. This sequence reflects a more gradual progression to protein malnutrition in chronic alcohol or drug injury.

(1) It is mainly due to the difference in turnover time for albumin compared with prothrombin time and the protein clotting factors.

(2) Clotting proteins have a short half-life of approximately 24 to 36 hours, and with acute injury they are rapidly depleted.

(3) Albumin with a half-life of approximately 14 days maintains its serum level for a longer period of time after the cessation or decrease in protein synthesis.

f. Thus, protein impairment in chronic disease is better reflected by changes in the albumin level, and in acute massive injury, by clotting factor changes.

3. Complete Blood Count

a. A good reflector of protein metabolism is the c.b.c., especially the hematocrit (HCT), red blood cell (R.B.C.) indices, and white blood cell (W.B.C.) count.

b. Anemia is almost always associated with interference of protein synthesis, especially with visceral-type protein malnutrition.

c. The most common hematological reflection of protein malnutrition is the presence of macrocytosis, which does not respond to vitamin B_{12} or folic acid.

(1) This is identified by low HCT and an increase in mean corpuscular volume (MCV) in the R.B.C. indices.

(2) Only after correction of the hypoalbuminemic state is the macrocytic anemia corrected.

(3) Response to treatment can be monitored by following the MCV of R.B.C. indices and HCT.

d. Suppression of W.B.C. count, due to an absolute decrease in lymphocytes, suggests impaired cell-mediated immunity associated with protein malnutrition.

4. Iron-Binding Capacity and Serum Transferrin Levels

a. Study of the iron-binding capacity provides an accurate means of identifying visceral protein malnutrition.

b. This can be done by measuring transferrin, a circulating serum protein.

c. Transferrin may be even more sensitive than albumin because it has a half-life of eight days.

E. Management

1. The management and correction of protein malnutrition in the alcoholic are dependent upon the clinical state of the liver.

2. Increased protein ingestion is beneficial and needed but will be detrimental if the individual is in impending hepatic failure (encephalopathy).

3. The total cessation of alcohol consumption is required, and the return to adequate dietary intake should be in a graded fashion.

4. The chronic alcoholic, depending upon the severity of his clinical disease, is akin to a person on long starvation. During the development of this malnourished state, the body has acclimated to a new milieu. The sudden return to a normal nutritional intake could be detrimental. The normal intake of a healthy adult may represent an excess protein load rather than the needed nutritional replacement.

5. Protein requirements can best be assessed clinically by determining the degree of muscle depletion and loss of calorie reserves and by determining the presence or absence of hepatic decompensation as illustrated in Tables 27–1 and 27–3.

6. Protein intake of approximately 1 to 1.5 g./kg./day will safely meet all requirements in cases of mild hepatic injury.

a. In those cases with hepatic decompensation, a reduction to less than 0.5 g./kg./day may be required to prevent the induction of hepatic encephalopathy.

b. As clinical recovery begins, a gradual protein increase of 10 to 20% can be given to a responding patient.

c. This can be continued until the patient has reached a 1.5 g./kg./day level.

d. It is important to point out, however, that 1 to 1.25 g./kg./day is adequate to allow gradual repair and that increased protein intake above 1.25 g./kg./day is not necessarily better and should not be pursued excessively without clinical conditions warranting it.

7. The effectiveness of therapy is best monitored by repeated determination of lean body mass as reflected by weight/height, arm circumference, muscle circumference, triceps skin fold, and serial studies of serum albumin, c.b.c., and transferrin levels.

Table 27-3. **Stages in the Onset and Development of Hepatic Coma**

Stage	Mental state	Tremor	EEG
I	Euphoria, occasionally depression Fluctuant, mild confusion Slowness of mentation and affect Untidy Slurred speech Disorder in sleep rhythm.	Slight	Usually normal
II	Accentuation of Stage I Drowsiness Inappropriate behavior Able to maintain sphincter control	Present (easily elicited)	Abnormal generalized slowing
III	Sleeps most of the time, but is rousable Speech is incoherent Confusion is marked	Usually present if patient can cooperate	Always abnormal
IV	Not rousable May or may not respond to noxious stimuli	Usually absent	Always abnormal

III. Management of Fat and Lipid Abnormalities

A. Indications

1. The most common lipid abnormality in alcoholics, drug users, and patients with acute toxicity syndrome is fatty liver. This usually occurs in the early stage of these disorders. However, systemic lipid abnormalities occur frequently in the later phases of chronic alcoholism.

B. Definition

1. For practical purposes, lipid malnutrition in these conditions can be defined as acute or chronic elevation of blood or tissue lipids.

2. It is most commonly induced by alcohol but is seen in pure drug addiction and in the acute toxicity syndrome.

3. In the majority of cases, it is related to decreased pancreatic function due to alcohol or drug injury.

C. Basic Principles

1. The accumulation of fat in the alcoholic liver can be due to:
   a. Direct effect of the ethanol itself
   b. Malnutrition alone
   c. Alcohol congeners
   d. Drugs
   e. Some combination of these

2. Lipids accumulate in the liver from three major sources.
   a. Dietary lipids, supplied as chylomicrons
   b. Adipose tissue lipids which are transported to the liver as free fatty acids
   c. Lipids synthesized in the liver itself

3. This accumulation occurs because of four major metabolic disturbances.
   a. Increased peripheral fat mobilization
   b. Decreased hepatic lipoprotein release
   c. Decreased lipid oxidation in the liver
   d. Enhanced hepatic lipogenesis

4. A high-protein diet during excessive alcohol intake does not prevent this fat accumulation.

5. The presence of pancreatitis and systemic hyperlipidemia is far more common than suspected.
   a. Its presence should be looked for in all chronic alcohol abusers.
   b. Steatorrhea (fecal fat excretion > 6 g./day) can be found in up to 33% of hospitalized chronic alcoholics.
   c. Milder forms (as detected by pancreatic lipase output after a stimulating test meal) can be found in up to 55% of hospitalized alcoholics.
   d. It is not uncommon to also find Type-IV or Type-V hyperlipoproteinemias present.

D. Criteria for Diagnosis

1. Serum Cholesterol Levels
   a. In both the early and intermediate stages of alcoholic liver injury and in the absence of hyperlipidemia, pancreatic disease, or diabetic state, one finds the serum cholesterol levels to be normal.

2. Serum Triglyceride Levels.
   a. Triglyceride levels are often abnormal but are of limited clinical usefulness.
   b. They are elevated in obstructive jaundice and in persons with severe alcoholic injury who have necrosis with fatty liver (alcoholic hepatitis) and with intrahepatic cholestasis.
   c. This might reflect the excessive mobilization of free fatty acids from adipose depots and the resulting re-esterification by the liver prior to transport back to the periphery.
   d. When cell function is severely depressed these values may be normal, reflecting the failure of this process.

3. Plasma Free Fatty Acids (Nonesterified Fatty Acids)
   a. These represent only 5% of the total plasma fatty acids.
   b. At low alcohol concentrations there is a fall in free fatty acid concentration. This is most likely due to acetate

which seems to cause a reduction in plasma free fatty acid concentrations.

c. When large doses of alcohol are consumed, a definite increase occurs in the concentration of free fatty acid.

d. This marked increase in plasma free fatty acids with high initial ethanol intake will diminish again if alcohol consumption is continued.

4. Serum Phosopholipid Levels (Lecithins)

a. These are presently of research interest only in the nutritional evaluation of the alcoholic.

5. Lipoprotein Electrophoresis

a. This can be used to detect the presence of hyperlipoproteinemias, which may be accentuated by alcohol consumption.

b. Type-IV hyperlipoproteinemia shows a striking increase in both the chylomicron and the pre-β lipoprotein concentrations. This disorder may be present or latent prior to the development of alcoholism.

6. Zeive Syndrome

a. Zeive syndrome is a hyperlipidemic state characterized by the association of increased serum lipids, hepatomegaly, and hemolytic anemia in the alcoholic.

b. These components may occur separately, and more than one mechanism may exist for each.

c. The hyperlipidemia may occur with the ingestion of large amounts of alcohol or may be associated with pancreatitis.

d. Although the term "Zeive syndrome" is useful in bringing these manifestations to clinical attention, the term itself is of limited usefulness.

E. Management

1. All of the acute lipid derangements associated with ethanol fatty liver, alcoholic hepatitis, fatty liver with cholestasis, and pancreatitis are potentially reversible.

2. The hyperlipidemias and pancreatitis will improve or return to the original state with an adequate diet and the cessation of alcohol consumption.

3. In most cases of pancreatic disease, function will have returned to normal after 4 to 6 weeks except for those with pancreatic calcifications.

4. The fatty liver lesions are corrected with normal dietary protein intake within 4 to 6 weeks, and their correction can be accelerated with the use of anabolic androgenic steroids.

5. Although these lesions are reversible, changes may occur very slowly. It is not unusual for the alcoholic fatty liver to remain present for up to 12 weeks after the cessation of alcohol consumption.

6. Treatment in these cases is always supportive, and the mainstay of therapy is the absence of ethanol.

7. Excessive changes in dietary lipids and excessive use of androgenic anabolic steroids and lipid-clearing drugs tend to complicate the clinical picture rather than assist it, and they should not be used except where there is a specific indication.

IV. Management of Carbohydrate Abnormalities

A. Definition

1. Carbohydrate abnormalities may be defined as abnormal changes in the circulating blood glucose levels.

2. There are two abnormal carbohydrate states, hyperglycemia and hypoglycemia.

3. Impaired carbohydrate tolerance is by far the more common presentation.

4. Despite high dietary carbohydrate intake, alcohol can produce hypoglycemia requiring immediate medical attention.

B. Basic Principles

1. Most alcoholics have dietary intake composed almost entirely of carbohydrates.

2. This excessive carbohydrate intake causes protein and other nutrient intake to be limited and also leads to loss of tissue protein, as a result of deficient protein intake.

3. Disturbances in carbohydrate metabolism are very common in the chronic alcoholic and in drug users who also drink excessively.

4. The liver is able to remove glucose from the blood stream, especially after a carbohydrate meal. It can also release glucose into the circulation during a fast or sustained exercise.

5. The hepatic portal vein obtains blood from the main absorptive area of the gastrointestinal tract and delivers it directly to the liver.

6. The portal vein communicates with the endocrine areas of the gut as well as the liver, the central organ of metabolic integration.

7. The transport of the glucose across the cell membrane is very rapid.

8. Glucose that is removed from the liver is converted to glycogen or to triglycerides by means of glycolysis or fatty acid synthesis.

C. Hyperglycemia

1. Abnormal increases in blood glucose level are often seen in chronic alcoholism.

2. Decreased pancreatic function and altered intracellular glucose metabolism are the two major causes.

3. Factors controlling glucose abnormalities

a. Degree of hepatocellular injury

b. Pancreatic and other carbohydrate hormone activity (i.e., insulin, glucagon)

c. Gastrointestinal absorption of carbohydrates

D. Hypoglycemia

1. Alcohol can also induce hypoglycemia, especially in cirrhotic individuals.

2. The hepatic glucose output is reduced, and alcohol inhibits the enzymes concerned with gluconeogenesis.

3. Ethanol intoxication enhances the transport of labeled glucose to the brain. This may reflect a defense response in the drinker, allowing more glucose to be available to a vital organ.

E. Criteria for Diagnosis

1. Hypoglycemia is suspect with blood glucose levels of less than 60 mg./dl.

a. Persons with alcohol hypoglycemia may present in a comatose or semi-comatose state and may manifest a variety of neurological signs. Trismus, conjugate eye movements, abnormal deep tendon reflexes, seizures, and hemiparesis have been seen.

b. Intervals of up to 30 hours may separate the last alcohol ingestion from the onset of hypoglycemia.

c. The hypoglycemic state is easily confused with inebriation.

2. Hyperglycemia states with blood glucose levels between 120 to 160 mg./dl. are often seen in the chronic alcoholic.

a. In alcoholics with hereditary diabetes, the alcohol consumed, together with a high-carbohydrate, low-protein diet, can aggravate the hyperglycemic state. Blood glucose levels as high as 600 to 800 mg./dl. have been seen.

b. Contrariwise, in secondary chronic pancreatitis-induced hyperglycemic states, blood glucose levels are seldom greater than 350 mg./dl.

F. Management

1. Discontinuance of alcohol with return to a normal diet will improve or return the hyperglycemic state to normal in most cases.

a. Exceptions include obese persons and those with chronic, calcific, or end-stage pancreatitis.

2. The hypoglycemia that follows alcohol ingestion can be found in persons whose blood alcohol levels do not exceed the range of intoxication.

a. It is often induced after prolonged periods of fasting and may persist despite adequate alimentation and prolonged rehabilitation in a controlled environment. It is not due to an enhanced peripheral utilization of glucose.

b. This type hypoglycemia cannot be terminated by glucagon.

c. Ketonuria and mild ketonemia frequently accompany alcoholic hypoglycemia, undoubtedly reflecting inadequate caloric intake.

3. Treatment of severe hypoglycemia is by intravenous administration of 35 to 50 ml. of 50% dextrose.

a. This will usually restore consciousness immediately; however, coma may recur if adequate carbohydrate is not administered.

b. Continuation of intravenous glucose (5 to 10% dextrose in water) should be maintained until a stable state is obtained.

4. During the recovery period, there often is evidence of glucose intolerance and at times, even after adequate alimentation, patients are unable to dispose of an oral glucose load.

a. This condition should be controlled by dietary means since such patients are often inordinately sensitive to small amounts of insulin or tolbutamide and to short-term starvation.

V. Management of Vitamin Abnormalities

A. Definitions

1. Vitamin deficiency is more difficult to define than carbohydrate, lipid, and protein deficiencies.

2. Serum levels of both fat- and water-soluble vitamins in most cases reflect the total body concentrations of vitamins.

3. Serum or plasma levels, however, may be increased with cellular injury or may seem to be normal in the presence of deficiency at the cellular level.

4. In some cases a low serum or plasma level may indicate a decreased body reserve and not a true deficiency at the cell level.

5. Essential vitamins, their normal blood levels, and the methods by which they are determined are shown in Table 27-4.

Table 27-4. **Essential Vitamins and Their Normal Blood Levels**

Vitamins	Normal Range
*Folic acid	5–24 ng./ml.
*B_{12} (cyanocobalamin)	115–800 pg./ml.
*B_1 (thiamine)	25–72 ng./ml.
*B_2 (riboflavin)	100–500 ng./ml.
*Niacin (nicotinic acid)	3.5–7 ng./ml.
*B_6 (pyridoxine)	30–80 ng./ml.
*Pantothenic acid	200–1000 pg./ml.
*Biotin	200–500 pg./ml.
†C (ascorbic acid)	0.4–1.5 mg./dl.
†A	25–75 mg./dl.
†E	0.6–1.2 mg./dl.
†D (25-Hydroxycholecalciferol)	10–40 ng./ml.

*Microbiological determination
†Chemical determination

B. Basic Principles

1. Since vitamins cannot be synthesized in the body, they must be provided in adequate amounts from dietary sources.

2. Adverse effects of alcohol significantly increase the requirements for both water- and fat-soluble vitamins.

3. Alcohol plays a major role in affecting vitamin nutrition because it interferes with their absorption, utilization, and excretion.

4. In addition to lowering intake by decreasing appetite, alcohol-induced gastrointestinal injury leads to impaired transport of vitamins across the gut.

a. This effect of alcohol has been shown to occur especially with vitamins B_1, B_6, B_{12}, and folic acid.

5. Concurrent protein depletion in the alcoholic with fatty liver, steatonecrosis, or cirrhosis also decreases vitamin absorption.

6. Folic acid deficiency is the most common deficiency seen in alcoholics, occurring in 50 to 60% of those with chronic alcohol consumption.

7. Thiamine, vitamin B_6, nicotinic acid, vitamin C, and vitamin A deficiencies quickly follow in decreasing frequency.

8. Multiple vitamin deficiencies are the rule in alcoholics.

C. Water-Soluble Vitamins

1. The water-soluble vitamins include folic acid, B_{12}, B_1, B_2, nicotinic acid, B_6, pantothenic acid, biotin, and C.

2. Folic acid is a required nutrient for DNA synthesis and, along with vitamin B_{12}, is required for active cellular generation and repair.

    a. Folic acid stores in the body are limited and are rapidly depleted with poor nutritional intake and defective absorption.

    b. Increased regeneration due to alcoholic or drug organ injury increases the need for these nutrients.

3. In contrast, vitamin B_{12} tends to be stored in excess quantities. It is increased in the peripheral circulation due to its cellular release during acute and chronic hepatocellular injury.

4. Evidences of folic acid and vitamin B_{12} deficiency are best reflected by abnormal hematopoesis.

    a. Deficiency is initially reflected by a decrease in the reticulocyte count, followed by an increased segmentation of polymorphonuclear leukocytes and, finally, macrocytosis and a macrocytic anemia.

5. Vitamin B_1 (thiamine)

    a. Alcohol induces intestinal damage and can cause a 50 to 60% reduction in the absorption of thiamine, even in the absence of liver injury.

    b. Thiamine deficiency is accompanied by an increase in circulating levels of pyruvic acid, reflecting the inability to utilize pyruvate for cellular energy production.

    c. Prolonged underutilization of pyruvate, due to thiamine deficiency, is accompanied by the development of two clinical syndromes.

        (1) Polyneuropathy or peripheral neuropathy (dry beriberi)

        (2) Cardiomyopathy (wet beriberi)

    d. Peripheral involvement is most common among alcoholics.

6. Vitamin B_2 (riboflavin)

    a. Like thiamine, the normal requirements of riboflavin depend on the overall metabolic activity of the person.

    b. Thyroid hormones play a major role in the control of the flavo-proteins.

    c. Deficiency is less common than with thiamine.

7. Nicotinic acid (niacin)

    a. Deficiency produces pellagra.

    b. This is not infrequent among alcoholics, with manifestations related to the skin, gastrointestinal tract, and central nervous system.

8. Vitamin B_6 (pyridoxine)

    a. This is necessary in a number of metabolic reactions with amino acids, including decarboxylation and transamination.

    b. Deficiencies can lead to changes in the skin, central nervous system, and in the production of red blood cells.

    c. Deficiency is frequent among alcoholics.

9. Pantothenic acid and biotin are important cofactors in fat metabolism.

    a. Since these vitamins are so ubiquitous, deficiencies are rarely seen except in the most severely malnourished persons.

    b. Specific syndromes can occasionally occur in the alcoholic who eats a pure carbohydrate diet, totally devoid of any other nutrients, for a prolonged period of time. Such a diet would consist of only refined sugars and ethanol, mainly whiskey.

10. Vitamin C (ascorbic acid)

    a. Its physiological and biological functions still are not completely known.

    b. While other vitamins have been demonstrated to be cofactors for specific enzymatic steps in biochemical reactions, ascorbic acid has not.

    c. Ascorbic acid appears to function in its reduced form in oxidation reduction reactions.

    d. Deficiency is common in the alcoholic.

D. Fat-Soluble Vitamins

1. The fat-soluble vitamins include A,

D, E, and K. Unlike the water-soluble vitamins, these may produce toxicity when taken in excess because they are not excreted in the urine but are stored in body fat depots.

2. Vitamin A

a. Among alcoholics it is the most common of the fat-soluble vitamin deficiencies.

b. Night blindness secondary to vitamin A deficiency has long been identified as a frequent development in alcoholics.

3. Vitamin D

a. The occurrence of osteoporosis in the alcoholic with severe hepatic disease and the role of vitamin D in the maintenance of normal calcium and phosphorus levels required for bone mineralization involve an interlocking relationship between liver's activation of vitamin D (D_3) and intestinal calcium absorption (see Chap. 25).

b. Chronic alcohol or drug injury to the liver can interfere with the biological conversion of vitamin D to its active form. This leads to gradual bone mineral imbalances and to the bone diseases commonly seen in alcoholics.

4. Vitamin E

a. Whether deficiency of this vitamin occurs in human nutrition is still an unsettled problem.

b. Deficiency is said to be present in about 15 to 20% of alcoholics, but its effects are unclear.

5. Vitamin K

a. Vitamin K is not measurable by a direct technique, but is determined by abnormalities in prothrombin production for which it is an essential cofactor.

b. It is often deficient in malabsorptive states associated with complete obstruction of the biliary tract.

c. Hypoprothrombinemias of the alcoholic generally are non-responsive to vitamin K because they are due to primary hepatocellular damage and interference with protein and prothrombin synthesis, rather than with vitamin K deficiency per se.

E. *Criteria for Diagnosis*
1. *Basic Principles*

a. All the vitamins, except K, can be determined by biochemical, bacterial, or protozoal methods.

b. In most cases, tissue, blood, and body fluid determinations can be made.

c. Clinical indicators are useful to verify laboratory findings and can be used as indicators of response to therapy.

2. *Water-Soluble Vitamins.*

a. Folic Acid and Vitamin B_{12}

(1) Deficiencies are reflected by decreased reticulocyte count, increased mean corpuscular volume, hypersegmentation of neutrophils, and a macrocytic hypochromic anemia.

(2) Clinically, in advanced cases, there is a swelling of the oral gums, atrophy of the filiform and the fungiform papillae of the tongue, and enlargement of the tongue with magenta or red surface.

b. Vitamin B_1

(1) The alcoholic polyneuropathy (peripheral neuritis or alcoholic neuritis) is manifested in the mild form by asymptomatic wasting of the leg muscles with depression of knee jerks and absence of ankle jerks. Calf muscles are tender, with patchy impairment of pain and touch sensation over toes and feet often present.

(2) In the severe form of polyneuropathy there is slow progressive development of paresthesias in toes, feet, and distal portion of legs described as pins and needles sensation or burning feet. Upper extremities are often involved in the more severe cases, with peripheral weakness of finger jerk and numbness of finger tips.

(3) The cardiovascular manifestations of B_1 deficiency are predominantly those of inadequate energy supply to the myocardium and an increase in cardiac output with eventual heart failure (high output failure).

(a) In the early stages, it stimulates a hypermetabolic state very similar to hyperthyroidism.

(b) The cardiac manifestations of thiamine deficiency are very uncommon in American alcoholics.

(4) Alcoholic cardiomyopathy without thiamine deficiency is the more common manifestation of chronic alcoholism.

(a) It can simulate the early stages of myocardial thiamine deficiency.

(b) It manifests itself as progressive cardiac failure with generalized cardiac enlargement.

(5) The central nervous system is affected by thiamine deficiency.

(a) Wernicke-Korsakoff syndromes are common and may simulate acute intoxication or withdrawal.

(b) Wernicke's encephalopathy is identified by an ophthamoplegia (lateral recti muscle weakness), nystagmus, ataxia, and mental changes.

(c) Mental changes vary in degree and include apathy, disorientation, and forgetfulness with occasional agitation, confusion, and hallucination simulating delirium tremens.

(d) This syndrome is often partially expressed and associated with Korsakoff's syndrome which includes polyneuritis, a characteristic recent memory loss, confusion, inconsistency of ideas, and an irritable depressed mood.

(e) The most well known feature is a tendency to confabulate.

(f) Wernicke-Korsakoff syndromes can develop, occasionally, secondary to head injury, intracranial hemorrhage, and expanding lesions, independent of alcoholism. These conditions therefore should be ruled out.

c. VITAMIN B₂ DEFICIENCY can be recognized by pathological changes in the cornea of the eye such as vascularization of the cornea and by cheilosis of the edge of the mouth.

(1) These findings can also be seen in non-alcoholics with cancer or those undergoing chemotherapy.

d. NIACIN DEFICIENCY OR PELLAGRA

(1) This disease has three major characteristics, diarrhea, dementia, and a dermatitis. One or all three may be present.

(2) The central nervous system involvement includes headache, insomnia, depression, dizziness, and difficulty with memory.

(3) The dermatological lesions, in their earliest manifestations, are red eruptions of the skin resembling a sunburn.

(a) This appears first on the back of the hands.

(b) Other areas which are exposed to light are subsequently involved.

(c) The lesions are symmetrical; they darken, shed skin, and eventually scar.

e. VITAMIN B₆ DEFICIENCY causes changes in the skin and the central nervous system and a reduction in red blood cell production.

(1) In more severe cases, skin lesions consist of seborrheic changes around the eyes, nose, and mouth, and swelling and redness of the tongue.

(2) With prolonged deficiencies, convulsive activities have been reported.

(3) The anemia which accompanies pyridoxine deficiency is microcytic hypochromic in type.

(4) A peripheral neuropathy similar to the one induced by thiamine can also be seen.

f. PANTOTHENIC ACID AND BIOTIN have produced, under special circumstances, a "burning legs" type peripheral neuropathy. This may simulate thiamine (B₁) or pyridoxine (B₆) neuropathy and occurs so rarely that it should be considered as the etiologic cause only when there is laboratory documentation.

g. VITAMIN C DEFICIENCY includes the development of changes in the capillary wall and hemorrhages into the space around the hair follicles, as well as areas of ecchymosis in the extremities.

(1) Vitamin C deficiency in adult

alcoholics is not associated with the interference with bone growth, separation of the periosteum from the cortex, and periosteal hemorrhage seen in children.

3. *Fat-Soluble Vitamins*

a. VITAMIN A

(1) The most common clinical symptom of vitamin A deficiency in the alcoholic is impaired adaptation to the dark.

(2) This plays a considerable role in the frequency of car accidents caused by alcoholics and is usually not a presenting complaint nor is it commonly detected except by those alerted to this frequent abnormality.

(3) This deficiency signifies prolonged dietary deficiency or malabsorption.

(4) The deficient dietary intake is aggravated by the presence of pancreatic, biliary, or gastrointestinal disease.

(5) More severe forms of the deficiency are associated with desiccation and alteration of the cornea and conjunctiva of the eye, keratinization and drying of the skin, and increased frequency of respiratory infections.

(a) The keratinization appears as a papular eruption which simulates goose pimples but which cannot be reversed by rubbing or warming of the skin.

(b) Careful observation can detect these skin findings in 15% of the alcoholics admitted to a general city hospital.

b. VITAMIN D

(1) Clinical evidence of vitamin D deficiency in the alcoholic is mainly related to bone involvement.

(2) Complaints of bone tenderness, back pain, early kyphotic or scoliotic changes should alert one to bone involvement in the alcoholic.

(3) Radiographs of bone may help, but bone biopsy, or determination of vitamin D, its metabolites, or parathyroid hormone may be needed.

c. VITAMIN E status is determined by biochemical testing. There are at present no known clinical signs or symptoms usable for the clinical diagnosis of its deficiency.

d. VITAMIN K status is best reflected by prothrombin time because there are no direct methods for its determination.

(1) The presence of multiple ecchymosis and early subcutaneous hemorrhages should lead one to consider a deficiency or malutilization of vitamin K.

F. *Clinical Management*

1. *Water-Soluble Vitamins*

a. The management of vitamin deficiencies in the alcoholic has, until recently, been one of a maternal approach, that is to say, "if a little is good, a lot must be better."

b. There is a large body of scientific knowledge which indicates that small quantities of vitamins will adequately correct these nutritional deficiencies.

(1) In the alcoholic with water-soluble vitamin deficiencies, low doses, such as thiamine 10 mg./day, riboflavin 25 mg./day, niacin 40 mg./day, pyridoxine 20 mg./day, folic acid 1 to 5 mg./day, vitamin C 300 mg./day, pantothenic 10 mg./day, biotin 0.1 to 0.3 mg./day plus vitamin B_{12} 100 μg./week (either by mouth or parenterally), will reverse rapidly most of the clinical manifestations.

c. There are many cases in which this vitamin replacement therapy will not be adequately absorbed orally and, therefore, to be effective, must initially be given intramuscularly.

d. A small number of chronic alcoholics will not respond even to intravenous or intramuscular therapy.

e. Doubling, at maximum, the stated doses without a response indicates an inability to utilize the vitamins in the form given.

(1) This is usually associated with the more severe cases of alcoholic liver injury or pancreatic disease.

(2) Correction of the underlying hepatic or pancreatic disorder subsequently is followed by increased utilization of the vitamins and finally reversal of the clinical symptomology.

f. In some cases, a nonreversible

stage is reached, in which vitamin therapy will no longer correct the abnormal clinical state.

g. Large quantities of vitamins, given in excessive doses, are of no significant value. They are mainly lost through urine excretion, or they may produce toxicity.

2. *Fat-Soluble Vitamins*

a. In treating fat-soluble vitamin deficiency disease, excess use or overdosage can produce toxicity, especially with vitamins A and D.

b. Overzealous treatment with preparations containing vitamin A can produce irritability, loss of appetite, and itchiness of the skin.

(1) Continued excessive administration leads to fatigue, myalagia, changes in body hair, and enlargement of the liver and spleen.

(2) Withdrawal of the vitamin leads to rapid regression of most of the symptoms.

(3) An exception is bony hyperostosis which develops on the extremities and in the occipital region of the skull.

(4) However, to induce this, treatment for 6 months or more with doses of 50,000 I.U. or greater per day must be given.

c. Vitamin A supplementation of 25,000 I.U./day for 1 to 2 weeks is adequate replacement for a deficiency state.

(1) This should be followed by daily oral injections of the recommended dietary allowance.

(2) This will prevent the possibility of overdosage.

d. The relationship between vitamin D deficiency and the osteoporosis/osteomalacia associated with alcoholic liver disease is not understood well enough to recommend specific vitamin D replacement.

(1) Since there is no way to predict the correct dose of vitamin D (as ergocalciferol, 0.25 mg. = 10,000 I.U.), it is suggested that one start with 0.25 mg. daily

and slowly increase the dose until there is symptomatic improvement.

(2) Serum calcium usually increases, and radiologic abnormalities may show improvement with or without changes in serum phosphorus or alkaline phosphatase.

(3) In the alcoholic with more severe hepatic injury, vitamin D analogues may be needed to bypass the need for hepatic metabolic conversion.

e. The response of the remaining vitamin deficiencies to treatment are best followed by laboratory determination of blood or tissue levels and correction of the clinical signs and symptoms.

VI. Management of Mineral and Trace Abnormalities

A. *Indications*

1. Mineral deficiencies occur in alcoholics and drug users with gastrointestinal and liver diseases. They play a significant role in the clinical syndromes seen in both.

B. *Definition*

1. All nutritionally required minerals and trace metals can be categorized in terms of their relative quantitative needs.

2. The more common, clinically referred to as electrolytes, have been named macrominerals and include potassium, sodium, chloride, phosphorus (phosphate), calcium, and magnesium.

3. The trace elements, such as cadmium, chromium, cobalt, copper, fluorine, iodine, iron, manganese, molybdenum, selenium, and zinc, are called microminerals.

C. *Basic Principles*

1. The roles of the macrominerals and some of the microminerals such as iron, iodine, fluorine, and cobalt in human nutrition are relatively well understood (see also Chap. 19).

2. Those of cadmium, chromium, cop-

per, manganese, molybdenum, selenium, and zinc are less defined, although chromium, copper, manganese, selenium, and zinc are known to be essential nutrients.

3. Because this is still a developing area, the recommendations made will be limited to those in which there is substantial clinical evidence of usefulness in the treatment of alcoholic and drug abuse nutritional problems. Emphasis will be mainly on the macrominerals and the microminerals, iron and zinc.

D. *Macrominerals*

1. *Potassium* deficiency is the most common macromineral deficiency in alcohol and drug users.

a. It is usually due to the gastrointestinal, pancreatic, and renal dysfunctions associated with alcoholism and drug addiction.

b. Potassium is lost by vomiting, diarrhea, gastrointestinal bleeding, and increased renal excretion which is frequently due to overuse of diuretics for the control of ascites and edema.

c. In addition, potassium requirement are a function of the metabolic rate of tissue cells.

(1) It is related to nitrogen balance, and its depletion often parallels that of nitrogen.

(2) It is required for the entry of glucose into the cell.

2. *Phosphate/Phosphorus Compounds* are the second most common macromineral deficiency in the alcoholic or drug user.

a. These elements play a central role in energy transformations within the body.

b. Oxidation of sugar requires phosphorus and lowers serum phosphate after carbohydrate ingestion.

c. An inverse relationship between serum phosphate and serum calcium usually exists.

d. Absorption of inorganic phosphorus is in part related to the amount of calcium in the diet.

e. Under ordinary conditions, feces contain about 30% of the dietary phosphorus.

f. Urinary phosphorus is largely inorganic phosphate and is related to the amount absorbed from the intestinal tract.

g. Catabolism of body tissue in starvation, acidosis, and the like, releases considerable phosphorus which is secreted by the kidney.

h. The alcoholic, therefore, has all the components—a high-carbohydrate diet, low in total calories, and a catabolic state, often with acidosis and diarrhea—which cause phosphate depletion.

3. *Magnesium* is the third most common macromineral deficiency found in the alcoholic.

a. It is most frequently associated with alcohol withdrawal and alcohol abstinence syndromes.

b. Earlier reports indicated that the correction of the magnesium deficiency caused amelioration of the withdrawal syndromes.

c. Disagreement exists over the effect of magnesium repletion and treatment because magnesium has a sedative and an anticonvulsant effect on the central nervous system.

d. No consensus exists about the pathogenic role that magnesium depletion plays in the symptomatology of delirium tremens.

e. Clear evidence of magnesium deficiency has been shown to cause hypomagnesemic tetany very similar to hypocalcemic tetany.

4. *Calcium* serum levels are often low in alcoholics and drug users.

a. Reductions in the serum calcium levels are correlated to reductions in serum albumin.

b. Sixty per cent of the serum calcium is ionized, depending upon protein concentration and *p*H.

c. The level of ionized calcium is important in maintaining the functional integrity of cells and, especially, normal neuromuscular irritability.

d. Calcium levels seldom fall to levels which cause neuromuscular symptoms except when secondary gastrointestinal malabsorption is present.

e. The exact role that phosphorus and calcium abnormalities play in the bone disease of the alcoholic is still under study.

5. *Sodium and Chloride* serum levels are frequently abnormally low in the alcoholic or drug user.

a. In 98% of the cases, low serum levels of sodium and chloride are due to intravascular dilution secondary to excessive water retention, in the presence of liver disease and protein depletion.

b. The presence of peripheral edema and ascites are invariably due to excessive sodium and water retention secondary to increased sodium reabsorption by the kidney.

E. Microminerals

1. Iron is an element required for life and is necessary for production of hemoglobin, myoglobulin, and certain essential enzymes.

a. The normal adult body contains 3 to 5 g. of iron, 53 to 60% in hemoglobin and 30 to 35% in storage forms.

b. Iron is held tenaciously by the body.

c. Normal loss of iron in urine, feces, sweat, and exfoliation of skin cells totals approximately 0.5 to 1.0 mg./day.

d. Iron loss in the alcoholic or drug addict is due, almost exclusively, to gastrointestinal bleeding secondary to gastritis, varices, ulcer, or drug-induced bleeding.

2. Zinc is the second most common micromineral depletion found in the chronic alcoholic, especially in those with liver damage.

a. Low serum zinc levels have been reported in up to 50% of alcoholic patients.

b. Chronic alcoholism leads to zincuria and reduced zinc concentrations in liver, red cells, and plasma, especially in those alcoholics with cirrhosis.

c. Zinc is needed for many enzymes, especially those dealing with RNA

metabolism and DNA synthesis, and plays a major role in the growth and repair of vital organs such as the liver.

d. Urinary loss of zinc is aggravated by a deficient dietary intake which is characteristic of the alcoholic and drug addict.

e. Zinc deficiency is a common finding associated with testicular atrophy, impotence, and decreased testosterone production in patients with alcoholic hepatitis and cirrhosis.

(1) Testosterone production in these patients is diminished but can be normalized by correcting the zinc depletion.

(2) After correction of zinc depletion, a failure to show improvement may reflect the absence of active hepatic cell regeneration due to other nutrient deficiencies.

3. The roles of copper, iodine, fluorine, cobalt, chromium, selenium, manganese, molybdenum, and cadmium have had only limited, if any, study in the alcoholic and drug user or are just now undergoing evaluation.

4. Intoxication by microminerals (especially iron, cobalt, and lead) can occur accidentally due to methods of fermentation.

a. Iron occurs in excessive amounts in some fermented beverages, especially when iron utensils are used in the process.

b. Cobalt added to beer to enhance quality and quantity of foam has resulted in serious myocardiopathy.

c. Moonshine whiskey made from lead-lined stills (automobile radiators) has resulted in lead poisoning.

F. Criteria for Diagnosis

1. It is essential for proper management of chronic alcoholics to have biochemical determination of the macro- and microminerals. These determinations are usually limited to blood and urine levels, but in some cases tissue levels can be obtained (see Table 27-5).

2. For practical purposes of day-to-day care, one should include determinations (blood or urine levels) of sodium, po-

tassium, chloride, calcium, phosphorous, magnesium, zinc, and iron. When historically warranted, lead and cobalt levels should also be determined.

    3. Macrominerals

      a. POTASSIUM depletion in the alcoholic is manifested by muscle weakness or paralysis, abnormalities of cardiac rhythm, conduction, and repolarization, usually consisting of arrhythmias, conduction defects, or ectopic contractions.

      (1) Potassium depletion is also associated with precipitation of hepatic coma in the alcoholic cirrhotic.

      (2) Clinical signs and symptoms of impending encephalopathy are listed in Table 27-3.

      (3) Respiratory hyperventilation, common in the alcoholic and drug addict, causes the shift of potassium into cells, due to respiratory alkalosis, and can lower serum potassium to critical levels.

      b. PHOSPHATE depletion has no specific identifiable clinical signs, but levels below 1.0 mg./dl. have been associated with weakness, periodic digital tingling, and malaise.

      c. MAGNESIUM. Clinical manifestations of magnesium deficiency are similar to alcohol withdrawal.

      (1) These include tremor, twitching, choreiform- and athetoid-type movements, convulsions, and, occasionally, frank tetany with carpal and pedal spasms.

      (2) Auditory and visual hallucinations and, occasionally, stupor and coma can be seen.

      d. SODIUM AND CHLORIDE

      (1) The presence of peripheral edema, ascites, and low urinary 24-hour sodium (< 10 mEq./day) are all indicators of excessive sodium retention independent of low serum sodium levels. This point cannot be emphasized enough.

Table 27-5. **Essential Minerals and Their Normal Blood and Urine Levels**

Minerals, Blood Level*	Normal Range
Potassium	3.5–5.0 mEq./L.
Phosphate	3.0–4.5 mg./dl.
Magnesium	1.8–3.0 mg./dl. (1.5–2.5 mEq./L.)
Sodium	136–145 mEq./L.
Chloride	96–106 mEq./L.
Calcium (total)	9.0–11.0 mg./dl. (4.5–5.5 mEq./L.)
Iron	75–175 mg./dl.
Zinc	90–116 mg./dl.
Copper, males	70–140 mg./dl.
Copper, females	85–155 mg./dl.

Minerals, Urine Level*	Normal Range
Calcium	250 mg./24 hrs.*
Chloride	110–250 mEq./24 hrs.*
Copper	0–30 μg./24 hrs.
Phosphorus	0.9–1.3 g./24 hrs.*
Potassium	25–100 mEq./24 hrs.*
Sodium	130–260 mEq./24 hrs.*
Zinc	500–700 μg./24 hrs.

*Varies with intake

(2) The presence of ascites or peripheral edema is de facto evidence of total body sodium excess.

e. CALCIUM

(1) Clinical signs of calcium deficiency occur most commonly in the chronic alcoholic with acute pancreatitis and can cause sufficient hypocalcemia to cause tetany.

(2) Recognition of associated magnesium deficiency is of equal importance.

(3) Clinical or radiological evidence of osteoporosis may not be correctable with calcium levels, but inadequate intake of calcium and protein are very likely the most important factors.

4. Microminerals

a. Iron

(1) Depletion can be identified by determining total iron, iron-binding capacity, the presence of microcytic hypochromic anemia, a low reticulocyte count, and a decreased mean corpuscular volume.

(2) There is good clinical evidence of the development of iron overload in severe chronic alcoholics.

(3) Liver biopsy tissue iron stain can help identify such patients.

(4) Excessive iron therapy and the avoidance of beverages with high-iron content is important.

b. Zinc deficiency is not clearly recognizable in adults clinically. History of decreased libido, impaired sexual function, the presence of hepatic cirrhosis, and poor wound healing should make one consider the diagnosis of zinc deficiency in the alcoholic.

c. The diagnosis of other micromineral deficiencies at this stage of development is dependent upon blood, urine, and tissue determinations, and these are still being investigated.

G. Management

1. Nutritional replenishment of some macrominerals may require immediate intravenous therapy.

a. Low-potassium-induced cardiac arrhythmias, muscular paralysis, and hepatic coma requires urgent treatment.

(1) Intravenous infusion of potassium chloride (KCl 40 to 80 mEq./L. in 1000 ml. 5% dextrose in water) should be administered until there is correction of the clinical signs and symptoms or stabilization of the serum potassium levels.

(2) Care must be taken in renal impairment or cellular acidosis not to produce hyperkalemia by overmedication.

b. Magnesium- or calcium-deficiency-induced convulsions or tetany also require immediate attention.

(1) Treatment with intramuscular or intravenous magnesium sulfate ($MgSO_4$) in divided doses can be given according to the method recommended by Flink*: Day 1—8 to 12 g. (67 to 97 mEq.); days 2, 3, and 4—4 to 5 g. (32 to 40 mEq.).

(2) Urinary output and blood magnesium levels should be monitored daily during this period.

c. Intravenous correction of low serum calcium levels in alcoholics (in the absence of tetany) is not indicated because they are most often decreased due to the lowered serum albumin.

(1) However, in the presence of acute tetany, 20 ml. of 10% calcium gluconate may be given slowly, intravenously and repeated if necessary.

(2) Alternatively, 30 to 60 ml. of 10% calcium gluconate in 1 L. of isotonic saline may be given over a 12- to 24-hour period.

d. Phosphate depletion can be supplemented intravenously in the form of potassium phosphate (40 mEq./L.) when necessary.

2. Nutritional replacement of all other macro- and micromineral deficiencies and abnormalities probably is best provided for in an adequate, well balanced, and

---

*Flink, E.B., Shane, S.R., Jacob, W.E., and Jones, J.E.: Some aspects of magnesium deficiency and chronic alcoholism. *In* Sardesai, V.M. (ed.): Biochemical and Clinical Aspects of Alcohol Metabolism, p. 256. Springfield, Illinois, Charles C Thomas, 1969.

nutritious diet (see also Chap. 21 and Chap. 19).

3. Management of nutritional disorders in the alcoholic and drug user should always be assessed according to the degree of hepatocellular, gastrointestinal, and pancreatic organ involvement.

DIET-DRUG INTERACTIONS

I. Basic Principles

A. The adequate delivery of essential nutrients in the case of drug addiction and drug toxicity syndromes requires a clear understanding of the metabolic basis of diet-drug interactions.

1. Although the importance of nutritional-pharmacological interactions is not fully recognized, a better understanding of the fundamental mechanisms of these potential interactions may have valuable clinical implications in the treatment of disease and malnutrition.

B. There are a number of drugs which may affect nutrient utilization, and, conversely, there are nutrients which may affect drug absorption and bioavailability.

C. Significant differences in the activities of drug-metabolizing enzymes, which ultimately affect drug toxicity, have been shown between adequate and deficient diets.

D. Numerous illicitly used drugs can potentially affect nutritional status through various means.

1. Some may alter food intake indirectly by producing side effects such as nausea, vomiting, and alteration of the sense of taste.

2. Others may inhibit nutrient synthesis.

3. Some drugs may interact with nutrients to reduce absorption, to alter their distribution, transport, utilization, or storage, or to increase excretion of nutrients.

E. How these interactions affect one's nutritional homeostasis is dependent largely on the body's reserve stores of the various nutrients, its compensatory adaptive mechanism in nutrient absorption and excretion, and on the relative adequacy of dietary intake of the nutrients.

1. When chronic persistent drug ingestion so affects the body that it is unable to adapt to these challenges, a gradual nutrient depletion occurs.

2. It is important to realize that continued drug addiction accentuates the coexisting subclinical malnutrition due to deficient dietary intake and coexisting disease.

II. Causes

A. The persistent use of illicit or addictive drugs may affect one's nutritional status by a number of mechanisms.

1. Appetite and Taste

a. The most widely recognized example of such a drug-nutrient relationship is that of the pharmacological effects of amphetamines.

b. These drugs may affect the physiological, emotional, psychological, cultural, social, and economic aspects of a person so as to impair both the appetite and food intake required to maintain a normal nutritional state.

2. Nutrient Synthesis

a. Drugs can influence synthesis of vitamins as a result of pharmacodynamic action in the cell or by impairing gastrointestinal absorption through interference with motility, as in the case of heroin and methadone.

3. Nutrient Absorption

a. Groups of drugs which may cause malabsorption include those that

(1) Affect the intestinal motility, such as laxatives and cathartics

(2) Interfere with the physiological activity of bile acids and bile salts needed for optimal absorption of fats and fat-soluble vitamins

(3) May induce cellular damage

to the intestinal mucosa or selectively block and interfere with transport mechanisms

(4) Can damage the exocrine pancreas and cause decreased synthesis or release of pancreatic enzymes with subsequent maldigestion of fat, proteins, and starch

4. Nutrient Distribution and Excretion

a. Drugs can displace nutrients from the plasma protein or tissue-binding sites by complexing the nutrient and thus detaching it from the binding sites.

b. They can also replace the nutrient on the protein-binding site.

c. There can exist a combination of these effects.

d. These interactions can promote renal excretion of the affected nutrients, which may be either free or complexed with the drug.

5. Nutrient Metabolism

a. Drugs can affect various aspects of carbohydrate, protein, and lipid metabolism.

b. In addition, they may prevent or impair the activation of vitamins and minerals and thereby prevent utilization at their target sites.

B. Although there is much investigative data suggesting altered nutritional status by drug-nutrient interaction, there have been relatively few clinical correlations identified that can be specifically related to the drug abuser or chronic illicit drug user.

C. Drugs are removed from or detoxified in the body by a group of nonspecific enzymes that are located predominantly in liver microsomes.

1. The metabolism and activity of this enzyme system are affected by acute starvation, undernutrition, protein depletion, and deficiencies or excesses of minerals, vitamins, and lipids.

2. The activity of these drug-metabolizing enzymes has been reported to decrease in diets deficient in calcium, zinc, magnesium, and ascorbic acid.

III. Criteria for Diagnosis

A. Most drug abusers present with clinical signs and symptoms related mainly to their drug addiction rather than to their malnourished state.

B. Identification of the illicit drugs used, by biochemical means, may give some clues to the type of nutritional impairment one is to look for.

C. Because most drug users abuse multiple drugs, it is difficult at best to assess the nutritional impact.

D. Assessment of hepatic, pancreatic, and gastrointestinal functions would be of greater value, as in the alcoholic.

E. Drug addicts with hepatitis often have impaired taste buds and sensory smell which interfere with their appetite even further.

1. Determination of impaired taste capability by using various concentrations of glucose, urea, and bitters can be done for more specific identification of the neurological taste abnormalities.

2. Some patients, for example, have an impaired urea tasting capacity which makes proteins taste like cardboard.

3. By changing dietary composition, one can correct for this defect and improve dietary intake of nutrients.

4. Protein taste impairments usually begin with meats, followed then by egg and cheese proteins. At times there may be an impairment of taste in all three areas.

IV. Management

A. Since calorie-protein depletion represents the major problem in drug addicts, reinstitution of an adequate, well-balanced, and nutritious diet is the mainstay of therapy.

1. Excess quantities of proteins may occasionally cause an unexpected case of hepatic encephalopathy if adequate total clinical evaluation has not been performed.

B. The major problem in drug addicts is the discontinuance of the addictive drugs and the mode of returning patients to an adequate dietary intake.

C. The residual effects of prolonged use of addictive drugs often leave the drug addict with secondary diseases such as chronic active hepatitis and pancreatic or gastrointestinal dysfunction which can affect nutritional status.

1. Prolonged use of narcotics impairs gastrointestinal tract motility, interferes with absorption, and occasionally leads to ileus of the small intestine and related complications.

2. In more severely involved cases, transient use of intravenous supplementation may be necessary.

3. In the majority of patients, the post-withdrawal period is associated with a return of appetite, and the patient only requires the availability of adequate food.

D. In general, carbohydrate, protein, fat, and vitamin replenishment in the drug addict and patients with acute toxicity syndrome are similar to those of the alcoholic without hepatic or renal failure.

E. The presence of renal or hepatic failure in acute toxicity syndromes presents special nutritional management problems.

1. The nutritional management of hepatic failure is discussed in Chapter 21.

2. Dietary therapy of renal failure is discussed in Chapter 15.

F. In the majority of alcoholics, drug addicts, and patients with acute toxicity syndromes, nutritional corrections can be handled orally. The use and need of intravenous hyperalimentation or elemental supplementation affect mostly patients with severe decompensated hepatic, biliary, or gastrointestinal disease.

G. The recommendations and indications contained in this chapter are primarily for the ambulatory alcoholic and drug addict. Frequently these nutritional depletions are first identified as inpatients during an acute illness. Prolonged follow-up, however, is always required for maximum effectiveness.

INDEX

Numbers in *italics* indicate a figure; "t" following a page number indicates a table.

Heart failure *(cont.)*
  congestive, in children,
      therapeutic approach, 87–88
  criteria for diagnosis, 135
  definition of, 134
  management, 135–136
Hedonic perceptions, cancer and, 259
Height, of adopted Korean children, 365
  daily allowances and, 12–13t
  I.Q. and, 364
  measurement of, 4
Height-weight index, accuracy of, 154
  errors in, 4
Hematocrit, alcoholism and, 372
  normal average values, 210t
Hematopoiesis, alcoholism and, 378
Heme, synthesis, pyridoxine and, 220
Hemochromatosis, iron and, 280, 281
Hemodialysis, nutrient loss and, 223
  pyridoxine deficiency and, 121
Hemoglobin, formation, anemia and, 211
  megaloblastic anemia and, 214
  normal average values, 210t
  pregnancy and, 34t
Hemolysis, megaloblastic anemia and, 214
Hepatic synthetic capacity, reduced, treatment of, 310–311
Hepatitis, drug abuse and, 388, 389
Hepatocellular damage, vitamin K and, 118–119
Hepatosplenomegaly, incidence of, 94
Hernia, hiatus,
  basic principles, 174–175
  definition, 174
  dietary management, 175
Heroin, nutrients and, 387
High-density lipoproteins, 139
  composition, 138t
High-protein diet, for clinical use, 182–183
Histidine, zinc deficiency and, 341
History, adolescent diets and, 93
  medical, nutritional status and, 3
  reproductive, nutritional risk and, 55
Homocysteine, vitamin B$_{12}$ and, 330
Homocystinuria, diet therapy, 87t
Hormonal response, to trauma or surgery, *152*
Hormone, antidiuretic, *see* Aldosterone
  metabolism in pregnancy and, 36, 37t
Host factors, dental caries and, 317–318
Howell-Jolly bodies, 216
Human chorionic gonadotropin, weight loss and, 254
Human placental lactogen (HPL), pregnancy and, 40
Hydralazine, pyridoxine and, 121, 329
Hydrogen, general considerations, 293
Hydrogen ions, sources of, 293
1α-Hydroxycholecalciferol, renal osteodystrophy and, 357
25-Hydroxycholecalciferol, anticonvulsant therapy and, 355–356
  formation of, 231, 352, 354–355

liver injury and, 310
  hypovitaminosis D and, 337
  uremia and, 356–357
18-Hydroxydeoxycorticosterone, hypertension and, 129
25-Hydroxyergocalciferol, formation, liver and, 352
Hydroxyproline, excretion of, 7
Hyperalimentation, *see also* TPN
  central venous, 161
  enteral,
      precautions, 164–165
      products available, 164
  intravenous,
      basic principles, 159
      complications of, 162t
      cyclic, 163
      indications for, 159–161
      methodology, 161–162
      special uses, 163
      use in children, 164
  orders for, 161t
  techniques using intralipid, 161–162
Hyperalimentation solutions, administration of, 300–301
  formulation, 300
Hypercalcemia, clinical neurologic features, 337–338
  dangers of, 117–118
  etiology, 277, 337
  laboratory tests, 338
  manifestations, 278
  nutritional therapy, 338
  prognosis, 338
  treatment, 278
Hypercalciuria, idiopathic, Vitamin D and, 353
Hypercarotenemia, skin and, 347
Hypercholesterolemia, diet and, 143
Hyperglycemia, alcoholism and, 376
  fetal, gestational diabetes and, 48
  hyponatremia and, 271
  TPN and, 302
Hyperkalemia, clinical neurologic features, 335–336
  etiology, 275, 335
  laboratory tests, 275
  manifestations, 275
  nutritional therapy, 336
  prognosis, 336
  treatment, 275–276
Hyperlipidemia, atherosclerosis and, 111
  correlation with hyperlipoproteinémia, 141t
  dialysis and, 228
  dietary treatment of, 144t, 146t, 147t–148t
      general considerations, 142–143
      type I, 143
      type II, 143
      type III, 143–144
      types IV an V, 144–145
  differential diagnosis, 142
  drug treatment of,
      indications, 145